INTERACTIONS BETWEEN
PLATELETS AND VESSEL WALLS

INTERACTIONS BETWEEN PLATELETS AND VESSEL WALLS

A ROYAL SOCIETY DISCUSSION

ORGANIZED BY
G. V. R. BORN, F.R.S., AND J. R. VANE, F.R.S.

HELD ON 20 AND 21 NOVEMBER 1980

LONDON
THE ROYAL SOCIETY
1981

Printed in Great Britain for the Royal Society
at the
University Press, Cambridge

ISBN 0 85403 164 2

First published in *Philosophical Transactions of the Royal Society of London*,
series B, volume 294 (no. 1072), pages 215–412

Published by the Royal Society
6 Carlton House Terrace, London SW1Y 5AG

PREFACE

One of the essential survival mechanisms of all animals is the arrest of loss of vital body fluid after injury. For this reason, haemostasis, the mechanism that arrests the loss of blood, has a long and fascinating evolutionary history. Haemostasis depends first on the adhesion and aggregation in vascular injuries of specialized circulating cells, the platelets or thrombocytes, and secondly on the clotting of the blood plasma. Platelets have only two properly established physiological functions: to form haemostatic plugs in injured vessels, and to provide a phospholipid material that greatly accelerates plasma coagulation. Therefore, the primary event that underlies the function of platelets is a change that results in their selective adhesion to damaged vessel walls and to each other to form aggregates.

The development of mechanisms for the selective adhesion of different types of cell has, of course, been essential for the evolution of multicellular organisms. Platelets are, however, highly specialized and extraordinarily efficient in this respect, which is not surprising in view of the fact that adhesion is their *raison d'être*.

What makes the interactions between platelets and vessel walls more interesting scientifically and important medically is their role in different diseases. The association of deficiencies of platelets, i.e. thrombocytopenia, with petechial haemorrhages suggests that platelets are somehow required for the functional integrity of small blood vessels. Something similar can also be inferred from the association of other haemorrhagic conditions with platelets that are defective functionally.

The commonest complication of atherosclerosis of arteries, which affects most people in this and many other countries, is acute thrombotic obstruction resulting in myocardial or cerebral infarction (respectively heart attacks and strokes). Extensive evidence indicates that arterial thrombosis is initiated by platelet aggregation, which thereby assumes very great importance as a problem in clinical and preventive medicine.

Most intriguingly, platelets are also liable to aggregate in extracorporeal circulations, such as those through artificial kidneys, oxygenators, and so on, the functioning of which can be nullified by the resulting thrombotic obstruction; and this in vessels the walls of which are made of various plastics and devoid of biological components.

It is therefore not surprising that interactions between platelets and vessel walls should arouse widespread interest and be the object of much research. This volume represents the proceedings of a Discussion Meeting on the topic held at the Royal Society in London on 20 and 21 November 1980. The contributions consider most of the major problems, from the question of why platelets show no tendency to adhere to normal vascular endothelium to those posed by the extreme rapidity of their adhesion and aggregation where endothelium is defective or deficient. On the basis of up-to-date presentations of facts, clinical, pathological and experimental, the various hypotheses are assessed that are at present in vogue for explaining the reactions involving platelets in haemostasis and in thromboses.

June 1981

G. V. R. BORN
J. R. VANE

CONTENTS
[Three plates]

CONTENTS

Phil. Trans. R. Soc. Lond. B **294**, 217–224 (1981)
Printed in Great Britain

Vascular injury: platelets and smooth muscle cell response

By M. B. Stemerman

*Department of Medicine, The Charles A. Dana Research Institute and The Thorndike
Laboratory of the Harvard Medicical School, Beth Israel Hospital, 330 Brookline
Avenue, Boston, Massachusetts 02215, U.S.A.*

The blood platelet appears to play an important role in the pathogenesis of the atherosclerotic plaque. Using a platelet specific antigen, platelet factor 4 (PF4), we have demonstrated that PF4 released from platelets enters the vessel wall. Smooth muscle cell (s.m.c.) proliferation *in vivo* was examined by using a new technique for measuring [³H]thymidine incorporation. With this technique, we have shown that a remote vascular injury can cause s.m.c. proliferation, presumably mediated by a humoral agent. Endothelial dysfunction, in turn, may be caused by a sustained, mild hypercholesterolaemia. This permeability dysfunction may provide circulating s.m.c. mitogens with access to the vessel, wall, thus allowing s.m.c. proliferation in areas of non-desquamated endothelium. These experiments form the basis for a modification of the hypothesis implicating platelets in atherogenesis.

The vascular smooth muscle cell (s.m.c.) and the blood platelet have been closely linked with atherosclerotic plaque formation. Although the contribution of platelets to atherosclerotic plaque build-up has been discussed for many years, it has only recently been suggested that platelets may play a causative role in vascular s.m.c. proliferation (Ross & Glomset 1976). This platelet effect is of particular importance, since the s.m.c. is the principal cell of the atherosclerotic plaque (Wissler 1968). The recent interest in this platelet–s.m.c. interrelation has been stimulated by the finding obtained from the propagation of vascular s.m.cs in cell culture. Cell culture experiments with the use of s.m.cs have demonstrated the s.m.cs ability to produce extracellular connective tissue including collagen and elastin, to metabolize lipoproteins and to be stimulated to grow by a mitogen carried by platelets.

The study of s.m.c. biology in culture is limited by the rapid metabolic changes that the cells undergo once placed in culture (Fowler 1977) and hence the potential change in their nature. On the other hand, characterization of s.m.c. growth *in vivo* has been hampered by difficult methodological problems. The use of autoradiography, for instance, is tedious and time-consuming. To overcome this problem, we have established an *in vivo* technique for determining s.m.c. proliferation based upon the incorporation of [³H]thymidine into s.m.c. DNA after de-endothelialization of the aorta by a balloon catheter (Stemerman 1973). The results of these experiments demonstrate that the method is rapid, quantitative and can be used to determine vascular s.m.c. growth.

The link between platelets and s.m.cs rests on the hypothesis that platelets carry an s.m.c. mitogen that can be released from the platelet α-granule and can enter the vessel wall at sites of injury (Stemerman 1979). Platelets do indeed attach to subendothelial connective tissue after endothelial desquamation, but little is known of the release of their intraplatelet contents and whether these materials can penetrate into the vessel wall. To trace the products of platelet release, we have purified a platelet-specific protein, platelet factor 4 (PF4) in rabbits and have raised an antibody against this antigen (Goldberg *et al.* 1980*b*). Using immunofluorescent microscopy, we have been able to detail the course of PF4 when released from platelets and have investigated potential inhibitors of the platelet release reaction *in vivo*.

SMOOTH MUSCLE CELL PROLIFERATION *IN VIVO*

For an examination of s.m.c. proliferation *in vivo*, rabbits were de-endothelialized by balloon catheter (Stemerman 1973) and injected with [^{3}H]thymidine, (0.5 µCi/g body mass) (20 mCi/mmol; New England Nuclear) intravenously (i.v.), followed 30 min later by an i.v. injection of 5 ml of Evans blue dye (Harvey Labs. Inc.). Evans blue was given to assure endothelial removal: the dye penetrates areas of intima not covered by endothelium. Rabbits were killed by cardiac exsanguination at 1, 8, 16, 24, 36 and 48 h and at 4, 5, 6, 7, 14, 28 and 48 days after initial injury; 5–12 rabbits were used at each interval sampled. Within 1 min after exsanguination, a thoracic segment (third to sixth intercostal arteries) and an abdominal segment (left renal to the aortic bifurcation) were removed, immediately frozen and stored at $-70\,°$C. These segments were used to determine DNA specific activity as outlined below. Adjacent thoracic and abdominal segments were not frozen but were immediately immersed in 2.5% glutaraldehyde (0.1 M cacodylate, pH 7.4, 20 °C) and processed for morphological and morphometric evaluation. The frozen segments from each rabbit were processed separately. The vessels were thawed and the adventitia was stripped away from each segment and discarded. The remaining intima–media tissues were homogenized and the Evans blue extracted by using heparin–Sepharose beads. DNA content was determined on the solubilized segments by the method of Burton. Samples of solubilized tissues were precipitated in parallel at 4 °C for 30 min in 10% trichloroacetic acid (TCA) and bovine serum albumin. Precipitates were trapped on a nitrocellulose filter, solubilized with methoxyethanol and their radioactivity determined in aquasol scintillation fluid (New England Nuclear). DNA specific activity was calculated for each sample, and the means ± standard errors were plotted against time (Goldberg *et al.* 1980*a*, 1979).

The fixed thoracic and abdominal segments were each cut into 1 mm rings, post-fixed in osmium tetroxide and stained with uranyl acetate for 30 min. The rings were dehydrated and embedded in Epon. Epon sections (1 µm) were cut from each of the thoracic and abdominal blocks of each animal and stained with methylene blue. These sections were evaluated for intimal cell nuclei and by radioautography for grain counts.

Results of the experiment indicate that the thoracic aorta, in comparison with the abdominal aorta, shows much less increase in DNA specific activity (figure 1) and likewise there is much less intimal s.m.c. accumulation (table 1). Thymidine incorporation into s.m.c. DNA does not begin until 24 h after de-endothelialization. At 24 h, a steady rise in DNA specific activity begins in both the abdominal and thoracic segments, peaking at days 2–4 and then gradually returning to the baseline by approximately 28 days. Radioautographic studies carried out in parallel with measurements of DNA specific activity show a correlation of $r = 0.77$.

These data indicate that, in response to a similar injury, s.m.cs from the abdominal aortic segment proliferate at a greater rate than those of the thoracic region. Segmental variation may therefore be a common feature of s.m.c. proliferation *in vivo* and may account, in part, for differences in growth of s.m.cs and hence the different sizes of plaques in different areas. In subsequent studies, de-endothelialization by balloon was carried out again at day 4 after the initial de-endothelialization. Injury was inflicted only on the abdominal aorta. Thoracic aortic segments (not subjected to the second injury) were analysed for [³H]thymidine incorporation into DNA after this injury at days 4.5, 5, 6 and 7. There is a marked increase in [³H]thymidine

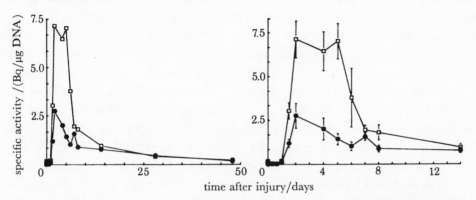

FIGURE 1. DNA specific activity curves for incorporation of [³H]thymidine into aortic smooth muscle cells. There is a latent period of 24 h followed by uptake of the label. Peak activity occurs 2–4 days after injury with a gradual decline in uptake. There is a marked difference in the DNA activity between thoracic (●) and abdominal (□) segments. This is seen most dramatically at days 2 and 4. Student's t-test comparing thoracic and abdominal segments showed a value of $p < 0.01$. (1 Bq = 60 disintegrations/min)

TABLE 1. INTIMAL CELL NUCLEI: ABDOMINAL AND THORACIC SEGMENTS

(Intimal cell numbers ± standard error; number of samples shown in parentheses.)

day	abdominal	thoracic
1	1.2 ± 0.20 (12)	0.81 ± 0.028 (9)
2	1.1 ± 0.17 (12)	0.21 ± 0.027 (12)
4	2.3 ± 0.39 (12)	0.66 ± 0.12 (12)
7	11.6 ± 0.74 (9)	7.38 ± 0.49 (17)
14	20.5 ± 0.75 (12)	11.0 ± 1.06 (11)
28	21.8 ± 1.71 (6)	11.3 ± 1.02 (6)
48	30.8 ± 0.46 (9)	13.9 ± 0.85 (9)

incorporation in the non-reinjured thoracic segment compared with the control animals. There is a peak specific activity at day 5 of approximately 30 Bq/mg DNA. These latter experiments indicate that a distal vascular injury, potentially freeing platelet materials into the circulation, can cause s.m.c. proliferation at a different vascular segment not experiencing the injury. This observation implicates a humoral material involved in smooth muscle cell proliferation that is effective *in vivo*. Whether this material is indeed platelet-derived is as yet unknown.

PLATELETS AND THE VESSEL WALL

To allow the course of materials released from platelets as they interact with the vessel wall to be followed, PF4 was purified from rabbit platelets. A monospecific antibody was raised in a goat against this antigen and used to detect the presence of rabbit PF4 antigen. Rabbit iliac arteries were denuded of endothelium with a low-pressure balloon catheter (Stemerman 1973). At 10 min, 30 min and 4 h after de-endothelialization, the animals were killed by exsanguina-

[3]

tion and portions of the injured artery were immediately frozen. These arteries were sectioned after freezing and were reacted with the anti-PF4 antibody by indirect immunofluorescent techniques adapted for the PF4 antigen (Goldberg *et al.* 1980*b*).

The PF4 antigen was identified at the luminal surface and in the tunica media of the artery 10 and 30 min after removal of the endothelium. Immunofluorescent platelets were seen on the vessel surface at 10 min. At this time, penetration of the antigen into the vessel wall was noted in the inner luminal one-third of the vessel. Platelets remained at the surface 4 h after injury and showed fluorescence, but there was virtually no immunofluorescent staining of the vessel wall by this time. Control arteries not injured showed no fluorescence in the vessel wall. The anti-PF4 serum was absorbed by incubation with purified PF4 protein. Application of the absorbed serum to vessel frozen sections produced no immunofluorescence. These results are consistent with those of morphological studies of platelet attachment to the vessel wall, and provide additional information about the reaction between platelets and the vessel wall several hours after injury. They also agree with the results of recent studies of ^{51}Cr label platelet turnover (Groves *et al.* 1979). In those studies, platelet interaction with the vessel wall was evaluated in rabbits whose endothelium was removed in the balloon catheter. It was shown that only 0.2 % of the circulating platelets attached to the damaged wall and that turnover was almost undetectable. Similarly, we have shown that secretion of antigen by platelets is a short-lived, self-limited phenomenon, with apparently little secretion occurring 4 h after injury.

Additional studies have been performed by using PF4 antigen as a probe for platelet release during a constant intravenous infusion of prostacyclin (PGI_2) (Adelman *et al.* 1980). Rabbits were given large doses (800 ng kg^{-1} min^{-1}) of PGI_2. In these rabbits, their platelets, tested by aggregometry, were non-reactive to collagen and adrenalin. Animals were killed 30 min after de-endothelialization by ballooning and the vessels removed and studied for the presence of PF4 antigen. A second group of rabbits was given a constant infusion of saline as control. The platelets in this second group adhered normally to the denuded subendothelium by light and electron microscopy and PF4 was identified by immunofluorescence within the vessel wall. In contrast, under a constant infusion of a large dose of prostacyclin, platelet adhesion to the vessel wall was greatly reduced and PF4 antigen was identified at occasional sites of attachment of rare, randomly distributed platelets on the subendothelium. Of importance is the observation that little if any PF4 antigen traversed the vessel wall. Large doses of prostacyclin inhibit release of PF4 antigen into the vessel wall.

ENDOTHELIAL INJURY

A basic tenet of atherogenesis states that endothelial cells (e.cs) protect against intimal proliferation by providing the vessel wall with a non-thrombogenic surface and a permeability barrier. The mechanism for the non-thrombogenic quality of the endothelium remains unclear but has been considered to be associated with the endothelial cells' ability to produce prostacyclin (PGI_2). The e.c. forms an effective barrier to penetration of materials into the vessel wall, limiting permeation into the underlying tissue to concentrations approximately one-hundredth that of materials in the plasma (Stemerman 1979). With removal of the endothelium, there is loss of this non-thrombogenic permeability shield, which (*a*) produces a haemostatic response to the now-exposed thrombogenic subendothelium, and (*b*) allows the unrestrained entrance of plasma constituents into the vessel wall. It has been considered that endothelial cells, when damaged, would be shed from their vascular surface. To test this hypothesis under a mild hypercholesterolaemic stress, we fed a cohort of rabbits a diet of their normal rabbit feed supplemented with whole eggs. The animals were fed this diet for 7 weeks, reaching a mean serum cholesterol level of 451 mg/dl. The animals were then killed by perfusion fixation (Stemerman 1973), but 1 min before perfusion they were given an intravenous infusion of horseradish peroxidase (HRP) (Sigma, type II), 80 mg/kg, over a 10 s period. The perfused

TABLE 2. INCREASE IN AREA OF INTIMA STAINED BY HORSERADISH
PEROXIDASE AFTER 7 WEEKS OF HIGH-CHOLESTEROL DIET

(Mean serum cholesterol increased from 59 ± 3.2 to 451 ± 29.8 mg/dl.)

diet	percentage area stained $\pm$ s.e.m.	number
normal	12.1 ± 5.0	6
egg-supplemented	45.6 ± 6.2	7

Comparison of group by Student's t-test: $p < 0.01$.

arteries were pinned out and reacted with diaminobenzidine–H_2O_2 in the dark. The surface was examined *en face* and showed 1–2 mm spots of brown at the endothelial surface indicating heightened permeability of the HRP permeability marker in these areas. The area of heightened permeability was calculated by morphometrics (Weibel 1973) and compared with a control group of rabbits not supplemented with eggs. As seen from table 2, there was a marked increase in the area of heightened permeability in the hypercholesterolaemic animals. These heightened permeability areas were examined by scanning electron microscopy (s.e.m.) and transmission electron microscopy (t.e.m.). S.e.m. showed some distortion of the linear arrangement of the endothelium; T.e.m. showed only increased penetration of the reaction product of the HRP but no qualitative changes in the e.c. ultrastructure. Neither t.e.m. nor s.e.m. showed loss of endothelium or platelet accumulation at the site of these permeability defects. The cause of the heightened permeability is not clear but it is apparent that loss of endothelium is not necessary for heightened permeability to occur. In the case explored, a mild elevation of serum cholesterol concentration caused a change in permeability of the vessel wall due to an 'endothelial dysfunction' without endothelial desquamation (Stemerman 1981).

A MODIFIED HYPOTHESIS

The studies provide a basis for modifying the current hypothesis that links platelets to s.m.c. proliferation. Basic to that hypothesis is the tenet that endothelial injury will lead to endothelial desquamation. After endothelial detachment, the desquamated surface is available to the blood as a thrombogenic surface. Platelets can adhere to this surface and can release intracytoplasmic constituents into the vessel wall. As seen by the above experiments, e.cs may become dysfunctional in the face of a sustained modest hypercholesterolaemia but do not desquamate. A dysfunctioning cell would allow the access of greater concentrations of circulating materials into the underlying vessel wall. Thus, mitogenic materials that might be constituents of plasma or might be released by platelets intravascularly, for whatever reason, could accumulate sufficiently in the vessel wall to initiate s.m.c. proliferation under an intact endothelium. It

[5]

appears, from our studies on segmental s.m.c. responses to injury, that certain s.m.c. beds are much more responsive than others Combined with an area of endothelial dysfunction, such areas may be more disposed than others to proliferate. Since our studies have demonstrated that a vascular injury can cause an s.m.c. proliferative response in a non-injured segment, this pathway may give rise to atherosclerotic lesions in susceptible areas over extended periods. A course of intervention in this sequence of events would be directed toward reduction of risk factors such as elevated serum levels of cholesterol, which cause endothelial dysfunction along with suppression of platelet function.

This work was supported in part by grants no. HL 25066 and HL 22602 from the National Institutes of Health, Bethesda, Maryland.

REFERENCES (Stemerman)

Adelman, B., Mannarino, A., Goldberg, I. D., Stemerman, M. B. & Handin, R. 1980 Prostaglandin I_2 prevents platelet interaction with injured vessels. *Clinical Res.* **28**, 489A.

Fowler, S., Shio, H. & Wolinsky, H. 1977 Subcellular fractionation and morphology of calf aortic smooth muscle cells. Studies on whole aorta, aortic explants and subculture grown under different conditions. *J. Cell Biol.* **75**, 166–184.

Goldberg, I. D., Stemerman, M. B. & Handin, R. I. 1980a Vascular permeation of platelet factor 4 after endothelial injury. *Science, N.Y.* **209**, 611–612.

Goldberg, I. D., Stemerman, M. B., Ransil, B. J. & Fuhro, R. I. 1980b *In vivo* aortic muscle cell growth kinetics: differences between thoracic and abdominal segments after intimal injury in the rabbit. *Circuln Res.* **47**, 182–189.

Goldberg, I. D., Stemerman, M. B., Schnipper, L. E., Ransil, B. J., Crooks, G. W. & Fuhro, R. L. 1979 Vascular smooth muscle cell kinetics: a new assay for studying patterns of cellular proliferation *in vivo*. *Science, N.Y.* **205**, 920–922.

Groves, H. M., Kinlough-Rathbone, R. L., Richardson, M., Moore, S. & Mustard, J. F. 1979 Platelet interaction with damaged rabbit aorta. *Lab. Invest.* **40**, 194–200.

Ross, R. & Glomset, J. 1976 The pathogenesis of atherosclerosis. *New Engl. J. Med.* **295**, 369–375.

Stemerman, M. B. 1979 Hemostasis, thrombosis and atherogenesis. In *Atherosclerosis reviews* (ed. A. M. Gotto & R. Paoletti), vol. 6, pp. 105–146. New York: Raven Press.

Stemerman, M. B. 1973 Thrombogenesis of the rabbit arterial plaque: an electron microscopic study. *Am. J. Path.* **73**, 7–26.

Stemerman, M. B. 1981 Effects of moderate hypercholesterolemia on rabbit endothelium. *Arteriosclerosis* **1**, 25–32.

Weibel, E. R. 1973 Stereologic techniques for electron microscopic morphometry. In *Principles and techniques for electron microscopy*, (ed. M. A. Hayat), vol. 3, p. 237. Rheinhold, N.Y.: Van Nostrand Press.

Wissler, R. W. 1968 The arterial medial cell, smooth muscle or multifunctional mesenchyme? *J. Atheroscler. Res.* **8**, 201–213.

Discussion

I. F. SKIDMORE (*Glaxo Group Research, Ware, Herts., U.K.*). Having mentioned the platelet-derived growth factor of Ross, would Professor Stemerman comment on the experiments of Gospodarowicz & Tauber (1980), which suggest that mitogenic factors present in serum but not in plasma, and thus presumably of platelet origin, are only required when smooth muscle cells are grown on synthetic surface, and that when smooth muscle cells are grown on extracellular matrix the mitogens contained in plasma are adequate. Secondly, the same workers have shown that HDL is mitogenic for vascular endothelial cells while LDL is toxic at physiological concentrations. Does Professor Stemerman think that this is significant in the response to vascular injury?

Reference

Gospodarowicz, D. S. & Tauber, J.-P. 1980 The control of vascular endothelial and smooth muscle cells by lipoproteins, FGF and the extracellular matrix. Presented at Symposium on Cellular Interactions, Cambridge, 23–26 September.

M. B. Stemerman. The experiments by Gospodarowicz & Tauber suggest that the cellular matrix provides the necessary information to eleviate the serum requirement for s.m.c. growth *in vitro*. Considerable s.m.c. growth was observed in the presence of plasma if an endothelial cell extracellular matrix was employed in the culture system. These experiments can be interpreted to suggest that the matrix is trapping serum-derived or platelet-derived growth factors. The ^{125}I-labelled FGF derivative used as a control in these studies is primarily basic myelin protein (BMP) as recently described, and if FGF can be iodinated among the BMP, the specific radioactivity of the ^{125}I-labelled FGF is probably very low. In addition, although ^{125}I-labelled FGF may be available, no evidence was presented to suggest that the ^{125}I-labelled derivative is biologically active while bovine brain FGF possesses an acidic pI, which eliminates it as a molecule for control. It is unfortunate that neither ^{125}I-labelled platelet-derived growth factor (PDGF) nor ^{125}I-labelled insulin-like growth factor-I (IGF-I) were used since both cationic hormones have been purified and the biological activity of the ^{125}I-labelled derivative assessed. The same logic applies to the question concerning HDL compared with LDL.

J. R. O'Brien (*Central Laboratory, St Mary's Hospital, Portsmouth, U.K.*). I was fascinated to see the amount of immunofluorescence in the sub-endothelium of the ballooned aortae indicating extensive PF4 deposition. Pepper and coworkers (Pumphrey *et al.* 1979) have shown that after minute doses of heparin IV, e.g. 500 U, there is a massive release of PF4 from some depot, but presumably not from platelets since there is no parallel release of βTB. An obvious depot was the endothelium or subendothelium. Accordingly I ask Professor Stemerman if animals were exposed to any heparin, and if not, what he thinks would happen to heparinized animals that were ballooned, or ballooned animals that were subsequently heparinized.

Reference

Pumphrey, C. W., Pepper, D. S. & Dawes, J. 1979 Heparin-PF4 pulsing as a measure of platelet endothelial cell reaction *in vivo*. *Thromb. Haemostas.* **42**, 43.

M. B. Stemerman. The animals described in our experiments were not given heparin. It is indeed possible that PF4 would bind to heparin and not enter the vessel wall; however, since no experimental data are yet available, we can only speculate on this.

Elspeth B. Smith (*Department of Chemical Pathology, University Medical Buildings, Foresterhill, Aberdeen, U.K.*). Caution is needed in interpreting endothelial injury in terms of allowing LDL to flood into the subendothelial space. In normal human aortic intima, the concentration of LDL, on a crude volumetric basis, is actually twice the concentration in the patient's plasma. Thus, removing the endothelium should in theory reduce the concentration of intimal LDL by allowing it to re-equilibrate with plasma.

May I ask Professor Stemerman a question about the [³H]thymidine labelling. There was a sharp bump in the specific activity curve just before the number of s.m.cs increased steeply and then settled at a constant high level. What happened to the actual rate of cell division? Did it remain high?

M. B. Stemerman. Recent studies by Dr Minick show that apolipoprotein B appears to be selectively trapped in areas that correspond to glycosaminoglycan deposition. The role of LDL in the pathobiology of smooth muscle cell proliferation *in vivo* remains unclear since its availability to the vascular s.m.c. is unknown. Therefore, not concentration of LDL but rather availability to the s.m.c. is the critical factor.

The growth rate of smooth muscle cells peaks at approximately day 7 (Goldberg *et al.* 1980*b*).

Phil. Trans. R. Soc. Lond. B **294**, 225–229 (1981)
Printed in Great Britain

The pathological basis and microanatomy of occlusive thrombus formation in human coronary arteries

By M. J. Davies and T. Thomas

*Department of Histopathology, St George's Hospital Medical School,
University of London, Cranmer Terrace, London SW17 0RE, U.K.*

[Plate 1]

Myocardial necrosis, usually called infarction, occurs in different patterns. A common form is necrosis of one segment of the left ventricle, i.e., anterior, septal, lateral or posterior. This regional infarction is consistently associated with an acute occlusive thrombosis of the artery supplying that region. Diffuse necrosis involving the whole circumference, usually the subendocardial zone, of the ventricle is not consistently associated with thrombi. Occlusive thrombi identified in post-mortem coronary arteriograms have been reconstructed in their entirety from serial sections at 150 μm intervals. Most occlusive thrombi were found to be associated with a dissection track into the intima at an atheromatous plaque. The break into the plaque usually extended over several millimetres, often in spirals, so that a mass of thrombus within the plaque compressed the original lumen. Previous accounts of plaque rupture or cracking greatly underestimated the magnitude of the dissection of blood into the intima.

The exact role of coronary thrombosis in producing the clinical features of ischaemic heart disease has been uncertain. The incorporation of microthrombi into the surface cap of atherosclerotic plaques almost certainly contributes to their slow growth towards the horizon for clinical expression of disease. Much larger thrombi form on plaques and occlude the arterial lumen as a sudden event to precipitate myocardial necrosis. This paper is concerned with the latter type of occlusive thrombus.

A historical review of pathological observations linking the finding of an occlusive thrombus to an area of myocardial necrosis reveals such variation that two opposing interpretations have emerged (Davies *et al.* 1979). One proposes that an occlusive thrombus is the cause of myocardial necrosis in the region supplied by the artery (Chapman 1974; Chandler 1974; Davies *et al.* 1976). The other is that myocardial necrosis is not related consistently to occlusive thrombi and that thrombosis is a secondary process in arteries in which flow is reduced (Silver *et al.* 1980; Roberts 1972, 1974). The observations are so discordant and their interpretations so opposed that explanations have been found in differences of definition and case selection. Many publications define the terms myocardial necrosis and infarction differently. Definitions of infarction range from a macroscopic area of necrosis several centimetres across and confined to one region of ventricular muscle, to microscopic foci of necrosis scattered throughout the myocardium. Another type of infarction consists of macroscopic areas of necrosis involving the whole subendocardial zone of the ventricle.

A recent investigation of ours on the relation of patterns of necrosis to occlusive thrombosis has gone some way towards resolving the differences (Davies *et al.* 1979). Myocardial necrosis was demonstrated in slices of heart by enzyme histochemistry. The technique increased the precision with which the margins of necrotic areas could be defined above that of simple visual inspection. Patterns of necrosis were classified into three groups; entirely regional, anterior, lateral or posterior; entirely diffuse, i.e. the whole circumference of the ventricle involved in a subendocardial necrotic zone; and complex mixtures of the other two patterns. There was a consistent association, namely in 70 of 71 cases, of regional infarction with occlusive thrombi. In contrast, diffuse necrosis was associated with widespread narrowing of the coronary arteries and not with occlusive thrombi.

Another major reason for the discrepancies has been a failure to distinguish between the terms sudden death and myocardial infarction. For myocardial necrosis to be demonstrable at autopsy the patient must survive at least 12 h after the onset of symptoms. When the patient survives only 6 h or less, infarction cannot be demonstrated. But it has been commonly assumed that an infarct would have been demonstrable after a longer period of survival. Clinical studies have now conclusively shown that patients who 'drop dead' and are resuscitated with instant defibrillation by emergency teams in an ambulance or on the street fall into two groups (Liberthson et al. 1974). Patients in the larger group do not develop any evidence, electro-cardiographic or other, of myocardial infarction. Patients in the smaller group, about 25%, develop myocardial infarction. Patients in the former, larger, group are now considered to have suffered from spontaneous ventricular fibrillation in an electrically unstable heart resulting from chronic ischaemia. Evidently the inclusion of such cases of sudden death without demonstrable necrosis will produce significantly lower figures of frequency of thrombi.

With the establishment of a constant association of regional infarction with occlusive thrombosis in the subtending artery, the microanatomy of the occlusive thrombi becomes of interest because it may throw light on the mechanisms of their formation.

MATERIALS AND METHODS

Twelve human hearts were studied in which acute regional infarction had been demonstrated by electrocardiography and the patient came to autopsy within a period of 2–5 days from the onset of chest pain. In all cases, strictly regional areas of myocardial necrosis were demonstrated by histochemistry of fresh slices of heart. The coronary artery orifices were cannulated and injected with a barium–gelatin suspension at pressures of less than 80 mmHg. The heart was X-rayed at 45 kV for 3.5 min, with the use of Industrex film. Then the coronary arteries were dissected free, decalcified in 10 % (by volume) acetic acid for 24 h, and X-rayed again. From these arteriograms the occluded segment was identified and removed intact. This arterial segment was cut serially at intervals of 150 μm into transverse sections 6 μm in thickness. The sections started proximal to the occlusion at a point where the barium outlined a normal luminal diameter and continued through the occlusion until the lumen was again patent. Each section was stained by a modified picro–Mallory trichrome method (Carstairs 1965), which differentiates red cells (stained yellow), fibrin (stained red), platelets (stained as purple punctate material) and collagen (stained light blue). The sections were projected and outline drawings made with a colour code for each type of tissue. Material was considered to be thrombus when it contained predominantly fibrin and/or platelets. From the series of transverse sections, the whole occluded segment of artery was reconstructed in longitudinal section.

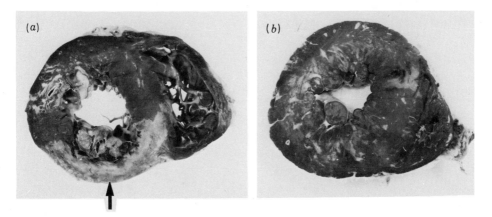

FIGURE 1. Transverse slice of human ventricular muscle stained to show succinic dehydrogenase activity (dark). In (*a*) an area of enzyme loss (pale) is confined to one region on the posterior wall (arrows) of the left ventricle. In (*b*) there are small focal pale areas throughout the whole circumference of the left ventricle.

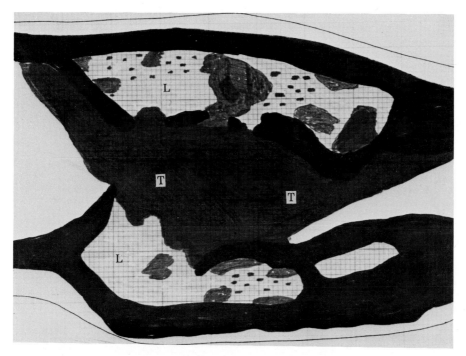

FIGURE 2. Reconstruction of a longitudinal section through an acute coronary occlusion. Thrombus (T) in the arterial lumen is in direct continuity with the lipid of the plaque (L) though numerous defects in the intima.

RESULTS

Twelve occlusive thrombi were reconstructed as described. Longitudinal sections of nine showed continuity between the thrombus occluding the lumen and thrombus deep within an atheromatous plaque. The breaks in the plaque cap allowing such continuity were often large, i.e. from 4 mm to about 15 mm long, and ran spirally along the artery. In three of the nine thrombi the barium proximal to the occlusion was continuous with that inside the plaque and could be identified in retrospect on the angiograms as a double lumen over several millimetres at the proximal end of the thrombus.

Thrombi deep within the atheromatous plaque extended proximally and distally from the tear into areas where on cross sections the plaque caps were intact. In two cases, lipid debris was extruded into the original lumen and admixed with thrombus distal to the tear. Thrombi in the vicinity of the tears and nearby in the plaques were rich in platelets. Thrombi extending proximally and distally in the arterial lumen were predominantly fibrin and red cells. Some thrombi had apparently increased the plaque volume, raising a flap of intima that narrowed the original lumen.

Three of the twelve occlusions had no demonstrable break in the intima underlying occlusive thrombi. These thrombi had apparently begun spontaneously at sites of gross stenosis and grown forward to the point of exit of a major branch.

DISCUSSION

Cracking, fissuring or breakage of the cap of atheromatous plaques was proposed some time ago as an immediate cause of occlusive thrombosis (Friedman & Van Den Bovenkamp 1966; Constantinides 1966; Ridolfi & Hutchins 1977). Subsequent confirmation was hampered by random sectioning of occlusive thrombi, whereby the breaks were not found consistently. The present investigation establishes that sections proximal and distal to plaques can show thrombus in the lumen but no intimal break. Random sectioning will therefore greatly underestimate the frequency of such breaks and will, moreover, give no impression of the shape or size of the breaks when present. Our work shows that these breaks are larger than the microscopic fissures described previously. The associated thrombi extended deep into the plaques and occlusion was probably preceded by extensive passage of blood into and dissection of the intima. This process has been aptly likened to internal haemorrhage from the artery (G. V. R. Born, personal communication).

While the contribution of plaque rupture has been confirmed, there were cases in which it could not be demonstrated even by serial sections. This suggests an alternative initiation of coronary thrombosis, presumably through abnormalities in the blood flow through greatly narrowed arterial segments. The investigation reported here does not allow accurate assessment of the comparative frequency of the two causes, because the tedious technique restricted the number of reconstructions.

If plaque fissure and intimal dissection are frequent antecedents of occlusive thrombosis, it becomes important to determine what factors are responsible for the fissuring. The destruction that takes place in fissured plaques effectively rules out any morphological interpretation of events, but all were large plaques containing extensive pools of lipid. If rupture of a plaque were a random event in patients with only isolated lipid-rich atheromatous lesions, thrombosis

227

may not occur again or at long time intervals, in keeping with the good prognosis of some patients who survive an acute myocardial infarction. On this assumption, patients with numerous lipid-rich plaques would run the risk of repeated episodes. Thrombosis without plaque fissure may be a manifestation of more diffuse coronary artery disease with widespread stenosis.

The microanatomy of the thrombi suggests that occlusion occurs over several hours or even 1–2 days. The initial crack allows blood to dissect the plaque with the formation of a platelet-rich thrombus, which may ultimately extend through the crack into the original lumen. From this occlusive platelet-rich thrombus, predominantly fibrinous thrombus extends proximally and also distally to the next major branch. This interpretation has been supported by evidence obtained from patients who were injected with radioactively labelled fibrinogen immediately after admission to hospital with chest pain (Erhardt 1976; Fulton & Sumner 1976). In those who came to autopsy, occlusive thrombi had no radioactivity in the centre, presumably where they originated in fissures, whereas the extensions in both directions were radioactive, presumably representing subsequent propagations.

REFERENCES (Davies & Thomas)

Carstairs, K. 1965 The identification of platelets and platelet antigens in histological sections. *J. Path. Bact.* **90**, 225–231.
Chandler, A. B. 1974 Coronary thrombosis in myocardial infarction. Report of a workshop on the role of coronary thrombosis in the pathogenesis of acute myocardial infarction. *Am. J. Cardiol.* **34**, 823–833.
Chapman, I. 1974 The cause–effect relationship between recent coronary artery occlusion and acute myocardial infarction. *Am. Heart J.* **87**, 267–271.
Constantinides, P. 1966 Plaque fissure in human coronary thrombosis. *J. Atheroscler. Res.* **6**, 1–17.
Davies, M. J., Fulton, W. F. M. & Robertson, W. B. 1979 The relation of coronary thrombosis to ischaemic myocardial necrosis. *J. Path.* **127**, 99–110.
Davies, M. J., Woolf, N. & Robertson, W. B. 1976 Pathology of acute myocardial infarction with particular reference to occlusive coronary thrombi. *Br. Heart J.* **38**, 659–664.
Erhardt, L. R., Unge, G. & Bowman, G. 1976 Formation of coronary arterial thrombi in relation to onset of necrosis in acute myocardial infarction in man. *Am. Heart J.* **91**, 592–598.
Friedman, M. & Van Den Bovenkamp, G. J. 1966 The pathogenesis of coronary thrombosis. *Am. J. Path.* **48**, 19–44.
Fulton, W. F. M. & Sumner, D. J. 1976 I^{125} labelled fibrinogen, autoradiography and steroarteriography in identification of coronary thrombotic occlusion in fatal myocardial infarction. *Br. Heart J.* **38**, 880.
Liberthson, R. R., Nagel, E. L., Hirschman, J. C., Nussenfeld, S. R., Blackborne, B. D. & Davis, J. H. 1974 Pathophysiologic observations in prehospital ventricular fibrillation and sudden cardiac death. *Circulation* **49**, 790–798.
Ridolfi, R. L. & Hutchins, G. M. 1977 The relationship between coronary artery lesions and myocardial infarcts: ulceration of atherosclerotic plaques precipitating coronary thrombosis. *Am. Heart J.* **93**, 1977–1986.
Roberts, W. C. 1974 Coronary thrombosis and fatal myocardial ischemia. *Circulation* **49**, 1–3.
Roberts, W. C. & Buja, L. M. 1972 The frequency and significance of coronary arterial thrombi and other observations in fatal acute myocardial infarction. *Am. J. Med.* **52**, 425–443.
Silver, M. D., Baroldi, G. & Mariani, F. 1980 The relationship between acute occlusive coronary thrombi and myocardial infarction studied in 100 consecutive patients. *Circulation* **61**, 219–227.

Discussion

J. McMichael, F.R.S. (*2 North Square, London NW*11 7*AA, U.K.*). This is an important demonstration of the complex situation at the site of occlusion. The contribution of mechanical damage is obvious and brings to mind steering wheel injuries, which can cause thrombosis of the arteries in the anterior wall of the heart. In more than 800 young men on military service who developed coronary occlusion, about one-third followed extreme physical exertion (Yater *et al., Am. Heart J.* **36**, 334, 481, 683 (1948)). Jogging also has its mortality.

P. D. RICHARDSON (*Brown University, Providence, R.I., U.S.A.*). The authors have provided an excellent description of plaque rupture and associated thrombus formation in coronary arteries. It would seem worth while to investigate mechanical factors associated with plaque rupture as this appears to be the immediate cause of thrombus formation. Relevant mechanical factors are, first, the mechanical strength of the cap which preserves the integrity of the plaque and, secondly, the fluid dynamic stresses induced on the plaque by the pulsatile flow of blood in the artery. The stresses are determined by the frequency of pulsation as well as by the pressure. Consequently it would be interesting to investigate the role of heart rate as well as blood pressure as a risk factor for myocardial infarction. It would also be useful to obtain information about the mechanical strength of plaque cap material.

Phil. Trans. R. Soc. Lond. B **294**, 231–239 (1981)

Printed in Great Britain

Vessel wall and blood flow dynamics in arterial disease

By R. J. Lusby†‖, H. I. Machleder†¶, W. Jeans‡, R. Skidmore§,
J. P. Woodcock§, P. C. Clifford† and R. N. Baird†

† *Department of Surgery, Bristol Royal Infirmary, Bristol BS2 8HW, U.K.*

‡ *Department of Radiodiagnosis, Bristol Royal Infirmary, Bristol BS2 8HW, U.K.*

§ *Department of Medical Physics, Bristol General Hospital, Bristol BS1 6SY, U.K.*

Recent developments in ultrasound techniques have made it possible to investigate patients with arterial disease non-invasively by using Doppler blood velocity signal analysis. Since January 1979, 189 patients with pre-stroke syndromes have been investigated by using pulsed Doppler and real-time B-mode ultrasound imaging and waveform analysis. The results were that both imaging systems were highly (more than 92 %) sensitive and specific when compared with conventional carotid arteriography. The ultrasound systems detected turbulence and could also be used to measure the distensibility of the arterial wall. The results show that varying grades of carotid stenosis can be demonstrated by two ultrasonic imaging systems, and that lateral scans are particularly helpful.

Introduction

Cerebrovascular disease is the third most frequent cause of death in England (Haberman *et al.* 1979) and Wales, with over 70 % of strokes being due to thromboembolism (Kannel *et al.* 1970). The contribution of extracranial atherosclerotic disease in the causation of stroke has been recognized only in the last 30 years (Fields *et al.* 1968; Fisher 1951; Yorks 1961). Recent investigation established that up to 88 % of patients have estcranial artery lesions (Hutchinson & Acheson 1975; Eisenberg *et al.* 1977), with the majority situated at the carotid artery bifurcation (Hass *et al.* 1968). Carotid artery lesions produce cerebral ischaemia by two mechanisms: (1) by subtotal stenosis or occlusion and (2) by platelet and cholesterol emboli generated on atheromatous plaques.

As there is no known treatment to limit or reverse cerebral infarction once it has occurred, effective prevention must depend on early recognition and treatment of high-risk groups with extracranial disease. Fortunately, not all strokes occur without warning and there are pre-stroke syndromes, namely transient ischaemic attacks (t.i.as), amaurosis fugax and asymptomatic bruits, which warrant investigation in an effort to prevent stroke. However, approximately half the patients with t.i.as and two-thirds with asymptomatic bruits will not proceed to stroke if left untreated. Critical to the selection for preventative measures is the identification of significant precursors of stroke. This can be achieved by more accurate characterization of the carotid lesions.

Recent developments in ultrasound techniques have made it possible to investigate patients with arterial disease non-invasively by using Doppler blood velocity signal analysis (Woodcock *et al.* 1972; Blackshear *et al.* 1979; Baird *et al.* 1980) and direct imaging of atheromatous lesions

‖ Present address: Department of Surgery, St Vincent's Hospital, Sydney, Australia.

¶ Present address: Department of Surgery, U.C.L.A. Medical School, Los Angeles, California 90024, U.S.A.

at specific sites (Fish 1972; Mozersky *et al.* 1971; Barnes *et al.* 1976; Baird *et al.* 1979; Lusby 1980; Sumner *et al.* 1979). We report the use of these techniques for detecting carotid artery lesions and for defining the factors that may contribute to cerebral infarction.

MATERIALS AND METHODS

Since January 1979, 189 patients with pre-stroke syndromes have been investigated in the vascular laboratory of the Bristol Royal Infirmary. Two ultrasound imaging systems have been used.

Pulsed Doppler system

MAVIS, a 30 channel, range-gated, 5 MHz pulsed Doppler system, was developed by Fish (1972). The 30 gates can be adjusted to a suitable depth and the movement of blood detected by the Doppler shift principle in any or all of the gates. By moving the probe manually across

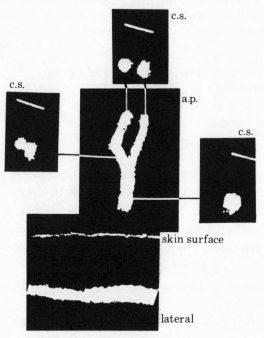

FIGURE 1. MAVIS pulsed Doppler projections in lateral, antero-posterior (a.p.) and cross-sectional (c.s.) planes.

the skin, an image of the moving column of blood is built up on a storage oscilloscope, a permanent record of which is made with a Polaroid photograph. The machine is directional, producing separate images of arterial blood moving towards the beam and venous blood moving away. Images can be produced in three orthogonal planes (figure 1). The resolution is of the order of 1 mm.

Real-time B-mode imaging

The Duplex real-time mechanical scanner produces a two-dimensional B-mode image from three 5 MHz transducers, which rotate in a plastic boot. The images obtained in longitudinal or cross-sectional planes are displayed on an oscilloscope. Superimposed on the display is a line corresponding to the location of a depth-sensitive pulsed 5 MHz ultrasound beam (figure 2), which can be adjusted to provide signals from selected sites for analysis. A photocopy of a frozen image is obtained for the permanent record. The Duplex scanner also has the facility for generating time–position M-mode scans. In this mode, echoes are recorded from moving structures such as the vessel walls and displayed as vertical deflexions (Lusby *et al.* 1981). The vessel wall distensibility with each pulse can therefore be displayed dynamically on the screen. By adding a scale, changes in vessel diameter with each pulse can be quantified. By using the B-mode scan the vessel to be observed was clearly identified and distensibility measured in the common carotid and at the origin of the internal carotid arteries.

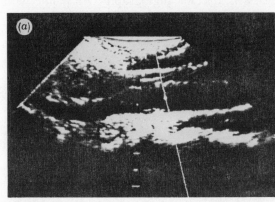 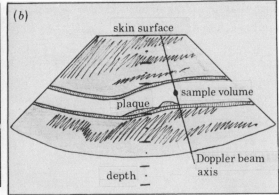

FIGURE 2. Duplex scan (*a*) of carotid artery with diagram (*b*) showing the pulsed Doppler beam and Doppler sample volume.

For more information about the dynamic properties of the carotid bifurcation, biplanar video tape recordings and cineangiography films at 50 frames per second were made during the injection of contrast into 12 carotid arteries of patients undergoing investigation for t.i.as. To ensure complete mixing of contrast material with blood and to limit boundary layer separation, the catheter tip was placed in the proximal common carotid artery near its origin from the aortic arch.

To evaluate the morphology of the carotid bifurcation and its relation to ultasonic and angiographic images, Perspex casts impregnated with barium were made from endarterectomy specimens of patients undergoing carotid surgery and from vessels obtained at post-mortem.

RESULTS

Ultrasonic imaging

Both imaging systems provided images of the vessels without discomfort or complication and were highly acceptable to the patients; 71 patients subsequently underwent angiography, at the discretion of the referring physician, with corroboration of the ultrasonic findings in 68 patients (90%). A detailed prospective evaluation of the systems was done on 78 vessels in which three planar angiography was performed, each being reported on independently without knowledge of the other findings (Lusby *et al.* 1980, 1981).

Pulsed Doppler imaging

Results with MAVIS imaging and angiography are compared in table 1. Of 43 lesions causing less than 50% decrease in vessel diameter, 39 (91%) were detected. There were four false negatives, i.e. lesions detected angiographically but missed on ultrasound imaging; two were associated with atheromatous plaques in bulbous origins of the internal carotid artery. The lateral scan was better at detecting lesions situated on the posterior wall and provided diagnostic information in 20 vessels (48%) with less than 50% decrease in diameter. All five occlusions of the internal carotid artery were detected.

Duplex B-mode imaging

Duplex imaging and angiography are compared in table 2. While 39 lesions (91%) were detected, four were given a classification of variance with that for angiography. All lesions with more than 50% diameter decrease were detected, but only four out of five of those that were totally occluded.

TABLE 1. MAVIS PULSED DOPPLER CAROTID BIFURCATION ASSESSMENT

angiographic findings	number of vessels	positive number	(%)	negative (%)	positive other† estimate
normal	16	1	—	94	—
less than 25%	26	22	85	4	—
25–50%	17	14	82	—	3 under
50–99%	14	12	86	—	2 under
occluded	5	5	100	—	—
total	**78**				

† Where a lesion was detected but the estimate of severity did not agree with that seen on angiography.

TABLE 2. DUPLEX B-MODE CAROTID BIFURCATION ASSESSMENT

angiographic findings	number of vessels	positive number	(%)	negative (%)	positive other† estimate
normal	16	1	—	94	—
less than 25%	26	19	73	4	3
25–50%	17	16	94	—	1
50–99%	14	13	93	—	1
occluded	5	4	50	1	—
total	**78**				

† Where a lesion was detected but the estimate of severity did not agree with that seen on angiography.

The essential difference between the two imaging systems is shown in figure 3, where in the lateral MAVIS scan the lesion is seen as a defect in the blood flow map, while the Duplex scan shows a vessel wall plaque encroaching on the lumen.

The ultrasonic classification of lesions was made solely on imaging although in producing the image the operator, with experience, was guided by the presence of turbulent flow in the Doppler audio signal to look further for a lesion not obvious at first. Several images were made of each vessel to confirm a persistent defect. The overall sensitivity in detecting all grades of lesion was 95% for the MAVIS pulsed Doppler and 93% for the Duplex system. The specificity for both was 94%.

Atheromatous plaque turbulence commonly occurred; an example is shown in figure 4. The profile of blood velocity in the common carotid artery was essentially normal proximal to a stenotic lesion; distally there were an increase in maximum velocity and a broader range of velocities, arising from turbulence and disorganization of normal laminar flow.

With the Duplex system it was necessary to confirm the presence of arterial flow. In five patients, soft thrombus completely occluded the internal carotid artery but the B-mode image failed to identify the occlusion due to the low acoustic impedance of thrombus which is similar to fluid blood. In four of the patients, failure to obtain a Doppler signal when the sample volume was placed in the vessel lumen indicated an absence of flowing blood even though the image appeared relatively normal; in the fifth, a patent external carotid artery was mistaken for the internal carotid artery.

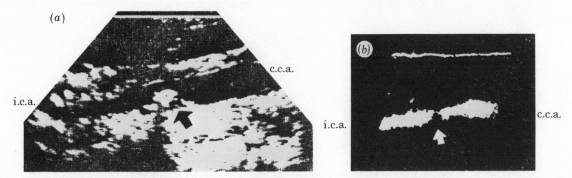

FIGURE 3. Lateral Duplex (*a*) and MAVIS (*b*) scans of carotid artery showing a lesion (arrowed). The Duplex scan shows encroachment onto the lumen of the lesion while the MAVIS scan shows a defect in the image of the moving column of blood. I.c.a., internal carotid artery; c.c.a., common carotid artery.

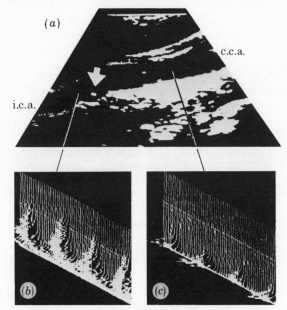

FIGURE 4. Duplex scan (*a*) of carotid artery, and Doppler velocity spectral analysis distal (*b*) and proximal (*c*) to a small lesion in the carotid bulb. There is a turbulent pattern with increased velocity just distal to the lesion.

Vessel distensibility

The real-time Duplex system showed up the systolic–diastolic changes in vessel wall distension. Recordings of contrast injection during angiography of 12 vessels showed that the internal diameter of the common carotid artery varied by $16.2 \pm 8.5\%$ (mean $\pm$ s.e.m.), and the bulbous origin of the internal carotid artery by $26.1 \pm 9.6\%$ ($p < 0.005$, Wilcoxon) (figure 5). In 10 patients time position M-mode scans showed that the average distensibility of the common carotid artery was $12.6 \pm 2.4\%$ (mean $\pm$ s.e.m.) and the bulbous origin of the internal carotid arteries $19.7 \pm 5.4\%$ ($p < 0.005$) (figure 6). In 23 vessels with bulbous origins, the average bulb internal diameter was 157% (range $120-246\%$) that of the distal internal carotid artery.

Correlation of ultrasonic and clinical observations

There were 189 patients referred to the vascular laboratory with symptoms suggesting episodes of transient cerebral ischaemia or amaurosis fugax. In 86% of them, vessel wall

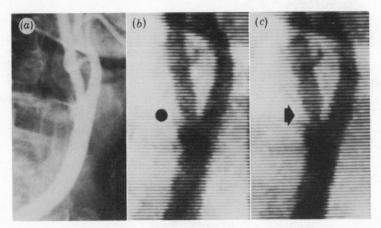

FIGURE 5. Single X-ray (a) and two video frames (b, c) of a carotid angiogram. The lesion arrowed is not so obvious in an earlier frame (dot) nor in the angiogram.

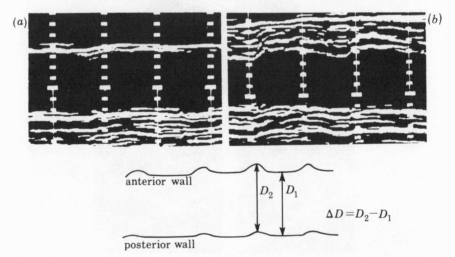

FIGURE 6. M-mode distensibility showing the movement in anterior and posterior walls of the carotid artery: (a) c.c.a.; (b) origin of i.c.a. An increase in percentage distensibility ($100\Delta D/D_1$) is noted at the origin of the internal carotid artery.

abnormalities were detected by ultrasound imaging. Among the 16% without evidence of lesions at the carotid bifurcation were patients known to have valvular disease of the heart, cardiac arrhythmias or evidence of subclavian or vertebral artery lesions.

Of patients with unilateral transient ischaemic attacks of amaurosis fugax, 45% had bruits in the neck over the corresponding carotid artery; 54% of bruits were associated with stenoses of more than 50% and the other 46% with lesser narrowings. There was no correlation between degree of stenosis and manifestation of transient ischaemic attacks or amaurosis fugax.

DISCUSSION

The aim of non-invasive investigations of carotid artery disease is the accurate character-ization of all grades of lesions. This report shows that varying grades of stenosis can be demon-strated by two ultrasonic imaging systems. The pulsed Doppler system with range-gating has the advantage that it can produce images in three orthogonal directions, thus providing three-dimensional information about the arterial lumen. In many cases where antero-posterior views failed to show a lesion it was detected on lateral scans. The predilection of atheroma for the posterior wall makes it necessary to obtain them in clear views, which are provided by the Duplex system and the lateral MAVIS scan. The techniques have provided similarly accurate detection of carotid artery lesions for others (Blackshear *et al.* 1979; Barnes *et al.* 1976; Sumner *et al.* 1979).

Carotid artery bruits are caused by vessel wall movements at high frequency in the audible range (McDonald 1974). There is evidence that particular frequencies cause changes in structural components (Gersten 1956; Bougner & Roach 1971) of the vessels walls, i.e. in collagen and elastin. These changes can lead to dilation, ulceration and exposure of wall components, e.g. collagen and basement membrane, which can activate platelets.

The variations in arterial diameter associated with pulsation appear much greater than appreciated before. In exposed intact vessels these variations are only 1–2% (Heath *et al.* 1973), whereas both M-mode and dynamic angiographies show them to be greater, confirming an early report (Arndt 1968) based on echo tracking. A new observation of ours is the great distensibility of the carotid bulb, even in the presence of atheromatous lesions. This disten-sibility is apparently due to a decrease in thickness of the media, which results in a structure similar to that of the pulmonary arteries (Heath *et al.* 1973).

Observed variations in distensibility probably indicate sudden differences in compliance, particularly at the origin of the internal carotid artery. These abrupt differences are associated with disruptive stresses in the walls, which may lead to dilation of the carotid bulb (Gonza *et al.* 1974; Eiken 1961; Baird & Abbott 1976). The same forces may also bring about fracture of atheromatous plaques, which is an immediate cause of obstructive thrombosis (Born 1978).

Turbulence is invariably present in lesions so large as to produce drops in pressure and flow to the brain (Blackshear *et al.* 1979). Distal to stenotic lesions, disorganization of laminar flow as detected with the pulsed Doppler and characterized by spectral analysis contribute to platelet thrombosis and embolism. These haemodynamically significant lesions frequently result in cerebral infarction and stroke (Machleder 1979). Increased velocity gradients and jet streaming effects may affect vascular endothelium (Fry 1968; Payling Wright & Born 1971). These investigations indicate that ultrasound and related techniques provide information about abnormalities in vessel walls and blood flow that determine thromboembolic events in arteries.

Dr H. I. Macleder was supported in part by the Fogarty International Centre, National Institutes of Health, U.S.A. (grant no. FO6 TW00525-01). Dr R. Skidmore was supported by the Medical Research Council (grant no. G.978/430). Mr P. C. Clifford was supported by the British Heart Foundation (grant no. 717).

REFERENCES (Lusby *et al.*)

Arndt, J. O., Klauske, J. & Mersch, F. 1968 The diameter of the intact carotid artery in man and its change with pulse pressure. *Pflügers Arch. ges. Physiol.* **301**, 230.

Baird, R. N., Abbott, W. M. 1976 Pulsatile blood flow in arterial grafts. *Lancet* ii, 948–950.

Baird, R. N., Lusby, R. J., Bird, D. R., Giddings, A. E. B., Skidmore, R., Woodcock, J. P., Horton, R. E. & Peacock, J. H. 1979 Pulsed Doppler angiography in lower limb ischaemia. *Surgery* **86**, 818–825.

Baird, R. N., Bird, D. R., Clifford, P. C., Lusby, R. J., Skidmore, R. & Woodcock, J. P. 1980 Upstream stenosis. Its diagnosis by Doppler signals from the femoral artery. *Arch. Surg.* **115**, 1316–1322.

Barnes, R. W., Bone, G. E., Reinerston, J. E., Slaymaker, E. E., Hokanson, D. E. & Strandness, D. E., Jr 1976 Non-invasive ultrasonic carotid angiography. Prospective validation by contrast angiography. *Surgery* **80**, 328.

Blackshear, W. M., Phillips, D. J., Thiele, B. L., Birsch, J. H., Chikos, P. M., Marinelli, M. R., Ward, K. J. & Strandness, D. E. 1979 Detection of carotid occlusive disease by ultrasonic imaging and pulsed Doppler spectral analysis. *Surgery* **86**, 698–706.

Born, G. V. R. 1978 Arterial thrombosis and its prevention. In *Proc. VIII World Congress of Cardiology*, Tokyo (ed. S. Hayase, S. Murao), pp. 81–91. Amsterdam, Oxford and Princeton: Excerpta Medica.

Bougner, D. R. & Roach, M. R. 1971 Effect of low frequency vibration on arterial wall. *Circuln Res.* **29**, 136.

Eiken, O. 1961 Pressure–flow relationship and thrombotic occlusion of experimental grafts. *Acta chir. scand.* **121**, 398.

Eisenberg, R. L., Nemsek, W. R., Moore, W. S. & Mani, R. L. 1977 Relationship of transient ischaemic attacks and angiographically demonstrable lesions of carotid artery. *Stroke* **8**, 483–486.

Fields, W. S., North, R. R. & Hass, W. K. 1968 Joint study of extracranial arterial occlusion as a cause of stroke. 1. *J. Am. med. Ass.* **203**, 955–960.

Fish, P. J. 1972 In *Blood flow measurement* (ed. V. C. Roberts), p. 29. London: Sector Publ.

Fisher, M. 1951 Occlusion of the internal carotid artery. *Arch. Neurol. Psychiat.* **72**, 182–204.

Fry, D. L. 1968 Acute vascular endothelial changes associated with increased velocity gradients. *Circuln Res.* **22**, 165.

Gersten, J. W. 1956 Relation of ultrasound effects to orientation of tendon in ultrasound field. *Arch. phys. med. Rehabil.* **37**, 201.

Gonza, E. R., Mason, W. F., Marble, A. E., Winter, D. A. & Dolan, F. G. 1974 Necessity for elastic properties in synthetic arterial grafts. *Can. J. Surg.* **17**, 1–5.

Greenfield, J. C., Tindall, G. T., Dillon, M. L. & Mahaley, M. S. 1964 Mechanics of the human carotid artery *in vivo*. *Circuln. Res.* **15**, 240.

Haberman, S., Capildeo, R. & Rose, F. C. 1979 Epidemiological aspects of stroke. In *Progress in stroke research*, vol. 1 (ed. R. Greenhalgh & F. Clifford Rose), pp. 3–14. Pitman Medical.

Hass, W. K., Fields, W. S., North, R. R., Kricheff, I. I., Chase, N. E. & Bauer, B. B. 1968 Joint study of extracranial arterial occlusion. 1. Arteriography, techniques, sites and complications. *J. Am. med. Ass.* **203**, 961–968.

Heath, D., Smith, P., Harris, P. & Winson, M. 1973 The atherosclerotic human carotid sinus. *J. Path.* **110**, 49–58.

Hutchinson, E. C. & Acheson, D. M. 1975 *Strokes: natural history, pathology and surgical treatment*. London: W. B. Saunders.

Kannel, W. B., Wolf, P. A., Verter, J. *et al.* 1970 Epidemiologic assessment of the role of blood pressure and stroke: the Framingham study. *J. Am. med. Ass.* **214**, 301–310.

McDonald, D. A. 1974 *Blood flow in arteries*, 2nd edn. London: Edward Arnold. Baltimore: Williams & Wilkins.

Machleder, H. I. 1979 Strokes, transient ischaemic attacks and asymptomatic bruits. *West. J. Med.* **130**, 205–217.

Mozersky, D. J., Bauer, D. W., Hokanson, D. E., Sumner, D. S. & Strandness, D. E. 1971 Ultrasonic arteriography. *Arch. Surg.* **103**, 663–667.

Mustard, J. F., Murphy, E. A., Rowsell, H. C. & Downie, H. G. 1962 Factors influencing thrombus formation *in vivo*. *Am. J. Med.* **33**, 621–646.

Lusby, R. J. 1980 Pulsed Doppler assessment of the profunda femoris artery. In *Diagnosis and monitoring in arterial surgery* (ed. R. N. Baird & J. P. Woodcock), pp. 39–46. Bristol: John Wright & Sons.

Lusby, R. J., Woodcock, J., Skidmore, R., Jeans, W., Clifford, P. C. & Baird, R. N. 1980 Carotid artery disease: a prospective evaluation of ultrasonic imaging in the detection of low and high grade stenosis. *Br. J. Surg.* **67**, 823.

Lusby, R. J., Woodcock, J. P., Skidmore, R., Jeans, W. D., Hope, D. T. & Baird, R. N. 1981 Carotid artery disease: a prospective evaluation of pulsed Doppler imaging. *Ultrasound Med. Biol.* (In the press.)

Lusby, R. J., Clifford, P. C., Bird, D. R., Skidmore, R., Woodcock, J. P. & Baird, R. N. 1981 Ultrasonic techniques in the study of graft survival. In *Haemodynamics of the limbs*, vol. 11 (ed. P. Puel). (In the press.)

Payling Wright, H. & Born, G. V. R. 1971 Possible effects of blood flow on the turnover rate of vascular endothelial cells. In *Theoretical and clinical haemorheology* (ed. H. H. Hartert & A. L. Copley), pp. 220–226. New York and Heidelberg: Springer.

Sumner, D. S., Russell, J. B., Ramsey, D. E., Hajjar, W. M. & Miles, R. D. 1979 Non-invasive diagnosis of extra cranial carotid arterial disease: a prospective evaluation of pulsed Doppler imaging and oculoplethysmo-graphy. *Arch. Surg.* **114**, 1222–1229.

Woodcock, J. P., King, D. H., Gosling, R. G. & Nueman, D. L. 1972 Physical aspects of the measurement of blood velocity by Doppler shifted ultrasound. In *Blood flow measurement* (ed. V. C. Roberts), ch. 1. London: Sector Publ.

Yates, P. O. & Hutchinson, E. C. 1961 Cerebral infarction. The role of stenosis of the extracranial cerebral arteries. In *Med. Res. Coun. spec. Rep. Ser.* no. 300. London: H.M.S.O.

Phil. Trans. R. Soc. Lond. B **294**, 241–250 (1981)
Printed in Great Britain

Aggregation of platelets in damaged vessels

By G. V. R. Born, F.R.S., P. Görög and M. A. A. Kratzer

Department of Pharmacology, King's College, Strand, London WC2R 2LS, U.K.

The only certain physiological function of platelets is their aggregation in injured vessel walls as haemostatic plugs. The association of thrombocytopenia with petechial haemorrhages suggests that platelets are somehow required for the functional integrity of small vessels, but no mechanism has yet been established. The pathological aggregation of platelets as thrombi in atherosclerotic arteries is commonly, if not always, initiated by haemorrhage. In artificial vessels, platelets tend to aggregate on the walls wherever blood flow is non-laminar. The mural aggregation of platelets is not prevented by unphysiologically high wall-shear forces. The facts suggest, on the contrary, that the process depends in some way on abnormal haemodynamic conditions.

This contribution is mainly concerned with questions about how haemodynamic conditions in and around vascular leaks affect arriving platelets that aggregate there, and about the chemical agents responsible for making the platelets reactive. The effects of these agents are known mainly from *in vitro* experiments in which aggregation can be quantitatively correlated with biochemical effects by simple and reproducible methods; the relevance to their reactions in haemostasis and thrombosis is uncertain. It is difficult to devise quantitative methods for analysing these processes *in vivo* because of the very low concentrations at which endogenous agents can activate platelets and haemostatic factors in the plasma; the rapidity with which platelets aggregate in a damaged blood vessel; and the complexity and inconstancy of the haemodynamic situation. All these facts must be accounted for in hypotheses of haemostasis. New experimental approaches towards analysing the haemostatic mechanism *in vivo* are described.

Introduction

Platelets aggregate in blood vessels that are damaged by injury, most commonly mechanical, or by disease, most commonly atherosclerosis. Mechanical injury causes aggregates to form both outside and inside any opening through the vessel wall. As these aggregates grow, they diminish and ultimately arrest haemorrhage, at least temporarily; such aggregates are therefore known as haemostatic plugs.

Platelet aggregates that form inside a vessel are thrombi, by definition (French & Macfarlane 1970). Atherosclerotic disease, which is confined to arterial vessels, can apparently induce thrombotic platelet aggregation either when a hardened plaque cracks so that there is haemorrhage into the vessel wall, or when lesions have deformed and constricted the arterial lumen and the flow of of blood is grossly abnormal.

One or other of these conditions initiate coronary and cerebral thrombosis, which manifest themselves clinically as heart attacks and strokes respectively. This paper analyses current evidence connecting haemodynamic effects in diseased arteries with the thrombotic aggregation of platelets in them. In analyses of these processes it is commonly assumed that the experimentally induced aggregation of platelets as haemostatic plugs is a relevant model of the clinical aggregation of platelets as arterial thrombi. The mechanisms may be similar in some respects. However, the haemodynamic conditions are probably very different (figure 1).

242   G. V. R. BORN, P. GÖRÖG AND M. A. A. KRATZER

Therefore, conclusions based on the haemostatic aggregation of platelets may not necessarily apply to their thrombotic aggregation, even when that is initiated by haemorrhage into the vessel wall; and it is important to beware of oversimplifications in hypotheses put forward to explain these complex processes.

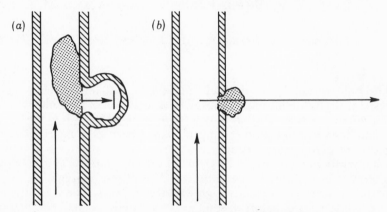

FIGURE 1. Haemodynamic conditions of (a) plaque fissure and (b) wall injury. In both arteries blood flow is fast. When a plaque cracks, blood makes its way through the fissure into the arterial wall. Flow slows down rapidly so that the extravasated blood becomes a reservoir of thrombogenic agents including presumably ADP, thromboxane A$_2$ and thrombin in varying proportions. Diffusion of these agents into the arterial lumen can account for the intravascular platelet thrombi that are observed under such conditions.

By contrast, when injury opens an artery the outflow of blood through the wall continues without the formation of such a reservoir. Thrombogenic agents appearing in the extravasated blood induce extravascular platelet aggregation, as observed under these conditions.

CLINICAL AND PATHOLOGICAL FEATURES OF ARTERIAL THROMBOSIS

Any hypothesis for thrombotic platelet aggregation must be able to account for the following facts. 1. Thrombi do not form in normal arteries. 2. Thrombi form in atherosclerotic arteries. 3. Arterial thrombi consist initially of aggregated platelets. 4. Atherosclerosis increases slowly, whereas thrombosis occurs rapidly and is individually unpredictable; therefore, atherosclerotic arteries must be subject to sudden, unpredictable events capable of initiating platelet aggregation. 5. Most occlusive thrombi are associated with fissures in underlying atheromatous plaques.

The erythrocyte-haemodynamics hypothesis (Born 1979a) proposes that the sudden unpredictable event that starts arterial (typically coronary) thrombosis is plaque fissure; haemorrhage through the fissure is associated with increased haemodynamic stress causing ADP (and other adenine nucleotides) to appear in the plasma; this ADP is principally responsible for activating platelets and their aggregation as mural thrombi.

Much progress has been made with support for this hypothesis (Born et al. 1976; Born & Wehmeier 1979).

Evidence includes the following. 1. In atherosclerotic arteries platelet thrombi form only when blood flow is sufficiently abnormal, i.e. as a result of haemorrhage into a fissure, or in tortuous and/or stenotic regions. 2. In artificial blood vessels mural thrombi of platelets grow where, and only where, flow is non-laminar. 3. In artificial vessels the formation of platelet thrombi in non-laminar flow depends on the presence of red cells. 4. Adhesion and aggregation of platelets on artificial surfaces increase with red cell concentration and are abolished by ADP-removing enzymes. 5. The haemodynamic stress associated with experimental haemorrhage is insufficient in duration and magnitude to activate platelets directly, but sufficient in both to induce release of red cell ADP (Born & Wehmeier 1979).

[26]

The thrombogenic adhesion of platelets to vessel walls therefore depends indirectly on the haemodynamic properties of the blood as it flows through arteries constricted and/or fissured by atherosclerosis.

Gross and histological appearances of arterial thrombi establish that their central mass consists mainly of aggregated platelets. What, therefore, is the mechanism responsible for rapid and extensive platelet aggregation in an artery as an apparently random event in time? Close serial sectioning of obstructed coronary arteries established some time ago that the platelet thrombus responsible is usually, if not invariably, associated with recent haemorrhage into an underlying atherosclerotic plaque (Friedman & Byers 1965; Constantinides 1966; Davies & Thomas, this symposium). The haemorrhages occur through fissures or fractures in the plaque, and it is a reasonable assumption that the sudden appearance of such a fissure or fracture is the random, individually unpredictable event affecting coronary arteries that has to be assumed to account for the clinical onset of acute myocardial infarction (Born 1979a). Why such a defect should develop at a particular moment is uncertain. Perhaps it is analogous to the sudden appearance of fine cracks in the wings of jet aircraft which is ascribed to the cumulative effects of variable stresses on metal known as metal fatigue (Gordon 1978; Frost et al. 1974). The chance event of plaque fissure can in principle be prevented only by preventing atherosclerosis, which is, as we know, still very problematical. Fortunately, the subsequent thrombotic process due to platelet aggregation is now understood to the extent that it may become preventable by drugs before long.

How does haemorrhage into a ruptured plaque start off platelet thrombogenesis? This can be regarded as part of the general question of how platelets are caused to aggregate through haemorrhage, most effectively from arteries. An explanation commonly put forward is that the process is initiated by platelets adhering to collagen exposed where damaged vessel walls are denuded of endothelium (Mustard et al. 1977; Packham & Mustard 1977). Adhering platelets then release other agents, including thromboxane A_2 and ADP, which in turn are responsible for the adhesion of more platelets as growing aggregates. This explanation is unlikely to be correct for the following reasons. First, haemostatic and thrombotic aggregates of platelets grow without delay and very rapidly (Hugues 1959). When an arteriole 200 μm in diameter is cut into laterally, the rate of accession of platelets to the haemostatic plug is of the order 10^4/s in the first seconds (Born & Richardson 1980). In contrast, the aggregation of platelets by collagen begins, even under optimal conditions for rapid reactivity, only after a delay or lag period of several seconds (Wilner et al. 1968). Secondly, platelets tend to aggregate as mural thrombi when anticoagulated blood flows through plastic vessels (Didisheim et al. 1972), for example in artificial organs such as oxygenators or dialysers (Richardson et al. 1976), which contain no collagen nor anything else capable of activating platelets similarly. This implies that there are conditions under which platelets are activated in the blood by something other than collagen or other constituents of the walls of living vessels. The plaque on which a thrombus grows has usually narrowed the arterial lumen. At constant blood pressure the flow of blood is faster through the constriction than elsewhere in the artery. Therefore, high flow and wall shear rates are no hindrance to the aggregation of platelets as thrombi (Born 1977). Indeed, the question arises of whether the activation of platelets, which precedes their aggregation, depends in some way on abnormal haemodynamic conditions.

Measurements of the haemodynamic forces required to activate platelets directly (Hellums & Brown 1977) indicate that the blood flow over atherosclerotic lesions in vivo is unable to do so (Colantuoni et al. 1977). The activation therefore must be indirect. Now, it has been known for many years that platelets can be activated by at least one agent, namely ADP, derived from the red cells, which outnumber and surround the platelets in the blood (Gaarder et al. 1961).

Clear evidence of increased platelet adhesiveness brought about by the operation of flow-mechanical factors on erythrocytes was provided by experiments in which blood was made to flow through branching channels in extracorporeal shunts (Rowntree & Shionya 1927; Mustard et al. 1962). Deposits of platelets formed consistently on the shoulders of a bifurcation in the flow chamber but nowhere else in the channels. In such divergent flow situations there is boundary-layer separation, which is accompanied by flow delays or stasis (Fox & Hugh 1966). This might by itself be expected to increase the probability of platelet aggregation. However, when the chambers were perfused not with blood but with platelet-rich plasma, no deposit was formed, showing that red cells were also essential.

The dependence of the deposition of platelets from flowing blood on the presence of red cells could be caused by physical or chemical mechanisms or, of course, by both acting synergistically. A *physical mechanism* would depend essentially on an increase in the *diffusivity* of platelets caused by the flow behaviour of the erythrocytes. Indeed, the diffusivity of platelets in flowing blood has been estimated to be two orders of magnitude greater than that calculated for platelets diffusing in plasma (Turitto et al. 1972; Turitto & Baumgartner 1975). This is consistent with the enhanced radial fluctuations of erythrocytes or of latex microspheres (2 μm in diameter) in flowing suspensions of red cell ghosts (Goldsmith 1972). High platelet diffusivity is required also to explain the growth of mural thrombi. This must depend on successful platelet–platelet collisions, the rate of which between platelets following streamlines near the walls would hardly be sufficient to account for the rapidity of growth observed *in vivo* (Begent & Born 1970; Richardson 1973; Born & Richardson 1980).

Is ADP involved in arterial thrombogenesis?

There is increasing evidence for a *chemical mechanism* in the increased adhesiveness of platelets in the presence of red cells, i.e. through their ADP. The concentrations of ADP required for activating platelets are small, probably less than 10^{-8} M (Frojmovic 1978) and ADP is also rapidly dephosphorylated in blood (Haslam & Mills 1967), so that its direct demonstration there under conditions relevant to thrombogenesis is difficult.

It has recently become possible to demonstrate the appearance of free ADP in blood *directly* in concentrations sufficient to activate platelets (Schmid-Schönbein et al. 1979). In specially designed apparatus, whole blood or resuspended red cells are exposed to controlled, different shear stresses for known time periods. The apparatus is designed to cover the range of these variables presumed to be relevant to the situations *in vivo*. The experiments show that ADP appears in the plasma in concentrations required for platelet activation (0.1–1.0 μM) but in direct proportion to free haemoglobin, indicating that platelet activation can result from small degrees of haemolysis due to haemodynamic stresses such as occur during haemorrhage, whether external or through a plaque fissure. It is not yet certain whether the appearance of free ADP is rapid enough to account for aggregation *in vivo*. This process appears to be faster than the release of ADP from the platelets themselves or of thromboxane A_2 produced by them which, in any case, induces aggregation via ADP (personal communications from B. Samuelsson and A. Marcus).

When blood vessels are injured so that they bleed, circulating platelets adhere to the damaged vessel wall and aggregate within the first seconds. The mechanism of the initial platelet aggregation remains uncertain. To investigate the initiation stage of haemostasis, the carotid arteries of rats were punctured with a 100 μm needle and free ATP, as an indicator of ADP, was measured in the emerging blood (Kratzer & Born 1981). This was brought into contact with luciferin–luciferase in a polyethylene tube, internal diameter 0.8 mm. The light produced at the blood–enzyme interface was measured with a sensitive photon-counting device which gave background counts of 1 photoelectron per second and could detect less than 10^{-8} M ATP in 2 μl blood.

When an artery was injured, the emerging blood contained about 10^{-7} M ATP in a first peak after about 2 s. After about 1 min the ATP concentration rose to a second peak of about 5×10^{-6} M. This was decreased by heparin or by chlorpromazine. The source of ATP accounting for the first peak remains uncertain; possibly this ATP is released from red cells undergoing high shear stress from the haemodynamic effects of haemorrhage. The observations suggest that the second peak represents ATP released from platelets.

The release reaction of platelets has been assumed to subserve a positive feedback mechanism responsible for their aggregation in haemostasis and thrombosis (Born 1965). This assumption is based mainly on *in vitro* experiments. Considerable uncertainty remains about the contribution of the release reaction to the initiation of haemostasis *in vivo*. The rapidity of the process and the presence of other tissues makes it impossible to follow the reaction quantitatively *in vivo* by methods that permit this *in vitro*. We have therefore applied quantitative electron microscopy to find out how quickly the concentration of dense bodies decreases in platelets during their haemostatic aggregation (Görög & Born 1981).

In mice, platelets were enriched in dense bodies by pretreatment with 5-hydroxytryptamine. Mesenteric arteries were incised with a sharp blade. Bleeding was stopped by a micromanipulator-operated device about 15 and 60 s after the cut. The cut segments were immediately fixed *in situ* with glutaraldehyde and postfixed. Serial sections were made for electron microscopy. Platelets isolated from peripheral blood of the same animal were prepared similarly. Electron micrographs were projected on to a television screen and numbers of dense bodies and total platelet areas were determined by an image analysing computer. After 15 s there were no significant differences in numbers of dense bodies in platelets from different parts of the haemostatic plugs ($8.31 \pm 0.57/100$ μm² (mean $\pm$ s.e.m.)) and in platelets from the blood 8.93 ± 0.38). On the other hand, after 60 s the parts furthest from the cut contained fewer dense bodies than the nearer parts and the overall dense body number (5.86 ± 0.05) was significantly smaller ($p < 0.001$) than that of platelets from the blood (14.45 ± 0.09). The results suggest that haemostatic aggregation of platelets does not initially depend on their release reaction. Furthermore, as the action of aspirin on platelets is inhibition of the release reaction these results also explain, in part at least, the comparative ineffectiveness of aspirin in clinical trials of the prevention of reinfarction.

Our observations suggest a new approach to the prophylaxis of arterial, e.g. coronary, thromboses (Born 1979b). This approach would require the demonstration that their incidence is diminished by drugs that, in clinically acceptable blood concentrations, do not inhibit platelet function directly but which inhibit the release of activating agent, presumably ADP, from red cells during rheological stresses such as occur in potentially thrombogenic arteries. Such a demonstration may then also explain the effect of dipyridamole or sulfinpyrazone in preventing increased utilization of circulating platelets under potentially thrombogenic conditions. This

[29]

cannot easily be accounted for by any direct action on platelets by either drug at its clinically effective concentration. Perhaps these drugs act mainly on the red cells to diminish their activating effect on platelets.

Some time ago one of us (G.V.R.B.) had the idea that drugs capable of counteracting haemolysis (Seeman 1972) might diminish this activating effect of red cells on platelets and so inhibit their aggregation as thrombi. Experimental evidence for this idea came with the demonstration (Born et al. 1976) that chlorpromazine added to anticoagulated human blood, in concentrations that in vitro diminish hypotonic haemolysis but have no direct effect on platelet aggregation (Mills & Roberts 1967), prolong the bleeding time from small holes in artificial vessels where extravasation is terminated, as in vivo, by aggregated platelets. More recent experiments (Born & Wehmeier 1979) support the conclusion that this effect is accounted for by the antihaemolytic action of chlorpromazine. This has led to the suggestion (Born et al. 1976, 1979a, b) that other drugs possessing this effect of chlorpromazine may diminish the incidence of arterial, particularly of coronary, thrombosis when it is induced by conditions of abnormal stress on the red cells, such as through haemorrhage into atheromatous lesions.

As already proposed (Born 1979b), evidence for or against this proposition could perhaps be obtained by comparing the incidence of acute coronary occlusions in populations on long-term treatment with chlorpromazine (or other drugs acting in this respect like chlorpromazine) with the incidence in control populations not on such drugs. The only conceivably relevant evidence of which we have been made aware up to now (through the courtesy of Dr J. A. Baldwin, Director of the Oxford University Unit of Clinical Epidemiology) is an investigation of mortality in Norwegian psychiatric hospitals during the period 1950–62 (Odegard 1967). This concluded that mortality from circulatory disease, predominantly 'coronary disease' and 'infarction', was higher in the mental hospital population than in the general population, although the excess was not as much as that from most other causes. Within the patient population, the excess mortality from coronary disease and infarction was less for schizophrenics than for all other psychoses. Furthermore, the excess mortality from circulatory disease diminished strikingly after 1957, particularly when compared with the period 1926–41, because the mortality did not rise to the same extent in the hospital as in the general population.

These conclusions, if confirmed, are of course open to different interpretations. Epidemiological considerations apart, chlorpromazine has many effects in the body, and also a large number of metabolites. Furthermore, the concentration of chlorpromazine in patients' plasma (Mackay et al. 1974) is one to two orders of magnitude lower than that required to prolong the ex vivo bleeding time described below. Therefore, if patients' blood were used for determining this bleeding time, a prolongation might be expected only if the drug or a similarly active metabolite were concentrated in red cell membranes. On the other hand, it has been observed that single clinical doses (5–20 mg) of chlorpromazine injected intramuscularly into apparently healthy volunteers cause the Ivy bleeding time to be significantly prolonged (Zahavi & Schwartz 1978).

Our experimental observations with chlorpromazine make it attractive to suggest that the general introduction of this drug for the control of schizophrenic in-patients from about 1955 onwards accounts for their relative protection against cardiac mortality at a time when it was increasing rapidly in Norway and elsewhere, including Britain. It would be interesting to learn of other information that may support or, just as important, invalidate this line of thought. It may be worth while to investigate appropriate populations from this point of view.

Are prostaglandins involved in arterial thrombogenesis?

A different explanation of arterial thrombosis has been widely canvassed (Gryglewski *et al.* 1976). This may be referred to conveniently as the prostacyclin–thromboxane hypothesis, and it proposes that: (1) whether or not thrombosis occurs in arteries depends on a local balance between prostacyclin (PGI_2), which inhibits platelets, and thromboxane A_2 (TXA_2), which aggregates platelets; (2) in normal arteries, thrombosis is prevented by prostacyclin in the blood where its sources are lungs and endothelium; (3) part of the 'endothelial' prostacyclin originates in endoperoxides transferred from adherent platelets; (4) the walls of atherosclerotic arteries synthesize less prostacyclin, and those of artificial blood vessels none at all. Platelets' endoperoxides are therefore utilized for thromboxane A_2 production, which is responsible for activating the platelets and their aggregation as thrombi.

In view of the extraordinary inhibitory potency of prostacyclin, this hypothesis appears attractive, but it is not entirely satisfactory because it does not explain:

(1) how platelets can produce endoperoxides for utilization by endothelium without the simultaneous formation of thromboxane A_2 by the platelets, which should aggregate them;

(2) that the haemostatic aggregation of platelets does occur under conditions in which it might be expected to be prevented by endothelial prostacyclin (Dejana *et al.* 1980).

(3) why platelet thrombi do not form in artificial blood vessels, i.e. in the absence of prostacyclin, except under particular haemodynamic conditions and in the presence of red cells;

(4) why arterial thrombosis does not occur continuously on all atherosclerotic lesions; and

(5) that the essential clinical characteristics of arterial thrombosis include an unpredictable and sudden onset, commonly in patients with either long-standing or minimal atherosclerotic lesions.

Evidence that the biosynthesis of prostaglandins is initiated by mechanical deformations of cell membranes (Piper & Vane 1971) does suggest a mechanism by which prostaglandins could be brought into thrombogenesis through haemodynamic effects. Platelets themselves produce the aggregating agent thromboxane A_2 (Hamberg *et al.* 1975; Svensson *et al.* 1976). The first step in its formation is the release of arachidonic acid from phospholipids in the cell membrane, catalysed by the enzyme phospholipase A_2 which is normally inactive; how the enzyme is activated physiologically is not known. Perhaps activation is initiated by small distortions of the outer membrane of platelets when they pass through regions in which the haemodynamic forces are greater than in the normal circulation, as during haemorrhage into a ruptured atherosclerotic plaque. This fluid-mechanical activation of platelets would not involve red cells, which apparently do not contain a thromboxane-forming system.

Is collagen involved in arterial thrombogenesis?

There has been ample confirmation of the observation (Didisheim *et al.* 1972) that 'thrombosis induced mechanically in a teflon shunt appears indistinguishable from thrombosis induced by mechanical or electrical injury in living vessels, despite the absence of endothelium, collagen and muscle from the teflon tubing'.

These observations do not support the assertion that haemostatic plugs or thrombi are initiated through the collision of platelets with exposed collagen. On the other hand, it has recently been shown that a nonapeptide sequence of collagen is a specific binding site for platelets (Legrand *et al.* 1980). If this binding depends on multiple interactions (Santoro & Cummingham 1979), these could also induce distortions in the platelet membrane sufficient to activate phospholipase A_2 and thereby the prostaglandin cascade, resulting in the release reaction as observed. This therefore represents yet another way in which prostaglandins could participate in thrombogenesis.

Our knowledge of arterial thrombogenesis is still sufficiently fragmentary that the most reasonable way to conclude is with two quotations that counsel caution: 'Un point de vue unique est toujours faux' (Paul Valéry); and 'The belief in a single truth and in being the possessor thereof is the root cause of all evil in the world' (Max Born).

We wish to thank the Minna–James–Heineman Stiftung of Hanover for a Research Fellowship for M.K., the Wellcome Trust and the British Heart Foundation for Research Fellowships for P.G., and the Fritz Thyssen Stiftung of Cologne for support.

Note added in proof (19 *May* 1981). Further evidence has now been obtained that ADP is involved in activating platelets *in vivo* (Krystyna Zawilska, G. V. R. Born & Nicola A. Begent, to be published). Novel techniques were developed for the reproducible determination of bleeding times from small arteries of rats and rabbits in the territory supplied by the superior mesenteric artery. One of its main branches was cannulated and infusions were made into the mesenteric circulation of two ADP-removing enzyme systems: either creatine phosphate (CP) with creatine phosphokinase (CPK) or phosphoenolpyruvate (PEP) with pyruvate kinase (PK). In both species these infusions increased the bleeding time significantly, suggesting that the increases were caused by decreases of free ADP in the blood. To confirm this conclusion, the same as well as other animals were infused with either substrate (CP or PEP) or enzyme (CPK or PK) alone. In neither species was the bleeding time prolonged by infusing enzyme alone. On the other hand, the bleeding times were significantly increased in rats and rabbits infused with substrate (CP or PEP) alone, suggesting that the ADP-removing systems were completed by endogenous enzymes. The plasma of both rats and rabbits were found to obtain CPK at concentrations higher than those in human plasma. In all experiments the arterial blood pressure, the blood platelet concentration and the haematocrit decreased moderately. The influence of these factors on bleeding time values was taken into account by appropriate controls.

These observations, which establish that infusion of different ADP-removing enzyme systems into arterial blood flowing towards fresh arterial injuries greatly increases the bleeding time from them, supports the conclusion that the activation of platelets for primary haemostasis depends on ADP.

REFERENCES (Born *et al.*)

Begent, N. A. & Born, G. V. R. 1970 Growth rate *in vivo* of platelet thrombi, produced by iontophoresis of ADP, as a function of mean blood flow velocity. *Nature, Lond.* **227**, 926–930.

Born, G. V. R. 1965 Platelets in thrombogenesis: mechanism and inhibition of platelet aggregation. *Ann. R. Coll. Surg. Engl.* **36**, 200–206.

Born, G. V. R. 1977 Fluid-mechanical and biochemical interactions in haemostasis. *Br. med. Bull.* **33**, 193–197.

Born, G. V. R. 1979*a* Arterial thrombosis and its prevention. In *Proc. VIII World Congress Cardiology* (ed. S. Hayase & S. Murao), pp. 81–91. Amsterdam: Excerpta Medica.

Born, G. V. R. 1979*b* Possible role for chlorpromazine in protection against myocardial infarction. *Lancet* i, 822.

Born, G. V. R., Bergqvist, D. & Arfors, K. E. 1976 Evidence for inhibition of platelet activation in blood by a drug effect of erythrocytes. *Nature, Lond.* **259**, 233–235.

Born, G. V. R. & Richardson, P. D. 1980 Activation time of blood platelets. *J. Membr. Biol.* **57**, 87–90.

Born, G. V. R. & Wehmeier, A. 1979 Inhibition of platelet thrombus formation by chlorpromazine acting to diminish haemodynamically induced haemolysis. *Nature, Lond.* **282**, 212–213.

Colantuoni, G., Hellums, J. D., Moake, J. L. & Alfrey, C. P., Jr 1977 The response of human platelets to shear stress at short exposure times. *Trans. Am. Soc. artif. intern. Organs* **23**, 626–631.

Constantinides, P. 1966 Plaque fissures in human coronary thrombosis. *J. Atheroscler. Res.* **6**, 1–17.

Dejana, E., Barbieri, B. & de Gaetano, G. 1980 'Aspirinated' platelets are haemostatic in thrombocytopenic rats with 'nonaspirinated' vessel walls – evidence from an exchange transfusion model. *Blood* **56**, 959–962.

Didisheim, P., Pavlovsky, M. & Kobayashi, I. 1972 Factors that influence or modify platelet function. *Ann. N.Y. Acad. Sci.*, **201**, pp. 307–315.

Fox, A. L. & Hugh, A. E. 1966 Localization of atheroma; a theory based on boundary layer separation. *Br. Heart J.* **28**, 388–399.

French, J. E. & Macfarlane, R. G. 1970 Haemostasis and thrombosis. In *General pathology* (ed. H. W. Florey), 4th edn, p. 273. London: Lloyd-Luke.

Friedman, M. & Byers, S. O. 1965 Induction of thrombi upon pre-existing arterial plaques. *Am. J. Path.* **46**, 567–575.

Frojmovic, M. M. 1978 Rheooptical studies of platelet structure and function. *Prog. Haemostas. Thromb.* **4**, 279–319.

Frost, W. E., Marsh, K. J. & Pook, L. P. 1974 *Metal fatigue.* (Oxford Engineering Science Series.) Oxford University Press.

Gaarder, A., Jonsen, J., Laland, S., Hellem, A. & Owren, P. A. 1961 Adenosine diphosphate in red cells as a factor in the adhesiveness of human blood platelets. *Nature, Lond.* **192**, 531–533.

Gryglewski, R. J., Bunting, S., Moncada, S., Flower, R. J. & Vane, J. R. 1976 Arterial walls are protected against deposition of platelet thrombi by a substance (prostaglandin X) which they make from prostaglandin endoperoxides. *Prostaglandins* **12**, 685–713.

Goldsmith, H. L. 1972 The flow of model particles and blood cells and its relation to thrombogenesis. In *Progress in haemostasis and thrombosis* (ed. T. H. Spaet), vol. 1, pp. 97–139. New York: Grune & Stratton.

Gordon, J. E. 1978 *Structures.* Harmondsworth: Penguin Books.

Görög, P. & Born, G. V. R. 1981 The time relation between the haemostatic aggregation of platelets and their release reaction in vivo. Presented at VIII Int. Congr. Thromb. Haemostas., Toronto, Canada, July.

Hamberg, M., Svensson, J. & Samuelsson, B. 1975 Thromboxanes: a new group of biologically active compounds derived from prostaglandin endoperoxides. *Proc. natn. Acad. Sci. U.S.A.* **72**, 2994–2998.

Haslam, R. J. & Mills, D. C. B. 1967 The adenylate kinase of human plasma, erythrocytes and platelets in relation to degradation of adenosine diphosphate in plasma. *Biochem. J.* **103**, 773–784.

Hellums, J. D. & Brown, C. H. 1977 Blood cell damage by mechanical forces. In *Cardiovascular flow dynamics and measurements* (ed. N. H. Hwang & N. A. Norman). Baltimore: University Park Press.

Hugues, J. 1959 Agglutination précoce des plaquettes au cours de la formation du clou hémostatique. *Thromb. Diathes. haemorrh.* **3**, 177–186.

Kratzer, M. A. A. & Born, G. V. R. 1981 Free ATP in blood during haemorrhage. Presented at VIII Int. Congr. Thromb. Haemostas., Toronto, Canada, July 1981.

Legrand, Y. G., Karnignian, A., Le Francier, P., Fauvel, F. & Chen, J. P. 1980 Evidence that the collagen-derived nonapeptide is a specific inhibitor of platelet–collagen interaction. *Biochem. biophys. Res. Commun.* **96**, 1579–1585.

Mackay, A. V. P., Healey, A. F. & Baker, J. 1974 The relationship of plasma chlorpromazine to its 7-hydroxy- and sulphoxide metabolites in a large population of chronic schizophrenics. *Br. J. clin. Pharmac.* **1**, 425–430.

Mills, D. C. B. & Roberts, G. C. K. 1967 Membrane active drugs and the aggregation of human blood platelets. *Nature, Lond.* **213**, 35–36.

Milton, J. G., Yung, W., Glushak, C. & Frojmovic, M. M. 1980 Kinetics of ADP-induced human platelet shape change: apparent positive cooperativity. *Can. J. Physiol. Pharmac.* **58**, 45–52.

Mustard, J. F., Murphy, E. A., Rowsell, H. C. & Downie, H. G. 1962 Factors influencing thrombus formation in vivo. *Am. J. Med.* **33**, 621–647.

Mustard, J. F., Moore, S., Packham, M. A. & Kinlough-Rathbone, R. L. 1977 Platelets, thrombosis and atherosclerosis. *Prog. biochem. Pharmacol.* **13**, 312–325.

Odegard, O. 1967 Mortality in Norwegian psychiatric hospitals 1950–62. *Acta genet. Statist. med.* **17**, 137–153.

Packham, M. A. & Mustard, J. F. 1977 Clinical pharmacology of platelets. *Blood* **50**, 555–573.

Piper, P. G. & Vane, J. R. 1971 The release of prostaglandins from lungs and other tissues. *Ann. N.Y. Acad. Sci.* **180**, 363–385.

Richardson, P. D. 1973 Effect of blood flow velocity on growth rate of platelet thrombi. *Nature, Lond.* **245**, 103–104.

Richardson, P. D., Galletti, P. M. & Born, G. V. R. 1976 Regional administration of drugs to control thrombosis in artificial organs. *Trans. Am. Soc. artif. intern. Organs* **22**, 22–23.

Rowntree, L. G. & Shionya, T. 1927 Studies in experimental extra-corporeal thrombosis. 1. Methods for the direct observation of extra-corporeal thrombus formation. *J. exp. Med.* **46**, 7–12.

Santoro, S. A. & Cummingham, L. W. 1979 Fibronectin and the multiple-interaction model for platelet–collagen adhesion. *Proc. natn. Acad. Sci. U.S.A.* **76**, 2644–2648.

Schmid-Schönbein, H., Rohling-Winkel, I., Blasberg, P., Jungling, E., Wehmeier, A., Born, G. V. R. & Richardson, P. D. 1979 Release of ADP from erythrocytes under high shear stresses in tube flow. [Abstract.] *Thromb. Haemostas.* (*Abstracts, VII Int. Congr. Thromb. Haemostas.*), p. 349.

Seeman, P. 1972 The membrane action of anaesthetics and tranquillisers. *Pharmac. Rev.* **24**, 583–655.

Svensson, J., Hamberg, M. & Samuelsson, B. 1976 On the formation and effects of thromboxane A_2 in human platelets. *Acta physiol. scand.* **98**, 285–294.

Turitto, V. T. & Baumgartner, H. R. 1975 Platelet interaction with subendothelium in a perfusion system: physical role of red blood cells. *Microvasc. Res.* **5**, 167–179.

Turitto, V. T., Benis, A. M. & Leonard, E. F. 1972 Platelet diffusion in slowing blood. *Ind. Engng Chem. Fundam.* **11**, 216–223.

Wilner, G. D., Nossel, H. L. & LeRoy, E. C. 1968 Aggregation of platelets by collagen. *J. clin. Invest.* **47**, 2616–2621.

Zahavi, J. & Schwartz, G. 1978 Chlorpromazine and platelet function. *Lancet* ii, 164.

Phil. Trans. R. Soc. Lond. B **294**, 251–266 (1981)

Printed in Great Britain

Rheological factors in platelet – vessel wall interactions

By P. D. Richardson

Division of Engineering, Brown University, Providence, Rhode Island 02912, U.S.A.

Rheological aspects of platelet–vessel wall interactions involve cell–cell encounters, platelet – vessel wall encounters and platelet–thrombus interactions. The cell–cell encounters are usually caused by convection of cells in shear flows rather than by Brownian motion; this is important in aggregation and in the enhancement of the diffusion of platelets by red cell motion. Platelet – vessel wall interactions can involve transient adhesion (lasting from a fraction of a second to a few minutes) as well as more permanent adhesion. Reaction rates between platelets and walls are generally very small except on damaged vessels and some artificial surfaces. Ultra-filtration through the vessel wall affects cell–wall interactions. Rheological analyses of thrombus formation have been made and show interesting relations to experimental observations. Some experimental results have indicated that platelets are capable of reacting within a small fraction of a second. Red cells may act as mechanoreceptors for increases in shear rate and facilitate the speed of response of platelets. Surface geometrical forms such as bumps and cavities tend to prolong residence times and facilitate thrombus formation.

1. Introduction

The interaction of platelets with the vessel walls is a dynamic process. The motion of the bloodstream and rheological factors must be considered. Indeed, according to some hypotheses concerning the processes leading to haemostasis, certain rheological events are essential factors. Like the biochemical processes now increasingly understood, rheological processes are invoked as necessary components in accounting for haemostasis and thrombosis.

This acknowledgement of rheological factors, the fluid dynamic events, is a departure from Virchow's triad. It is an amplification rather than a contradiction, posing new questions and the development of new techniques in the study of platelet – vessel wall interactions. The recognition of rheological factors is by no means new: Mustard *et al.* (1962), is an extensive review of thrombus formation *in vivo*, point out that the opinion that mechanical factors have a role can be traced back into the late nineteenth century (Welch 1887).

A major stimulus for study of platelet–wall interactions has been the observation that many myocardial infarctions follow the development of major thrombus tied to an atheromatous plaque in a coronary artery, that related processes in carotid vessels lead to strokes, and that thrombi develop at vessel–prosthesis anastomoses and at junctions in extracorporeal blood circuits. Indeed, the development and use of artificial heart valves, artificial kidneys and prosthetic blood vessels since about 1960 has coincided with a period of intense study of platelet behaviour. It has also coincided with a renewed interest in blood rheology, and it has become increasingly clear that flow phenomena on the scale of the cells in blood have needed more attention than had been previously given. The name 'microrheology' has been given to the study of flow at the scale of the blood cells, and the name 'macrorheology' to the study of bulk flows in which the blood is considered to have simple averaged properties. Both representations are important in the understanding of rheological effects in platelet–wall interactions. The period of intense study of platelet behaviour has also coincided with the introduction of several new and refined techniques such as scanning electron microscopy and high-pressure liquid chromatography.

Studies of platelet biochemistry, of thrombus micropathology, of blood rheology, of artificial organs and of clinical control of risk factors for myocardial infarction and stroke have coincided in time but they have not been closely coordinated. In providing an account of the role of rheology, the development of some significant stages in thrombosis research will be examined in relation to studies of fluid dynamics and convective transport.

2. DEVELOPMENT OF THE FEEDBACK HYPOTHESIS

Mustard *et al.* (1962) pointed to injury to the vessel wall as a mechanical factor predisposing to thrombus formation, and suggested that atheromatous lesions may be consequences of antecedent mural thrombi; further, they point to the effects of flow distribution such as bifurcations and small ridges in producing thrombotic deposits. Most significantly, in discussing the growth of a thrombus, they infer that the rate of growth of a thrombus should in some way be proportional to the size of the thrombus, and that it might not be surprising to find something like an exponential growth.

At the same time, the technique of aggregometry was introduced (Born 1962), and this method for observing platelet response to applied factors by measuring light transmission through a small tube of platelet-rich plasma was found to be a powerful tool for research *in vitro*. The small cuvette has a stirrer creating a rotation – a shear flow field – which raises the inter-platelet collision frequency well above that which would occur by Brownian motion. The flow field is not uniform and has a range of shear rates rather than a single value. Because of this it is not practicable to use the instrument to measure collision efficiency (the fraction of encounters between platelets that result in aggregation of the encountering cells), as this is expected to vary with the shear rate, but the instrument has shown itself to be a fine device for the study of factors that promote aggregation and those that inhibit it. The average time interval between platelet collisions is of the order of 3 s, and this allows the device to respond quickly and to complete a test in a few minutes. It has been shown subsequently that factors that promote platelet aggregation in platelet-rich plasma (p.r.p.) also promote it in whole blood, and that inhibitors of aggregation in p.r.p. act similarly in whole blood. Indeed, it has been demonstrated (Richardson *et al.* 1976) that regional application of drugs that inhibit aggregation in p.r.p. can be used to reduce thrombus formation in artificial organs through which whole blood passes. In this sense, the necessary absence of the red cells from the aggregometer is not misleading in assaying the effects of chemical factors on platelet aggregation. However, it has been found that thrombus growth rates are affected by the presence of red cells, an effect attributed at first to enhancement of platelet diffusivity by red cell motion – a purely rheological effect – but now considered to involve the red cells biochemically as well. This is discussed further later.

Two aggregometer systems were developed subsequently to make aggregation measurements under conditions of well-defined flow. Chang & Robertson (1976) used a rotating concentric cylinder system, and were able to deduce collision efficiencies. Rieger (1976), working in the laboratory of Schmid-Schönbein in Aachen, used a rotating cone-and-plate system (sweeping

[36]

through shear rates of 4.5–115 s^{-1} in 12 min) and obtained data on the effect of shear rate in a continuous rather than discrete manner. Both systems have relatively large surface:volume proportions.

Animal models provided opportunities for observation of thrombus growth. In the micro-circulation (e.g. hamster cheek pouch, mouse mesentery, rat mesentery, rat cremaster and bat wing) it was possible to record thrombus growth on an injured vessel site by using a 1 mA

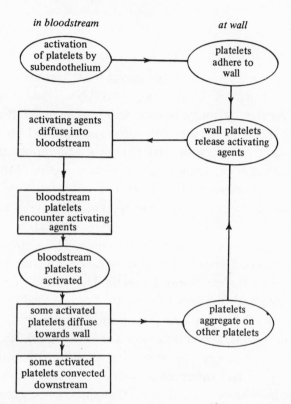

FIGURE 1. Hypothesis (*ca.* 1970) concerning the interaction between the bloodstream and the vessel wall, leading to thrombus formation. Events in the bloodstream are shown in the left column; events on the wall are shown on the right. Rectangles enclose events that are predominantly physical in nature, while ovals enclose those predominantly biochemical.

discharge or a laser to induce vessel damage. A model involving a larger vessel was provided by the rabbit aorta de-endothelialized by balloon; basement membrane was exposed and platelet-dominated thrombi grew on the denuded vessel wall (Baumgartner 1973).

Numerous studies demonstrated the importance of calcium and of fibrinogen as essential factors in platelet adhesion and aggregation; platelet adhesion to collagen was also shown. The aggregometer and electron microscope showed how platelets are activated by an adequate concentration of adenosine diphosphate, with morphological changes leading quite rapidly to the development of pseudopodia. After the work of Bangham & Pethica (1960) it was per-ceived that the pseudopodia would facilitate adhesion of the cell membrane, e.g. by reducing the effect of Coulomb repulsion forces. It was also realized that the deployment of pseudopodia would increase the effective cell radius and thereby increase the collision frequency in a shear flow. Later after platelet activation there is the release reaction (specifically inhibited by ASA) in which platelet granules discharge into the plasma factors that themselves activate platelets (ADP serotonin).

These observations were put together to support a thrombosis hypothesis incorporating feedback. It is illustrated in figure 1. This hypothesis was a natural sequel to the suggestion of Mustard *et al* (1962). The figure has been drawn to give distinguish between processes that are predominantly physical or predominantly biochemical. Some of the physical processes are controlled by blood flow.

3. THROMBUS GROWTH RATE AND THE ACTIVATION DELAY TIME

A significant step was the experimental measurement of thrombus growth rates. An animal model was developed by Begent & Born (1970), who showed that it was possible to stimulate thrombus growth in venules by iontophoretic application of ADP in the tissue space just outside the vessel. The thrombus attached to the vessel wall and grew by capture of passing platelets. The model was reversible; with cessation of the stimulus the thrombus embolized and no further thrombus formed at the site unless ADP was reapplied. Morphologically, the vessel wall appeared to preserve an intact endothelium.

Begent & Born applied intravital morphometry to observe the growth rates of the thrombi that they induced. Each thrombus, developing in the vessels of about 50 μm internal diameter, was found to increase in volume exponentially with time. This showed that the speculation of Mustard *et al.* (1962) was well founded. Begent & Born went further by observing the effect of different blood flow rates on the exponential growth. They found that the time constant of the exponential growth varied with the blood flow rate. At low blood flow rates, the growth rate factor increased with blood flow rates until it reached a maximum. At higher blood flow rates the growth rate factor decreased, and at the extreme it went to zero. Richardson (1973) analysed this problem in terms of the theory of aggregation in shear flow (due to Smoluchovski and described by Levich (1962)) and interpreted the low flow-rate results as indicating that the thrombus was enlarged by capture of all platelets that approached it closely enough as they were swept along in the blood flow. To explain the higher flow rate results, Richardson proposed that platelets have a finite time delay between activation and development of a sufficient adhesive force to allow successful aggregation. It was assumed that for each platelet the clock is started on the first moment of encounter with the thrombus. If platelets reached the end of the thrombus in a time less than the activation delay time, they would not adhere to it (although they might adhere somewhere downstream). With a shear flow in the vessel, the platelets approaching the wall most closely generally experience the longest contact times. The activation delay time was deduced to be 0.1–0.2 s from the hamster cheek-pouch experiments.

More recently, Predecki *et al.* (1980a, b) have used an entirely different technique *in vitro* to assess the activation delay time of human platelets and have deduced it to be 0.3–0.5 s. Their technique used pulsating flows of physiological solution through porous plates supported in whole blood; by controlling the frequency of pulsations they could limit the duration of contact between blood cells and each porous plate, and examination of the plates for adherent platelets allowed the activation time to be assessed.

These estimates for activation delay time (which may vary between species, and also with drugs and so on) are on a timescale that is not readily measurable in cell–cell encounters in aggregometers because of the relatively long time between collisions and also the finite time required for the injection of an activating agent (such as ADP) into the cuvette and mixing with the p.r.p.

Born & Richardson (1980), in examining the activation delay time further, pointed out that the theory indicates that the thrombi formed at the higher flow rates would be less thick (for specific length in the direction of flow) than those formed at lower flow rates, and found that this was demonstrated by the observations.

4. THROMBUS GROWTH AND RED CELL INVOLVEMENT

The thrombi whose growth rates have been measured in microcirculatory experiments have been quite small, about 50–100 μm in length. The mean spacing between platelets in blood is of the order of 15 μm, so that the thrombi do not differ much in size from the mean spacing between platelets, especially in the early stages of thrombus growth. If one compares the frequency of platelet–platelet encounters by convection in a shear flow with the frequency of encounter by Brownian motion, the ratio of these frequencies (the Smoluchovski number) is of the order of 10^4 for the experiments of Begent & Born (1970). These numbers indicate that, for the small thrombi, an analysis that assumes the convective transport of platelets is dominant and one that ignores diffusion of platelets (associated with their Brownian motion) is reasonable. However, if thrombi can grow much larger, 1–10 mm or so, then the depletion of platelets from the blood passing immediately over a thrombus will be compensated for by a net diffusive flux of platelets towards the regions where the free platelet concentration is low, and thrombus growth downstream can be dominated by the diffusive flux. Thrombi of this size can be formed in flow chambers built for the purpose (as well as in coronary arteries). Experimental data on thrombus growth rates in such chambers have indicated that growth could occur faster than would be expected from ordinary diffusive transport of platelets, and it was inferred that the red cells in blood were serving somehow to enhance the diffusivity of platelets, and indeed by a factor of 10^2 or so. This rheological process has been confirmed in several ways.

The augmentation of diffusivity by red cell motion has been demonstrated by observing the motion of specific cells as they move through a tube (Goldsmith & Karino 1966) and by carrying out a Taylor interface diffusion experiment with flow in a tube (Turitto et al. 1972). The self-diffusion coefficients of spherical and disc-like particles in a shear flow of suspensions of particles of various volume fractions have been measured by Eckstein et al. (1977) with the use of a concentric cylinder cuvette apparatus. Fischer & Richardson (1980) have illustrated how small tracer particles introduced in a steady shear flow around an isolated red cell experience lateral movements (in the direction across the shear flow) when they come close to the red cell. These lateral displacements provide a mechanism for augmenting diffusion. The particle motions are similar in form to the streamlines described by Poe & Acrivos (1975) for flow around a sphere and a cylinder in a shear flow. As the volume fraction of the suspension is increased, the interval between lateral displacements induced for each particle should be reduced, so that the effective diffusivity is increased. At the large particle volume fractions in blood (i.e. at normal haematocrits) it is not clear how much mutual interference arises to limit the degree of enhancement of diffusion. The experiments of Eckstein et al. and of Goldsmith & Karino indicate there is a limit at high particle concentrations. In any case, the rheological phenomenon of enhancement has been demonstrated clearly.

The fact that there is platelet diffusion enhancement in a shear flow does not mean that thrombus growth is equally enhanced. Very small thrombi do not benefit from it. The process of attachment of a platelet to a surface bounding the fluid flow is controlled partly by the reaction rate between platelets and the surface. It is controlled partly by the diffusion process, which brings platelets close to the surface and which determines the concentration available in the blood in contact with the surface. In some circumstances the principal limitation in attachment is the reaction rate between the platelets and the surface, and whether or not the platelet diffusivity is enhanced is then of no account. Robertson & Chang (1974) took this approach in making an analysis of the behaviour of blood passing through a bead column, for which platelet retention is affected strongly by the presence of red cells.

There are many pieces of evidence pointing to a chemical involvement of red cells in thrombus formation and platelet adhesion. Some of the evidence suggests that there is a release of intracellular ADP, which activates the platelets. Born *et al.* (1976) investigated the bleeding time at cuts made in thin plastic tubing through which anticoagulated blood was flowing. The bleeding time was very long when p.r.p. was used and red cells were absent. It was much shorter when the haematocrit was normal. It was prolonged when apyrase (which catalyses the dephosphorylation of ADP to AMP) was present. It was prolonged when chlorpromazine had been added to the blood: it is known that chlorpromazine at the concentrations used increases the mechanical resistance of red cells to hypotonic haemolysis while it does not affect platelet aggregation. (In some recent experiments on adhesion of human platelets, it was found also that chlorpromazine did not alter adhesion rates.) Born (1977) has summarized other experiments that indirectly indicate an involvement of red cells in platelet adhesion via ADP.

This has led to the development of a newer hypothesis for thrombosis at cut vessels, which invokes an essential rheological factor: under conditions where blood leaks through a cut, there is a sudden increase in shear close to and in the cut, which can cause enough change in the red cells that they release, *inter alia*, ADP. This hypothesis in illustrated in figure 2, and the next section takes up the testing of the hypothesis in detail.

5. CELLS UNDER SHEAR: CHEMICAL CONSEQUENCES

The experiments of Born *et al.* (1976) provide a critical challenge to previous hypotheses about thrombus formation. The most critical aspect of the observations lies in the following facts. When blood is pumped steadily through the plastic tube, and the tube is free of cuts or holes, the blood flows steadily through and exits from the end without forming a haemostatic plug. For that matter, the effluent blood is free of platelet aggregates. When a cut or hole is made in the side of the tube, there is a disturbance in the flow so that after a period of blood loss, a haemostatic plug forms and seals the hole; in the blood that flows on through the tube to its end there are some platelet aggregates that have probably embolized from the lumen of the tube in the vicinity of the site of the cut. With the *in vitro* system used, there is no possibility of invoking effects of collagen exposed by the cut, or of the absence of protective endothelial cells, or even the possibility of communication to proximal blood flow via extravascular tissue. The flow is steady rather than pulsatile so that there is no possibility of upstream convection of activating factors as might occur during a pulsatile motion. It would therefore seem that the flowing blood reacts to the stimulus of the cut through mechanical effects created in the vicinity of the cut, and that red cells are strongly involved in that reaction.

The nature of the reaction is the subject of hypothesis and testing. One hypothesis is that the red cells are subject locally to haemolysis, and release intracellular adenine nucleotides with

ADP in sufficient proportion to activate the platelets: it is a convenient feature of steady tube flows that the highest shear stresses are closest to the wall. Another hypothesis is that the red cells may be deformed sub-haemolytically yet sufficiently to release adenine nucleotides through pores opened in the red cell membrane by the deformations associated with increased shear. Yet another hypothesis is that the shear stress in rising transiently causes a transient potentiation

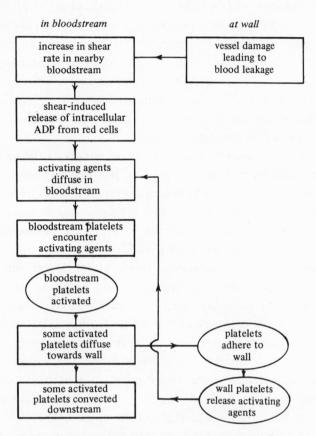

FIGURE 2. Hypothesis (*ca.* 1975) concerning the interaction between the bloodstream and the vessel wall, leading to thrombus formation, especially after arterial puncture. Symbols as in figure 1.

of platelets for adhesion and aggregation presumably by membrane events, e.g. the transfer of a potentiator from the red cell to the platelet when the red cell is stressed enough. These hypotheses are not mutually exclusive.

Two approaches have been taken to testing these hypotheses. One approach is to establish controlled rheological conditions, without thrombus formation, and to measure the chemical effects. The other approach is to try to measure adenine nucleotides present during the formation of a thrombus. Neither approach serves to test the last hypothesis mentioned above.

Controlled rheological conditions have demonstrated the deformability of red cells under steady shear. The combination of normal and shear stresses serve to elongate the cell and make the membrane rotate around the cell contents in a tank-tread motion (Fischer *et al.* 1978). The concept that the red cell may act as a mechanoreceptor for shear more effectively then can the platelet itself is tied to the simple rheological fact that in a given shear flow the stresses induced around the red cell are much greater because of its larger size. After experience with microporous tubing in a hybrid artificial organ (Chick *et al.* 1975) in which ultrafiltration through the tube wall was significant, an experiment was developed in which a red cell suspension was pumped steadily through the lumen of a microporous tube and the ultrafiltrate that passed through the tube wall was collected for chemical analysis (Schmid-Schönbein *et al.* 1979). This ultrafiltrate was drawn from the region in the tube flow where the red cells were under the highest shear and should therefore contain any adenine nucleotides leaked from the red cells. It proved difficult to demonstrate whether the concentration of ADP in the ultrafiltrate was greater than that associated with the slight degree of haemolysis that occurred even when the maximum shear in the tube was below that required for haemolysis. In experiments that take the alternative approach of looking for adenine nucleotides effluent during the formation of a thrombus, Born & Kratzer (1981) have used the luciferin–luciferase system to identify ATP (and also by the use of pyruvate kinase, ADP) in the effluent from a freshly cut artery and a freshly punctured tube with blood flowing through. The early post-cut effluents do not show the presence of impressive amounts of nucleotides.

It has become clear that experiments to test the hypothesis about the nature of the chemical response of red cells under shear are difficult to perform because the amounts of adenine nucleotides being looked for are rather small. The results do not yet appear definitive.

There is an additional aspect of the experiment of Born *et al.* (1976) that merits consideration. This aspect is that there is very little time for the reaction to occur. It is possible to estimate for a typical experiment the extent over which there is an increase in wall shear in the region of the tube immediately upstream from the puncture: this is about 65 μm, and cells moving with their centres 2.5 μm from the wall will reach the lip of the hole in less than 25 ms, and (if there is no local region with closed streamlines formed) will take less than 1 ms in transit through the puncture. These times are short compared with the activation delay times discussed earlier. The experiments to determine the activation delay times were conducted at relatively low shear conditions, and it is possible that potentiation in flows at relatively high shear (as in the cut artery) may reduce the activation time. However, the potentiation and adhesive reactions have very little time to occur before the cells are swept away from the site of the cut, an aspect which may add weight to the hypothesis that the chemical effects involve the cell membranes rather than intracellular substances because the membranes are more readily available to act in such short times.

The extent of damage to platelets is also affected by the duration of the stress. Colantuoni *et al.* (1977) reported that with exposure times of the order of 10^{-3} s there were no significant changes measured in the platelets for stresses below 0.07 N/cm^2, that higher stresses lead to monotonic increases in plasma serotonin and that stresses above 0.15 N/cm^2 lead to diminution of the platelet count and to plasma LDH activity, interpreted as being due to lysis. For shorter exposure times, 10^{-4} s, stresses of the order of 0.4 N/cm^2 are needed to produce evidence of changes in platelets.

Drugs can affect the response of platelets to mechanical stress. For example, Hardwick *et al.* (1980) have shown that incubation of platelets with prostaglandin E_1 and theophylline before exposure to mechanical stress reduced shear-induced aggregation, but above roughly 1 mN/cm^2 there was increased serotonin release and lysis compared with controls. Effects of shear on leucocytes are less well known. McIntire *et al.* (1980) have shown that levels of shear 1–3 mN/cm^2 cause development of phagocytic vacuoles and loss of cytoplasmic granules in PMN leucocytes; they also found that incubation with 3 μM prostaglandin E_1 and 1 μM RA233 (a phosphodiesterase inhibitor related to dipyridamole) for 10 min before shear greatly reduced the mechanical damage suffered.

6. INTERACTIONS BETWEEN INDIVIDUAL CELLS AND WALLS

So far this review of rheological factors in cell – vessel wall reactions has concentrated on events surrounding thrombus formation because of the significance of the phenomenon. It is important to stress that most interactions between platelets (and red cells) and walls do not result in thrombus formation and consist of transient osculations rather than adhesion. Rheologists have known for some time that flow of slurries – dense suspensions of particles in fluids – often occurs with a relatively particle-free layer of fluid, the skimming layer, close to the wall in tubes with diameters many times the particle size. This phenomenon occurs also with blood flows. This might be thought to reduce or eliminate blood cell–wall contacts, but the skimming layer is a macrorheological phenomenon and at the microrheological level one finds frequent osculatory collisions between blood cells and the walls, and these collisions can be accompanied by exchange processes, as demonstrated by uptake of radioactive labels from the wall by red cells (Keller & Yum 1970). These collisions can therefore alter cells but usually in minor ways, and the changes are not like the all-or-nothing changes associated with platelet involvement in thrombus formation. The diffusion of cells to and from a wall is affected by the augmentation process described in §4.

Evidence is now growing that degrees of reaction can occur between platelets and walls that are intermediate between simple collision and permanent adhesion and aggregation. Richardson *et al.* (1979) have studied the adhesion of platelets to foreign surfaces and have observed that many platelets depart after adhesions lasting 2–3 min, and moreover that sites previously occupied by platelets were preferred for adhesion by platelets (passing subsequently) compared with unused adhesion sites. Adams & Feuerstein (1980) observed fluorescently labelled platelets in shear flow over a wall and reported that there were transient adhesions lasting up to 0.5 s, but that platelets adhering longer than that tended to remain for a relatively long time. Richardson *et al.* (1979) have observed that individual platelets that adhere and then come free often adhere again downstream, and that circumstances can prevail with this turnover process that the platelet adhesion density (platelets per unit area) becomes progressively larger downstream, suggesting that platelets can become more adhesive as they progress downstream after adhesion–detachment events. It is not clear whether repeated adhesions and detachments are necessary to augment the adhesiveness, or whether it occurs with the passage of time after a damaging event as illustrated by the results of Feuerstein *et al.* (1980) for serotonin release from the mechanically injured platelet.

A significant factor in controlling the interaction between individual cells and walls is the existence of an ultrafiltration flow through the wall. Forstrum *et al.* (1975) investigated formed element deposition onto porous walls for red cells and for platelets when ultrafiltrate leaves the blood stream. Noting that cells would experience a drag force towards a surface because of the ultrafiltration, they showed that when the value of a deposition parameter

$$\lambda \nu^{\frac{1}{2}} U_{\mathrm{f}} / R^2 S^{\frac{3}{2}}$$

(where U_{f} is the ultrafiltration velocity, λ is a function of the particle volume concentration, R is the particle radius, ν is the kinematic viscosity of the suspending phase and S is the wall shear rate) exceeds a certain value, cells will deposit at the wall even when there is no adhesion. For red cells the critical value of the parameter is about 0.15 and for platelets the critical value (which showed experimental scatter) ranged from 0.01 to 0.15. A corollary of this is that if ultrafiltration occurs through a wall in the opposite direction, i.e. into the bloodstream, it can prevent adhesion to a surface to which platelets would otherwise adhere, as demonstrated by Predecki *et al.* (1980 *a*).

7. FLOWS AROUND OBSTACLES, IN CAVITIES, AND INTO HOLES

Mural obstacles and cavities, such as those formed when atheromatous plaques fracture, assist thrombus formation. There are flow-controlled effects on lipid deposition processes near blood vessel bifurcations. These observations have led to interest in flows around obstacles, in cavities, and into holes branching from a vessel or duct. The experiments of Born *et al.* (1976), where a cut or hole is made in the side of a tube, provide another example of the latter type of flow. Unfortunately the flows are rather complicated, with streamlines taking paths that are sometimes very tortuous.

Baker (1979) has shown that a small cylindrical mural obstacle alters the structure of a simple shear flow by inducing formation of horseshoe-shaped vortex structures with the curved part of the shoe draped around the upstream side of the obstacle. These flows increase the residence time near the obstacle of the fluid entrained in these structures. This may help to provide time for fibrin polymerization in slow flows, or retention of platelets to times beyond their activation-delay times in faster flows. In any case, the experimental evidence shows clearly that the disturbance created is sufficient to enhance adhesion and thrombus formation. Flows in cavities have a large degree of recirculation so that residence times can be very long indeed. Flows at tube junctions have been studied with ranges of values of the Reynolds number, ratios of branch diameter to main tube diameter, ratios of branch flow rates to main supply flow rates, branch angles and so on. Rodkiewicz & Roussel (1973) have investigated conditions for large arteries with experimental Reynolds numbers in the range 700–5000, for example, and Karino & Goldsmith (1980) those for smaller Reynolds numbers (10–350). Both groups observed that the flow down the side branch had a double-helicoidal structure (reminding one of the secondary motion in curved tube flow) and that there were local regions of flow separation and reattachment. Of the flow which enters the side branch, some turns directly from the main flow while another fraction of it overshoots and then executes a 270° turn to reach the side branch rather like road traffic using a clover-leaf turn to gain access from one highway to another. Karino & Goldsmith found that the radius of curvature of the wall surface at the junction of the branch to the main tube had a profound effect on the extent to which separated flow zones were generated, with the smoother, more curved transitions generating less flow separation. The flow structures look vortical in places, such as the cloverleaf turn, but are open streamline flows and do not markedly increase residence times for most of the flow.

The studies mentioned above were carred out with steady flows in stiff-walled chambers. Some differences in the flows occur especially if the flow is pulsatile, and to some degree if the walls are compliant. Even without the modifications associated with such changes in conditions, the flow is complex enough to negate the prospects of simple analysis, but its description helps to provice a background against which transport of platelets to local portions of the wall can be compared.

8. ROLE OF PLASMA PROTEINS

It is well known that the rheology of whole blood is influenced by plasma proteins; most particularly, the viscosity of blood in steady shear flow is affected by the concentration of fibrinogen. The possible rheological role of plasma proteins in thrombosis has ben overwhelmed by their biochemical role, as fibrinogen is an essential constituent in platelet aggregation. On foreign surfaces the adhesion of platelets is mediated through plasma proteins that have adsorbed to the surface, and it would seem that to some degree the thrombogenicity of a surface is related to the degree to which it binds fibrinogen, and its passivity is related to the binding of albumin.

The alignment of long molecules such as proteins in a shear flow involves time constants for

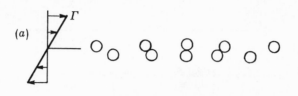

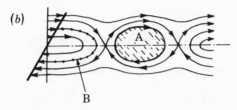

FIGURE 3. Cell–cell interactions. (a) Five successive views of two cells undergoing collision in shear flow with velocity gradient Γ. The rotation rate of cells is approximately $\frac{1}{2}\Gamma$. (b) Flow induced by red cell A in a shear flow. The points on streamline B show a relatively small particle or cell at successive intervals of time and illustrate how the flow induced by A can cause augmentation of the diffusion of particles across the mid-plane (shown as chain line).

relaxation, and in a pulsatile flow there is some question as to the extent to which the relaxation has occurred and therefore how much the long molecules affect the flow.

9. DISCUSSION AND CONCLUSIONS

In most flows of practical interest for platelet–vessel wall interactions the cell–cell encounters are caused dominantly by shear-flow encounters rather than by Brownian motion. The fraction of collisions leading to aggregation is known as the collision efficiency; for platelets this is affected by the shear rate and by the degree of activation such as that caused by ADP. The apparent collision efficiency of platelets may be enhanced by the morphological changes (development of pseudopodia) that follow activation, as these morphological changes may increase the effective radius of the platelets. Red cells, which are of course larger than platelets, induce flows around themselves when they are in shear flows, and a consequence is to cause a considerable enhancement of platelet diffusivity in the direction of the velocity gradient. This effect increases with haematocrit when the haematocrit is very small, but is only weakly dependent on haematocrit if at all at normal physiological values. There is some possibility that the red cells serve as mechanoreceptors for increases in shear rates; such increases occur near sites of vascular injury. The response of the cells, through mechanical deformation, may be to provide a chemical signal sensitizing the platelets and leading to enhanced aggregation. This effect is not certain but has been proposed as the explanation of an oft-repeated experimental phenomenon. Cell–cell interactions are illustrated in figure 3.

The interaction of platelets with vessel walls can involve simple collision, collision with some transient adsorption or adhesion with some mutual changes occurring between platelet and wall, or relatively permanent adhesion. Transient interactions, while involving changes in platelets, do not have activation of the all-or-nothing sense associated with them. Platelet–wall interactions can often be characterized in terms of a rate constant. Cell–wall interactions are affected by ultrafiltration through the wall, ultrafiltration from the blood stream being

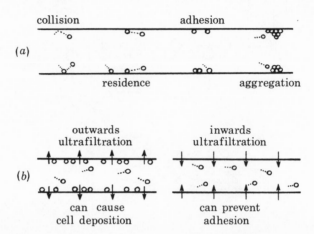

FIGURE 4. Platelet–wall interactions. (a) Successive illustration of a simple collision, residence (where collision is followed by a generally brief period of residence of the platelet with subsequent departure), adhesion (from which the platelet does not depart) and aggregation. (b) Effects of ultrafiltration through vessel walls.

capable of causing cell deposition without adhesion while ultrafiltration into the bloodstream is capable of preventing adhesion. Platelet–wall interactions are illustrated in figure 4.

The magnitude of the forces that can be exerted between platelets and a wall is not well known, although this is obviously important in determining the stability of adhesion under a pulsating flow and the maximum shear rate in which specific aggregates can be safe from shear-driven embolization. It does appear that there is an activation time delay for platelets to be able to exert sufficient force to sustain adhesion; this is a fraction of a second.

It has proved possible to develop a rheological theory for the growth of small mural thrombi (typically 50–100 μm long) that predicts the exponential growth of volume with time found in experiment and which relates the exponential coefficient to the shear rate in a way that corresponds with experiment when the effects of the activation delay time are taken into account. For long mural thrombi (more than 1 mm) it has been found that the growth rate can be limited by either the surface reactivity for platelets or the diffusion of platelets from the bloodstream, the latter being affected by the enhancement provided by red cells in a shear flow, as noted earlier.

Timescales have shown themselves to be important. On the one hand, at short times, there are the effects of the platelet activation delay time in limiting thrombus growth rates at high shear rates, and the evidence that the haemostatic reaction for vessel damage and for the experiment of Born et al. (1976) occurs in a small fraction of a second. On the other hand, additional time is provided for reactions to occur by bumps on walls and by cavities due to the fluid motions associated with these wall geometries. These extra-time situations are illustrated in figure 5.

(a)

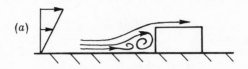

(b)

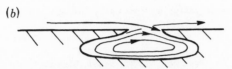

FIGURE 5. Situations leading to additional time being spent by portions of a blood stream in local regions near a surface. (a) Flow near an excrescence by which vortices are formed. The vortices drape themselves around the obstacle in the form of a horseshoe when viewed from above, and particles or cells entering each vortex are eventually swept downstream. (b) Flow over and in a cavity. While there is some exchange of fluid between the stream and the cavity, the residence time in the cavity is relatively long.

REFERENCES (Richardson)

Adams, G. A. & Feuerstein, I. A. 1980 Visual fluorescent and radio-isotopic evaluation of platelet accumulation and embolization. *Trans. Am. Soc. artif. intern. Organs* **26**, 17–22.

Baker, C. J. 1979 The laminar horseshoe vortex. *J. Fluid Mech.* **95**, 347–367.

Bangham, A. D. & Pethica, B. A. 1960 The adhesiveness of cells and the nature of chemical groups at their surfaces. *Proc. phys. Soc. Edinb.* **28**, 43–52.

Baumgartner, H. R. 1973 The role of blood flow in platelet adhesion, fibrin deposition and formation of mural thrombi. *Microvasc. Res.* **5**, 167–179.

Begent, N. & Born, G. V. R. 1970 Growth rate *in vivo* of platelet thrombi, produced by iontophoresis of ADP, as a function of mean blood flow velocity. *Nature, Lond.* **227**, 926–930.

Born, G. V. R. 1962 Aggregation of blood platelets by adenosine diphosphate and its reversal. *Nature, Lond.* **194**, 927–929.

Born, G. V. R. 1977 Fluid-mechanical and biochemical interactions in haemostasis. *Br. med. Bull.* **33**, 193–197.

Born, G. V. R. & Kratzer, M. 1981 Contribution of blood platelets to the pathogenesis of myocardial infarction. *Revue méd. Brux.* **2**, 157–160.

Born, G. V. R. & Richardson, P. D. 1981 Response time for platelet activation. *J. Membr. Biol.* (In the press.)

Born, G. V. R., Berqvist, D. & Arfors, K.-E. 1976 Evidence for inhibition of platelet activation in blood by a drug effect on erythrocytes. *Nature, Lond.* **259**, 233–235.

Chang, H. N. & Robertson, C. R. 1976 Platelet aggregation by laminar shear and Brownian motion. *Ann. biomed. Engng* **4**, 151–183.

Chick, W. L., Like, A. A., Lauris, V., Galletti, P. M., Richardson, P. D., Panol, G. Mix, T. W. & Colton, C. F. 1975 A hybrid artificial pancreas. *Trans. Am. Soc. artif. intern. Organs* **21**, 8–14.

Colantuoni, G., Hellums, J. D., Moake, J. L. & Alfrey, C. P. 1977 The response of human platelets to shear stress at short exposure times. *Trans. Am. Soc. artif. intern. Organs* **23**, 626–630.

Eckstein, E. C., Bailey, D. G. & Shapiro, A. H. 1977 Self-diffusion of particles in shear flow of a suspension. *J. Fluid Mech.* **79**, 191–208.

Feuerstein, I. A., Marzeo, U, & Bernstein, E. F. 1980 Serotonin kinetics in the mechanically injured platelet. *Trans. Am. Soc. artif. intern. Organs* **26**, 172–177.

Fischer, T. F. & Richardson, P. D. 1980 Blood cell interactions in shear flow and consequences for diffusion and aggregation. In *Advances in bioengineering 1980* (ed. V. C. Mow), pp. 305–308. American Society of Mechanical Engineers.

Fischer, T. F., Stöhr-Liesen, M. & Schmid-Schönbein, H. 1978 The red cells as a fluid droplet: tank tread-like motion of the human erythrocyte membrane in shear flow. *Science, N.Y.* **202**, 894–896.

Forstrum, R. J., Bartelt, K., Blackshear, D. L. & Wood, T. 1975 Formed element deposition onto filtering walls. *Trans. Am. Soc. artif. intern. Organs* **21**, 602–607.

Goldsmith, H. L. & Karino, T. 1977 Microscopic considerations: the motions of individual particles. *Ann. N.Y. Acad. Sci.* **283**, 241.

Hardwick, R. A., Hellums, J. D., Moake, J. L., Peterson, D. M. & Alfrey, C. P. 1980 Effects of antiplatelet agents on platelets exposed to shear stress. *Trans. Am. Soc. artif. intern. Organs* **26**, 179–183.

Karino, T. & Goldsmith, G. L. 1980 Disturbed flow in models of branching vessels. *Trans. Am. Soc. artif. intern. Organs* **26**, 500–505.

Keller, K. H. & Yum, S. I. 1970 Erythrocyte–tube wall interactions in laminar flow of blood suspensions. *Trans. Am. Soc. artif. intern. Organs* **16**, 42–47.

Levich, V. G. 1962 *Physicochemical hydrodynamics*. Prentice-Hall.

McIntire, L. V., Stockwell, D. J., Martin, R. R. & Sybers, H. D. 1980 Leukocyte response to mechanical trauma – antiplatelet drug effects. *Trans. Am. Soc. artif. intern. Organs* **26**, 289–293.

Mustard, J. F., Murphy, E. A., Rowsell, H. C. & Downie, H. G. 1962 Factors influencing thrombus formation in vivo. *Am. J. Med.* **63**, 621–647.

Poe, G. G. & Acrivos, A. 1975 Closed-streamline flows past rotating single cylinders and spheres: inertia effect. *J. Fluid Mech.* **72**, 605–623.

Predecki, P., Life, L. & Newman, M. M. 1980a Prevention of platelet adhesion to porous surfaces. *J. biomed. Mater. Res.* **14**, 405–415.

Predecki, P., Life, L., Russell, P. A. & Newman, M. M. 1980b Measurement of the activation time for platelet adhesion to foreign surfaces. *J. biomed. Mater. Res.* **14**, 417–426.

Richardson, P. D. 1973 Effect of blood flow velocity on growth rate of platelet thrombi. *Nature, Lond.* **245**, 103–104.

Richardson, P. D., Galletti, P. M. & Born, G. V. R. 1976 Regional administration of drugs to control thrombosis in artificial organs. *Trans. Am. Soc. artif. intern. Organs* **22**, 22–28.

Richardson, P. D., Mohammed, S. F., Mason, R. G., Steiner, M. & Kane, R. 1979 Dynamics of platelet interaction with surfaces in steady flow conditions. *Trans. Am. Soc. artif. intern. Organs* **25**, 147–151.

Rieger, H. 1976 Zur Physiologie und Pathophysiologie der Blutplättchen unter rheologischen Aspekten. Habilitationsschrift der Medizinischen Fakultät der RWTH Aachen.

Robertson, C. R. & Chang, H. N. 1974 Platelet retention in colums packed with glass beads. *Ann. biomed. Engng* **2**, 361–391.

Rodkiewicz, C. M. & Roussel, C. L. 1973 Fluid mechanics in a large arterial bifurcation. *Trans. Am. Soc. mech. Engrs: J. Fluids Engng* **95**, 108–112.

Schmid-Schönbein, H., Born, G. V. R., Richardson, P. D. Rohling-Winkel, I., Blasberg, P., Cusack, N., Wehmeyer, A. & Jüngling, E. 1979 ADP release from red cells subjected to high shear stresses. In *Basic aspects of blood trauma* (ed. H. Schmid-Schönbein & P. Teitel), pp. 322–340. Martinus Nijhoff Publ.

Turitto, V. T., Benis, A. M. & Leonard, E. F. 1972 Platelet diffusion in flowing blood. *Ind. Engng Chem. Fundam.* **11**, 216–223.

Welch, W. H. 1887 The structure of white thrombi. *Trans. path. Soc. Philad.* **13**, 25.

Discussion

D. B. Longmore (*National Heart Hospital, London, U.K.*). The results presented in this important paper possibly may not reflect what happens in life. Studies with clear fluids in artificial systems fail to take into account two fundamental factors.

First, blood is an extremely complex non-Newtonian fluid. Its mechanical properties change with the physical environment and with flow patterns. It has been rightly pointed out that when blood is flowing above a critical velocity in a vessel, there is an axial stream of cells. The blood in contact with the vessel walls consists mainly of plasma, which consists in part of a range of plasma protein molecules. Some of these plasma proteins are highly deformable if stressed or put in shear. The normally barrel-shaped coiled molecules can deform to become long spirals or nearly straight. There is a profound change in viscosity when this occurs. No artificial blood has yet been made with these unique properties. Furthermore, when whole blood is pumped through artificial circuits the plasma proteins soon lose these properties.

The second important difference between any experimental model and life relates to the development of the cardiovascular system in the embryo. The mesoderm forms the cardiovascular system and the blood from one material. During the development of the embryo, the central liquifying blood-forming elements ebb and flow, and then flow through the vascular plexus, which is to form the adult tree. The detailed internal architecture of the vascular system is therefore at least partly moulded by the very blood that is flowing through it. As the foetus develops, the network of vessels soon develops into a definitive vascular tree possibly because of the fluid logistics of the system. Small biasing streams in a network deflect the whole flow in one direction.

Because blood has variable physical properties and it flows through vessels moulded by its flow, does Dr Richardson think it likely that we will obtain most information from studies of blood flow *in vivo*? Range gated pulsed Doppler instruments can show us more than just the anatomy of vessels, the flow rates and the velocity profiles within them. They can detect the difference between laminar flow and energy consuming turbulent flow.

Bibliography

Bass, R. M. & Longmore, D. B. 1969 *Nature, Lond.* **222**, 30–33.

P. D. RICHARDSON. I wish to thank Mr Longmore for his discussion, in which he has brought out five main points: the non-Newtonian rheological properties of blood, the role of plasma proteins, axial streaming of cells in tube flows, embryonic blood flow, and measurement of velocity profiles in whole blood flow. These points I should like to address briefly.

The non-Newtonian rheological properties of blood have been well documented, and the higher values of effective viscosity at smaller values of the shear rate are attributed to the aggregation of red cells into rouleaux. It is expected that there are larger rouleax near the centre of a tube carrying a blood flow than there are near the wall, because the shear stress is smaller near the centre than it is near the wall. Recently we have been able to demonstrate this by ultrasound (Abts *et al.* 1979). There is, however, a finite timescale for aggregation of rouleaux and also for disaggregation of rouleaux upon experiencing higher shear. Consequently some differences may be found between the bulk rheological properties of blood in steady flows and in flows with oscillations with time scales of the order of (or less than) the rouleaux relaxation timescales. As Mr Longmore points out, long-chain molecules can cause non-Newtonian properties in a fluid, and indeed these can be found with very dilute suspensions; however, here again there are characteristic timescales associated with the alignment of the long chains in a shear flow and with stretching of coils, and the rheological response at high enough frequencies of oscillation can be different from that in steady flows. Not enough is yet known about the quantitative details of the constitutive equations that represent this behaviour for blood. Mr Longmore is correct to observe that a coloured Newtonian liquid is not a rheologically perfect substitute for blood. It is only fair to point out that blood is not a simple fluid; even with a patient who undergoes heart–lung bypass as an adjunct to surgery, the blood in his circulation may start with a haematocrit of more than 40 % but can be reduced by haemodilution to 25 %, cooled, and partly depleted of plasma proteins by passage through the extracorporeal circuit, not to mention other changes, so that substantial alterations in the rheological properties can occur even during such a procedure. Changes also occur during life, and there are significant differences for different species.

Axial streaming is an interesting phenomenon, and there is not room here to treat it broadly. It should be noted, however, that the 'cell-poor' layer (or 'skimming' layer) near the wall is affected by axial development length, vessel curvature and pulsatility of the flow. Its relative significance depends on the vessel size.

Embryonic blood flow is a fascinating subject. Physiologists and biomechanicians alike are very conscious of the importance of convective transport of nutrients to tissue masses too large to be supplied adequately by diffusion alone from their peripheries, and the development of embryonic blood flow is interesting for this and for other reasons. The development of pulsatile action in the embryonic heart, even before the chambers are distinctly formed, may be important for augmenting transport because pulsatile motions can induce steady secondary motions that provide a vehicle for convection. Platelet – vessel wall interactions are poorly known in these circumstances.

In his final point, Mr Longmore raises the question of measurement of velocity profiles in whole blood flow. I agree wholeheartedly with his view that one should try to obtain measurements with real blood rather than with a substitute liquid. There are serious problems in obtaining accurate measurements in whole blood, especially if accurate measurements of velocity gradients are desired. Invasive measurements (e.g. hot-film anemometry) are not widely suited to different vessels; optical methods such as laser velocimetry run into problems as the vessel size rises above 50 μm or so because of absorption and scattering from the red cells, although it is possible to achieve good spatial resolution (Melling *et al.* 1976). Pulsed Doppler ultrasound has the ability to obtain measurements in larger blood vessels but generally lacks the spatial resolution to determine accurately the velocity gradient in the important region close to the wall. The incidence and structure of turbulence are somewhat hard to measure in human physiological flows because turbulence can be spatially patchy and temporally cyclic in large vessels and in extracorporeal circuits. This obviously complicates the platelet – vessel wall interactions.

References

Abts, L., Richardson, P. D. & Schmid-Schönbein, H. 1979 Ultrasound detection of aggregation of red cells in blood flow. In *Proc. 7th North East Bioengineering Conference*, pp. 228–231. Pergamon.
Melling, A., Richardson, P. D. & Whitelaw, J. H. 1976 Development of laser anemometry for blood-velocity measurement in small-diameter tubes. In *Proc. 4th New England Bioengineering Conference*, pp. 243–246. Pergamon.

Phil. Trans. R. Soc. Lond. B **294**, 267–279 (1981)

Printed in Great Britain

The role of Willebrand factor in platelet – blood vessel interaction, including a discussion of resistance to atherosclerosis in pigs with von Willebrand's disease

By E. J. W. Bowie, V. Fuster, D. N. Fass and C. A. Owen, Jr

Hematology Research, Mayo Clinic and Mayo Foundation, Rochester, Minesota
55901, U.S.A.

Von Willebrand pigs have all the manifestations of the severe human disease. The role of Willebrand antigen (VIII R:AG) and ristocetin cofactor (VIII: RWF) was assessed in these pigs by (1) transfusion and (2) 'in vitro' bleeding time assay. The skin bleeding time became normal when the level of transfused Willebrand factor (VIII R:AG/RWF) was raised in the plasma above 30 U/dl. After single or repeated transfusions, skin capillary endothelium and platelets were still distinguished from normal by VIII R:AG deficiency. When incisions in excised porcine skin (*'in vitro'* bleeding time) were perfused with blood and plasma fractions, haemostasis occurred when plasmatic Willebrand factor exceeded 30 U/dl whether the skin or platelets came from normal or from von Willebrand pigs. The platelet plug occluding the skin incision contained VIII R:AG by immunofluorescence. Willebrand factor appears to coat surfaces and to serve as a platelet attachment protein.

These bleeder pigs are resistant to atherosclerosis. If platelets are involved in early atheroscolerotic lesions, the role of Willebrand factor in platelet – blood vessel interaction may be important.

Von Willebrand's disease

In 1926, Professor Erik von Willebrand described a bleeding disease (von Willebrand 1926) and found that prolongation of the bleeding time was the main haemostatic abnormality. Since that time, a variety of haemostatic defects have been described in his eponymous disease and it has been the subject of research by many groups in many countries. The disease affects not only the coagulation portion of the haemostatic mechanism but also the interaction of the platelet and the blood vessel wall. Research into this disease is leading to a greater understanding of the haemostatic defect and is also making fundamental contributions to our knowledge of the haemostatic mechanism. More recently, the disease has assumed even greater importance because of the observation that severely affected pigs are resistant to the development of atherosclerosis.

Patients with von Willebrand's disease, like patients with classic haemophilia, have a decrease factor VIII coagulant activity; but they differ from haemophiliacs because their bleeding time is prolonged. Von Willebrand himself suggested that the abnormality in the disease was related to the capillary and the platelet. Subsequent experiments with the use of an instrument known as a capillary thrombometer showed that the thrombosing time, a correlate of platelet function was abnormally long (Morawitz & Jurgens 1930). Further evidence of a functional abnormality of platelets was proposed by Borchgrevink, who showed that considerably more platelets escape from skin incisions in von Willebrand's disease than in normal people (Borchgrevink 1961). An *in vitro* test was then developed using glass bead columns, the 'platelet retention' test. It was found that, in von Willebrand's disease, fewer platelets were retained in the column (Salzman 1963; Zucker 1963; Bowie *et al.* 1959). A further abnormality of platelet function was demonstrated by the use of the antibiotic ristocetin. Ristocetin was shown to aggregate platelets in normal platelet-rich plasma but failed to aggregate them in the platelet-rich plasma of patients with von Willebrand's disease (Howard & Firkin 1971).

Testing of platelet function and electron microscopy failed to produce any convincing evidence of an intrinsic abnormality of the platelet. There was suggestive evidence that the abnormality of platelet function in von Willebrand's disease was due to the decrease or abnormality of some factor in the plasma, because the platelet retention test was corrected by the addition of normal plasma (Bowie *et al.* 1969; Meyer & Larrieu 1979). Our group then showed that the abnormality of platelet retention could be corrected by the addition of concentrates of factor VIII (Bowie *et al.* 1959); this was the first demonstration that the functional abnormality of the platelet and the decrease of factor VIII were in some way connected (Bowie *et al.* 1969). These findings were subsequently confirmed by Weiss & Rogers (1972) and Bouma *et al.* (1972).

The next observation about platelet function was that normal or haemophilic plasma and factor VIII preparations would allow ristocetin to produce aggregation of von Willebrand platelets (Firkin & Howard 1971; Howard & Firkin 1971; Howard *et al.* 1973; Weiss *et al.* 1973; Meyer *et al.* 1974; Olson *et al.* 1975).

Subsequently, it was found that an antibody made against factor VIII detected a protein that was present in normal quantities in patients with haemophilia and absent, or decreased, in patients with von Willebrand's disease (Zimmerman *et al.* 1971). Further observations of the chemistry of factor VIII have demonstrated that the factor VIII molecule is a complex structure composed of two non-covalently linked proteins, one of which has the coagulant property and is missing or abnormal in haemophilia and the other a large polymeric protein that is missing or abnormal in von Willebrand's disease. It is this latter protein that can be detected immunologically by precipitating rabbit antibodies (the so-called factor VIII related antigen). This protein is also probably responsible for the ability of ristocetin to agglutinate platelets (the ristocetin Willebrand factor or the ristocetin cofactor).

This introduction has been a brief summary of the complex series of investigations that led to the discovery of Willebrand factor. At this point the disease can be even more concisely summarized by stating that it is due to the decrease or abnormality of a protein in the plasma (Zimmerman *et al.* 1971), which can be detected immunologically by immunoelectrophoresis (Zimmerman *et al.* 1971) or immunoradiometric assay (Ruggeri *et al.* 1976) and functionally by its ability to allow ristocetin to cause aggregation of washed platelets (Howard *et al.* 1974; Olson *et al.* 1975).

WILLEBRAND FACTOR IN HAEMOSTASIS

Studies in humans

Willebrand factor appears to be synthesized in the endothelial cell (Jaffe *et al.* 1973, 1974; Booyse *et al.* 1977) and perhaps also in the megakaryocyte (Nachman *et al.* 1977). The protein is also present in the platelet (Glagov 1973) and, of course, it circulates in the plasma. In cultures of endothelial cells from pig aortas, the protein is to some extent extracellular and it may be fibrillar or associated with a fibrillar protein (Booyse *et al.* 1977).

Examination of partly purified and highly purified preparations of Willebrand factor by electrophoresis in sodium dodecyl sulphate (SDS) suggest that the protein circulates in plasma as a series of polymers (van Mourik *et al.* 1974; Counts *et al.* 1978; Fass *et al.* 1978; Perret *et al.* 1979; Weinstein & Deykin 1979; Ruggeri & Zimmerman 1980). The protein is extremely large and in the pig the polymers range in relative molecular mass from 10^6 to 21×10^6 (Fass 1978) and in the human from 0.86×10^6 to 9.9×10^6 (Ruggeri & Zimmerman 1980). This large polymeric protein therefore exists in a series of biological compartments; one of the important investigations in the physiology of haemostasis is to elucidate the role of Willebrand factor in these various areas.

There is increasing evidence that the level of plasmatic Willebrand factor plays an important role in platelet – blood vessel interaction and the eventual production of haemostasis. Platelets from patients with von Willebrand's disease adhered poorly when exposed to the subendothelium of the de-endothelialized everted segments of rabbit aorta in a perfusion chamber (Tschopp *et al.* 1974; Weiss *et al.* 1975; Fuster *et al.* 1980). The type of anticoagulant used in these experiments is important and when higher citrate concentrations were used, the adhesion defect was more pronounced (Weiss *et al.* 1977). When an antibody to human factor VIII (Baumgartner *et al.* 1977) was used to deplete normal plasma of Willebrand factor, there was also defective adhesion of platelets to subendothelium.

An interesting finding in all of these studies was that the difference between normal and von Willebrand blood depended upon the shear rate, and was greater at higher shear rates. In more recent studies, the perfusion system has been modified to allow the examination of native human blood, and subsequent studies have confirmed the shear rate dependent decrease of adhesion in von Willebrand's disease. These experiments have been criticized because they were not done with tissue from the same animal species; human blood was used in conjunction with rabbit aorta. Sakariassen and colleagues, however (Sakariassen *et al.* 1979), have now adapted the Baumgartner perfusion chamber to use human tissues only by substituting renal arteries, obtained at post-mortem, for the rabbit aortas. These workers labelled platelets and Willebrand factor radioactively and their study suggested that Willebrand factor bound to the subendothelium induced platelet adhesion and that it was the plasma protein alone that was necessary for normal platelet adhesion. Recent work in our own laboratory, with the use of a porcine system, is entirely consistent with these results (Bowie *et al.* 1978; Kimura *et al.* 1979).

Studies in pigs

At the Mayo Clinic, we have maintained for several years a breeding colony of pigs with von Willebrand's disease (Bowie *et al.* 1973). The term for a collection of pigs is actually a 'sounder' – a particularly appropriate designation, as pigs are rather vocal animals. The Mayo Clinic 'sounder' shares the observed impairment of primary haemostasis and other haemostatic abnormalities of the severe form of the disease in humans (Mannucci *et al.* 1976; Bowie & Owen 1979). The animals are afflicted with a serious bleeding tendency (Bowie *et al.* 1973; Fass *et al.* 1976a) that is autosomally transmitted (Owen *et al.* 1974; Fass *et al.* 1979) and is manifested by a long bleeding time, reduced platelet retention, an almost complete absence of factor VIII related antigen (0.025 % by immunoradiometric assay) and a lack of Willebrand factor in the plasma. Like the human protein, porcine Willebrand factor purifies with and is probably identical to the factor VIII related antigen (Fass *et al.* 1976b).

The availability of such an animal model has allowed us to conduct experiments on the role of Willebrand factor in haemostasis, with tissues from the same animal species. We have developed a technique known as the '*in vitro*' bleeding time. A small piece of excised porcine skin is attached to the channel in the base of a flow cube, and heparinized porcine blood or plasma is allowed to flow through a 5 mm incision in the skin at a constant hydrostatic pressure The technique is described in detail by Kimura *et al.* (1979). The volume of blood or plasma exuding from the incision is measured and the incision site examined microscopically after haemostasis has occurred.

When normal blood or platelet-rich plasma was allowed to flow through the skin incision, there was a gradual decrease in the volume of blood and the bleeding eventually stopped whether the skin came from a normal or a von Willebrand pig. When the incision in the skin was examined microscopically, a platelet clump was found to occlude the epidermal end of the incision, and it was shown to stain positively for Willebrand factor by immunofluorescence. If blood or platelet-rich plasma from a pig with von Willebrand's disease was used, the bleeding continued and haemostasis did not occur. The delayed haemostasis was corrected to normal by the addition of normal plasma or cryoprecipitate. The addition of an antibody to Willebrand factor to normal pig blood caused a gradual increase in the bleeding time, which became indefinite when the Willebrand factor had been completely inhibited by the antibody. From these experiments, it was concluded that plasmatic Willebrand factor played an essential role in haemostasis in this *in vitro* system.

Transfusions of plasma and concentrates of Willebrand factor into the living animal have shown a remarkable correlation with these *in vitro* experiments. Haemostasis in these studies was evaluated by a new technique, the 'ratio bleeding time' developed by one of us (D.N.F.), which is fully described elsewhere (Bowie *et al.* 1980). In a series of experiments involving the administration of 20 transfusions of plasma cryoprecipitate and a partly purified preparation of Willebrand factor, the role of Willebrand factor in the plasma, platelet and endothelial cell was evaluated. Platelets and endothelial cells (skin biopsies) were examined at intervals after the transfusion of a large quantity of cryoprecipitate. Although the ratio bleeding time was completely corrected, there was never any evidence of Willebrand factor in the platelets or in the endothelial cells. In these studies, the bleeding time was found to be normal when the level of Willebrand factor in the plasma was above 30 %, about the same level as was found with the '*in vitro*' bleeding time.

Although the brief correction of the bleeding time after transfusion can be correlated with the brief residence of Willebrand factor in the plasma, there is evidence that the level of plasmatic Willebrand factor is not the whole story. One line of evidence comes from studies on the bleeding time. The Duke bleeding time may be normal in some patients with von Willebrand's disease in whom the Ivy bleeding time is prolonged (Nilsson *et al.* 1959; Cornu *et al.* 1963; Larrieu *et al.* 1968). Moreover, after transfusion the Duke bleeding time is more easily corrected than the Ivy bleeding time (Nilsson *et al.* 1959; Cornu *et al.* 1964; Silwer & Nilsson 1964; Larrieu *et al.* 1968). Capillary pressure is increased in the Ivy bleeding time test, in contrast to the Duke bleeding time, and the consequent increased shear rate may be enough to impede haemostasis in the Ivy test when compared with the Duke test (Jaffe *et al.* 1974). After transfusion, the level of plasmatic Willebrand factor in the Duke and Ivy tests would be the same, which suggests that for completely normal haemostasis, Willebrand factor must be present in the platelets and endothelial cells as well as in the plasma.

Another line of evidence comes from the study of patients with variant forms of von Willebrand's disease. It is becoming clear that von Willebrand's disease is a heterogeneous group of diseases, and in one type of the disease, normal Willebrand factor may be decreased or absent in the plasma, platelet and endothelial cell. In a second type the Willebrand factor may be abnormal (Mannucci 1977; Ruggeri & Zimmerman 1980). In a third type the level of Wille-brand factor in the plasma may be extremely low, but there are normal or increased levels in the platelet and endothelial cells. In this last type of the disease, it would appear that the Willebrand factor is not being released from its sites of synthesis; it is this variant form of the disease that may give us a clue as to the role of Willebrand factor in haemostasis. Pigs and people who have no Willebrand factor in plasma or platelets or endothelial cells have a severe haemorrhagic diathesis. As we shall point out later, our pigs periodically bleed to death. On the other hand, humans with the third variant type of von Willebrand's disease have a mild bleeding diathesis although they have extremely low levels of plasmatic Willebrand factor. One explanation for their haemostatic competence would be the presence of Willebrand factor in the platelets and endothelial cells. It is, of course, possible that we are dealing with another factor – a bleeding time factor – which is hinted at in earlier work summarized by Blombäck et al. (1964). The bleeding time factor, however, has not been isolated and has not been clearly differentiated from Willebrand factor.

From these studies, we can conclude that plasmatic Willebrand factor plays an essential role in the haemostatic mechanism but that for entirely normal haemostasis Willebrand factor must be present both in the platelet and endothelial cell. It seems likely that plasmatic Willebrand factor coats surfaces and serves as an attachment protein for the platelet (Bowie et al. 1978; Nyman 1980).

RESISTANCE TO ATHEROSCLEROSIS IN PORCINE VON WILLEBRAND'S DISEASE

Our current understanding of the haemostatic mechanism gives a central role to the platelet, which forms the haemostatic plug and also makes an essential contribution to the coagulation mechanism and the subsequent formation of fibrin. Furthermore, the platelet may be the main reason why the haemostatic mechanism is localized to an injured area because all the reactions involved in haemostasis may take place on its surface membrane.

It is paradoxical that the platelet, which may preserve life by staunching bleeding, may cause death by initiating atheroma. It has been suggested by many investigators (Stemerman & Ross 1972; Ross et al. 1974; Fishman et al. 1975; Mustard 1975; Harker et al. 1976; Lewis & Kottke 1977) that the platelets adherent to the damaged endothelium may promote the intimal hyperplasia seen in the early atherosclerotic plaque. The early lesion of atherosclerosis is a nodule of hyperplastic smooth muscle in the intima as a result of the hyperplasia of medial smooth muscle that has migrated into the intima through fenestrae in the internal elastic lamina. Platelets are believed to release a mitogenic factor or factors – the platelet-derived growth factor – that stimulate the proliferation of smooth muscle cells and, in fact, smooth muscle cells cannot grow in tissue culture when the serum is derived from platelet-free plasma. Serum derived from fatty platelet-rich plasma is effective in supporting cell growth (Ross et al. 1974).

Harker et al. (1976) have observed that in experimental homocystinaemia, platelet consumption correlated with the formation of intimal lesions. When platelets were inhibited by the administration of dipyridamole, the increased platelet consumption was prevented as well as the formation of the intimal lesions. The studies of Moore et al. (1976) and of Friedman et al.

(1977) showed that thrombocytopenia prevented the arteriosclerosis induced by aortic catheters. Cohen & McCombs (1968) found that ^{32}P-induced thrombocytopenia prevented arteriosclerosis in rabbits fed on an egg yolk diet, but they showed increased arterioclerosis in rabbits with thrombocytosis induced by phlebotomy (Cohen & McCombs 1967). More recently Pick *et al.* (1979) have found that the development of coronary atherosclerosis in cynomologus monkeys (*Macaca fascicularis*) fed on an atherogenic diet was inhibited by the administration of aspirin.

In the light of these studies, therefore, the demonstration that von Willebrand pigs may be resistant to atherosclerosis (Fuster *et al.* 1980) was extremely interesting because of the possibility that it was related to the abnormality of primary haemostasis in these animals. The observation assumed even greater importance because the pig appears to be an ideal animal model of human atherosclerosis. Porcine atherosclerotic lesions are similar in distribution and development to the human lesions, and they are big enough to be easily measured macroscopically and microscopically. In addition, porcine atherosclerosis may be induced by a high cholesterol diet in less than 6 months. A number of studies were therefore initiated to compare the development of atherosclerosis in von Willebrand pigs with that in normal pigs.

As already mentioned, the von Willebrand pigs have a severe bleeding diathesis and bleed to death periodically from exsanguinating gastrointestinal haemorrhage and severe epistaxis. For unknown reasons, the epistaxis always starts in the posterior nose, and because porcine turbinates are convoluted, the bleeding site cannot be visualized. At post-mortem, it was observed that there was negligible aortic atherosclerosis (Bowie *et al.* 1975). This observation was interesting and unexpected because, as already mentioned, pigs have an arterial system closely resembling that of man (French *et al.* 1965), and they usually develop atherosclerotic lesions early in life (Getty 1965). Following the post-mortem observations, a retrospective study of spontaneous atherosclerosis was started in 1974. The incidence of spontaneous aortic atherosclerosis in von Willebrand pigs was compared with the incidence in normal pigs obtained from the slaughterhouse. The normal pigs were of the same breed as the von Willebrand pigs – a cross between Poland–China and Yorkshire–Hampshire. The aortas of 11 normal pigs were examined, and 6 were found to have multiple raised fatty or fibrous atherosclerotic plaques (Fuster *et al.* 1978). Measurement of the intima showed an increased thickness over the plaques ranging from 63 to 130 μm in contrast to the normal areas, where the intima measured 20–64 μm. In the 11 von Willebrand pigs very little atherosclerosis was seen. None of the aortas had multiple plaques, four had single plaques, but only one was more than 2 mm in diameter.

Although the von Willebrand pig aortas appeared to be macroscopically normal, seven showed evidence of extensive fat deposition after staining with Sudan IV. Subendothelial infiltration of fat in the intima was found on microscopic examination. Measurement of the intima showed no evidence of significant thickening and ranged from 27 to 81 μm. Areas of the aorta that were influenced with fat were called non-atherosclerotic flat fatty lesions.

This first study therefore showed that there was a striking difference between the normal pig and pigs with von Willebrand's disease in the incidence and extent of atherosclerotic lesions in the aorta. However, the study had a number of shortcomings: it was retrospective, the body mass of the controls was higher than that of the pigs with von Willebrand's disease, and we did not have exact information about the diets of the normal pigs. We therefore decided in the following year to initiate a prospective study in which the pigs were matched for breed, age and sex and the diet was strictly controlled (Fuster *et al.* 1978): 18 newborn pigs were fed with maternal milk supplemented with cows' milk until 3 months of age at which time they received an atherogenic high-cholesterol diet (approximately 500 g/40 kg body mass, containing 2 % cholesterol) for a period of 6 months. Seven pigs (four male and three female) had homozygous von Willebrand's disease and there were eleven normal control pigs (five male and six female). At 3 and 4 months, respectively, two pigs bled to death and control animals were killed. At autopsy, the mean body mass was 94 kg (± 21 kg s.d.) for the von Willebrand pigs and 105 kg (± 30 kg s.d.) for the normal pigs. The 11 control pigs all developed raised fatty or fibrous atherosclerotic plaques on the aorta. Between 13 and 34 % of the aortic surface was involved in 9 of the pigs, and in the remaining 2 pigs the involved areas measured 2 and 5 %. The plaques were located mainly in the aortic arch and at the trifurcation of the aorta. Measurement of the intimal thickness showed a range of 50 to 390 μm over the plaques in contrast to the intima in the normal areas, which ranged from 18 to 40 μm. In the von Willebrand pigs there was a striking contrast: four pigs developed no atherosclerotic lesions at all, two developed athero-sclerotic lesions effecting 6 and 7 % of the aortic surface, and in the seventh, 13 % of the aortic surface was involved.

It was again noted that on staining with Sudan IV, the aortas of the pigs with von Wille-brand's disease showed large areas of non-atherosclerotic flat fatty lesions. Six of the von Willebrand pigs had 2–23 % of the aortic surface involved with these lesions. In these areas, it was again found that there was subendothelial infiltration of fat without intimal thickening.

Dietary-induced atherosclerosis may, of course, be different from the spontaneously occur-ring variety, so a prospective study of spontaneous atherosclerosis was also undertaken (Fuster 1979 a). Twelve newborn pigs were fed with maternal milk supplemented with cows' milk until 3 months of age, at which time they received a non-atherogenic diet for a period of 4 years. Six pigs (four male and two female) had homoxygous von Willebrand's disease and six were normal control pigs (all female). At 5 and 6 months, two von Willebrand pigs bled to death and were excluded from the study. The other two von Willebrand pigs bled at 23 and 26 months and at these times control animals were also killed. The mean body masses at the time of death were 261 kg (± 94 kg s.d.) for the four pigs with von Willebrand's disease and 284 kg (± 68 kg s.d.) for the six normal control pigs.

On macroscopic examination, the aortas of five of the six control pigs showed raised athero-sclerotic plaques involving 2–8 % of the surface. The distal trifurcation was primarily involved, and the lesions were large, irregular and elongated. In contrast, two of the four pigs with von Willebrand's disease had no atherosclerotic lesions, one had 1 % of the aortic surface involved and the other 2 %. When the aortas were stained with Sudan IV, again non-atherosclerotic flat fatty lesions were seen in three of the von Willebrand pigs.

These three studies, therefore, are evidence that pigs with von Willebrand's disease are resistant to the development of atherosclerosis. There are a number of possible explanations for these findings, and one of them may lie in the abnormal platelet – blood vessel interaction seen in von Willebrand's disease (Booyse et al. 1977). The explanation that we shall now develop is speculative, but it is supported at many of the steps by experimental observation.

The explanation starts at the endothelial cell which, in normal pigs, is known to be damaged by haemodynamic factors (Wesolowski et al. 1965; Fry 1969; Caro et al. 1971; Somer et al. 1972; Texon 1972; Glagov 1973; Cornhill & Roach 1976; Reidy & Bowyer 1977) and also by diets high in cholesterol (Imai & Thomas 1968; Frost 1969; Shiamoto et al. 1971; Chvapil et al. 1976; Ross & Marker 1976). Following the endothelial injury, the platelet then adheres to the damaged endothelial surface or the exposed subendothelial tissue (Stemerman & Ross 1972; Fishman *et al.* 1975; Lewis & Kottke 1977). This platelet – arterial wall interaction is enhanced by the von Willebrand factor in the plasma (Fass *et al.* 1976*a*; Bowie *et al.* 1978), platelets and the arterial wall (Jaffe *et al.* 1974). The earlier discussion of our studies with the use of transfusions and the *in vitro* bleeding time technique suggests that the level of Willebrand factor in the plasma plays an important role in this platelet – blood vessel interaction (Bowie & Owen 1979; Kimura *et al.* 1979). There is also evidence that adherence of platelets to the arterial surface in the normal animal may help to repair the endothelium and reduce its permeability (Gimbrone *et al.* 1969; Wojcik *et al.* 1969; Fry *et al.* 1976; Reidy & Bowyer 1977). In a normal pig, therefore, the continual endothelial damage results in platelet blood vessel adherence mediated by Willebrand factor and the restoration of endothelial integrity. In addition, the platelet-derived growth factor may, in some instances, result in intimal smooth muscle hyperplasia and the beginning of atherosclerosis.

In the von Willebrand animal, in contrast, although endothelial damage occurs as in the normal animal, the platelet cannot adhere because of the lack of Willebrand factor. Endothelial integrity is therefore not restored, and there is increased endothelial cell permeability. This increase of permeability allows fat to accumulate in the intima and results in the non-atherosclerotic flat fatty lesions. The intima in the areas of fatty infiltration have increased permeability, because intravenous injection of Evans blue dye 3 h before killing resulted in an intense blue staining of these areas. Scanning electron microscopy showed that the blue-stained areas were completely denuded of endothelium (Fuster *et al.* 1978). Some of the aorta was stained less intensely; in these areas, scanning electron microscopy showed endothelial damage. In pigs with von Willebrand's disease, platelets cannot adhere effectively to the subendothelial surface (Weiss *et al.* 1975; Baumgartner *et al.* 1977) so that the animals are functionally thrombocytopenic like the animals that are resistant to atherosclerosis after the experimental induction of thrombocytopenia. Furthermore, if such adherence is a necessary first step in the generation of atherosclerosis (Stemerman & Ross 1972; Ross *et al.* 1974; Harker *et al.* 1976), the life-threatening haemostatic defects of these pigs may be a life-preserving vascular phenomenon.

It is important to recognize that there may be explanations other than impaired platelet function for the resistance to atherosclerosis described in von Willebrand pigs. We considered the possibility that the level of platelet-derived growth factor in von Willebrand platelets might be decreased. Fass *et al.* (1977, 1981) showed that porcine von Willebrand's platelets contain the same amount of factors mitogenic for 3T3 cells as normal platelets. They also have shown for the first time that normal and von Willebrand porcine aortic endothelial cells contain a potent mitogenic activity that appears to be different from the mitogenic activity in platelets. The description of a mitogenic activity in endothelial cells is an observation of great significance and suggests new areas for investigation in the initiation of the early arteriosclerotic lesion.

It was also noted that the level of serum cholesterol was slightly higher in the control pigs than in the von Willebrand pigs (Fuster *et al.* 1978). During the time of administration of the high cholesterol diet, however, the levels of serum cholesterol were not different in the two groups of animals. There was also no significant difference in blood sugar and the haematocrit. We have no observations on blood pressure because, for accurate readings in pigs, it is necessary to cannulate the arteries; this would be a hazardous undertaking in our bleeder animals

We have also considered the possibility that the aortas of the pigs are genetically less responsive to the development of atherosclerosis than the aortas from normal pigs. The cross-aortic transplantation study was, therefore, begun to test this hypothesis (Fuster *et al.* 1979*b*) and 5 cm segments of abdominal aorta, 1 cm proximal to the aortic trifurcation, were excised from each pig. Aortic segments of two normal control pigs were cross-transplanted with the aortic segments of two von Willebrand pigs. The appropriate control operations were also done, and we have actually performed 18 such procedures. The von Willebrand pigs were infused with 60 ml of normal pig cryoprecipitate about three hours before the procedure, to improve haemostasis. Ten days after operation, at which time the effect of cryoprecipitate had disappeared, the pigs began to receive an atherogenic high-cholesterol diet. The diet was continued for 6 months, the pigs were killed, and the aortas were removed, examined and measured for gross atherosclerotic plaques. It was found that atherosclerosis developed in the aortic segments from the von Willebrand pigs that were transplanted into normal control pigs. Endothelial von Willebrand factor was identified by immunofluorescence in the vasa vasorum of these transplanted von Willebrand aortic segments, although, of course, it was originally absent. The aortic segments from control pigs that were transplanted into von Willebrand pigs did not develop atherosclerotic plaques; in addition, it was shown by immunofluorescence that they lost their Willebrand factor (Fuster *et al.* 1979*b*). By transplanting aortas from pigs of opposite sexes, we are attempting to discover whether the transplanted segment becomes covered with the endothelial cells from the host or whether it retains its own. The study is turning out to be more complicated than we surmised because the sex chromosomes of pigs do not fluoresce, and it is necessary to make cultures of the endothelial cells to identify their sex. At the moment, however, we can say that the development of atherosclerosis seems to be related to the presence of Willebrand factor in the transplanted segments.

Finally, we should consider how these studies may relate to the incidence of atherosclerosis in von Willebrand's disease in man. There have been few studies on this subject apart from the paper published by Silwer *et al.* (1966), who found that the incidence of atherosclerosis in von Willebrand's disease in man was the same as in normal subjects. Silwer's findings are, perhaps, not surprising because the severe type of von Willebrand's disease that is found in our pigs is extremely rare in humans (Mannucci *et al.* 1976). Most humans with von Willebrand's disease have detectable levels of normal or abnormal Willebrand factor in their plasma, and the levels may be high enough to cause a sufficient platelet – endothelial cell interaction to initiate atherosclerosis. The heterozygous pigs that carry von Willebrand's disease have approximately 40 % of Willebrand factor in their plasma, and our recent study of the incidence of diet-induced atherosclerosis in these carrier animals has shown that they do not appear to be resistant to the development of atherosclerosis (Fuster *et al.* 1979*c*). There is also a form of variant von Willebrand's disease in our pigs, and we are about to initiate a study of diet-induced atherosclerosis in these animals. This last study may be of more relevance to the incidence of atherosclerosis in human von Willebrand's disease than the carrier studies described.

The study of von Willebrand's disease has given us important new information about the physiology of haemostasis as well as a new avenue for investigation of atherosclerosis. There is a great deal of ambivalence nowadays about the importance of animal models in investigation of human disease. In our view, animal experimentation has provided information about human physiology and pathology that could not have been discovered by other means. Von Willebrand's disease in pigs is an excellent example of how an animal model can lead to important advances in our understanding of human disease.

REFERENCES (Bowie *et al.*)

Baumgartner, H. R., Tschopp, T. B. & Meyer, D. 1977 Shear rate dependence of platelet adhesion to collagenous surfaces in Willebrand factor-depleted blood. [Abstract.] *Thromb. Haemostas.* **38**, 50.

Blombäck, M., Blombäck, B. & Nilsson, I. M. 1964 Response to fractions in von Willebrand's disease. In *The hemophilias* ed. K. M. Brinkhous), pp. 236–294. Chapel Hill: University of North Carolina Press.

Booyse, F. M., Quarfoot, A. J., Bell, S., Fass, D. N., Lewis, J. C., Mann, K. G. & Bowie, E. J. W. 1977 Cultured aortic endothelial cells from pigs with von Willebrand's disease: *in vitro* model for studying the molecular defect(s) of the disease. *Proc. natn. Acad. Sci. U.S.A.* **74**, 5702–5706.

Borchgrevink, C. F. 1961 Platelet adhesion *in vivo* in patients with bleeding disorders. *Acta med. scand.* **170**, 231–243.

Bouma, B. N., Wiegerinck, Y., Sixma, J. J., van Mourik, J. A. & Mochtar, I. A. 1972 Immunological characterization of purified anti-haemophilic factor A (factor VIII) which corrects abnormal platelet retention in von Willebrand's disease. *Nature, new Biol.* **236**, 104–106.

Bowie, E. J. W. & Owen, C. A., Jr 1979 Von Willebrand's disease. *C.R.C. handbook series in clinical laboratory science,* (*Hematology*) (ed. R. M. Schmidt), vol. 1, pp. 471–501. Boca Raton, Florida: C.R.C. Press.

Bowie, E. J. W., Fass, D. N. & Owen, C. A., Jr 1980 The hemostatic effect of transfused Willebrand factor in porcine von Willebrand's disease. *Hemostasis* **9**, 351–365.

Bowie, E. J. W., Fuster, V., Owen, C. A., Jr & Brown, A. L. 1975 Resistance to the development of spontaneous atherosclerosis in pigs with von Willebrand's disease. [Abstract.] *Thromb. Diathes. haemorrh.* **34**, 599.

Bowie, E. J. W., Kimura, A., Owen, C. A., Jr & Fass, D. N. 1978 Willebrand factor in hemostasis. [Abstract no. 809.] *Circulation* **58**, II-208.

Bowie, E. J. W., Owen, C. A., Jr, Thompson, J. H., Jr & Didisheim, P. 1969 Platelet adhesiveness in von Willebrand's disease. *Am. J. clin. Path.* **52**, 69–77.

Bowie, E. J. W., Owen, C. A., Jr, Zollman, P. E., Thompson, J. H., Jr & Fass, D. N. 1973 Tests of hemostasis in swine: normal values and values in pigs affected with von Willebrand's disease. *Am. J. vet. Res.* **34**, 1405–1407.

Caro, C. G., Fitz-Gerald, J. M. & Schroter, R. C. 1971 Atheroma and arterial wall shear observations, correlation and proposal of a shear dependent mass transfer mechanism for atherogenesis. *Proc. R. Soc. Lond.* B **177**, 109–159.

Chvapil, M., Stith, P. L., Tillema, L. M., Carlson, E. C., Campbell, J. B. & Eskelson, C. D. 1976 Early changes in the arterial wall of chickens fed a cholesterol diet. *Atherosclerosis* **24**, 393–405.

Cohen, P. & McCombs, H. L. 1967 Platelets and atherogenesis. I. Augmentation of cholesterol atherogenesis in the rabbit by a phlebotomy programme designed to induce thrombocytosis. *Br. J. exp. Path.* **48**, 346–356.

Cohen, P. & McCombs, H. L. 1968 Platelets and atherogenesis. II. Amelioration of cholesterol atherogenesis in in rabbits with reduced platelet counts as the result of 32p administration. *J. Atheroscler. Res.* **8**, 398.

Cornhill, J. F. & Roach, M. R. 1976 A quantitative study of the localization of atherosclerotic lesions in the rabbit aorta. *Atherosclerosis* **23**, 489–501.

Cornu, P., Larrieu, M. J., Caen, J. & Bernard, J. 1963 Transfusion studies in von Willebrand's disease: effect on bleeding time and factor VIII. *Br. J. Haemat.* **9**, 189–202.

Counts, R. B., Paskell, S. L. & Elgee, S. K. 1978 Disulfide bonds and the quaternary structure of factor VII von Willebrand factor. *J. clin. Invest.* **62**, 702–709.

Fass, D. N., Bowie, E. J. W., Owen, C. A., Jr & Zollman, P. E. 1979 Inheritance of porcine von Willebrand's disease: study of a kindred of over 700 pigs. *Blood* **53**, 712–719.

Fass, D. N., Brockway, W. J., Owen, C. A., Jr & Bowie E. J. W. 1976*b* Factor VIII (Willebrand) antigen and ristocetin–Willebrand factor in pigs with von Willebrand's disease. *Thromb. Res.* **8**, 319–327.

Fass, D. N., Didisheim, P., Lewis, J. C. & Grabowski, E. F. 1976*a* Adhesion of porcine von Willebrand (VWD) platelets. [Abstract no. 454]. *Circulation* **54**, II-116 (suppl. 2).

Fass, D. N., Downing, M. R., Meyers, P., Bowie, E. J. W. & Witte, L. D. 1978*a* Cell growth stimulation by normal and von Willebrand pig platelets and endothelium. *Circuln Res.* (Submitted for publication.)

Fass, D. N., Knutson, G. J. & Bowie, E. J. W. 1978 Porcine Willebrand factor: a population of multimers. *J. Lab. clin. Med.* **91**, 307–320.

Fass, D. N., Meyers, P., Pederson, D. C. & Witte, L. D. 1981 Growth factor from endothelial cells: mitogens in normal and von Willebrand pig platelets and endothelium. (Submitted for publication.)

Firkin, B. & Howard, M. A. 1971 Ristocetin – a new approach to the investigation of von Willebrand's disease. [Abstract.] *Aust. N.Z. Jl Med.* **1**, 278.

Fishman, J. A., Ryan, C. G. & Karnovsky, M. J. 1975 Endothelial regeneration in the rat carotid artery and the significance of endothelial denudation in the pathogenesis of intimal thickening. *Lab. Invest.* **32**, 339–351.

French, J. E., Jennings, M. A. & Florey, H. W. 1965 Morphological studies on atherosclerosis in swine. *Ann. N.Y. Acad. Sci.* **127**, 780–799.

Friedman, R. J., Stemerman, M. B., Wenz, B., Moore, S., Gauldie, J., Gent, M., Tiell, M. L. & Spaet, T. 1977 The effect of thrombocytopenia on experimental arteriosclerotic lesion formation in rabbits. *J. clin. invest.* **60**, 1191–1201.

Frost, H. 1969 Zur Pathogenese obliterierender Arterienprozesse bei Hypercholesterinämie. *Thromb. Diathes. haemorrh.* **22**, 351–359.

Fry, D. L. 1969 Certain chemorheologic considerations regarding the blood vascular interface with particular reference to coronary artery disease. *Circulation* **40**, 38–57 (suppl. 4).

Fry, G., Maca, R. D. & Hoak, J. C. 1976 Enhancement of endothelial contiguity by human platelets. [Abstract.] *Clin. Res.* **24**, 570A.

Fuster, V., Bowie, E. J. W. & Fass, D. N. 1979c Atherosclerosis in homozygous and heterozygous von Willebrand pigs fed a high cholesterol diet. [Abstract no. 1062.] *Circulation* **60**, II-272.

Fuster, V., Bowie, E. J. W., Fass, D. N. & Owen, C. A., Jr 1979a Long-term prospective study on spontaneous atherosclerosis in normal and von Willebrand pigs. [Abstract no. 1061.] *Circulation* **60**, 11–271.

Fuster, V., Bowie, E. J. W., Josa, M., Kaye, M. P. & Fass, D. N. 1979b Atherosclerosis in normal and von Willebrand pigs: cross-aortic transplantation studies. [Abstract no. 1018.] *Thromb. Haemostas.* **42**, 425.

Fuster, V., Bowie, E. J. W., Lewis, J. C., Fass, D. N., Owen, C. A., Jr & Brown, A. L., Jr 1978 Resistance to arteriosclerosis in pigs with von Willebrand's disease. *J. clin. Invest.* **61**, 722–730.

Fuster, V., Dewanjee, M. K., Kaye, M. P., Fass, D. N. & Bowie, E. J. W. 1980 Evaluation of platelet deposition following selective endothelial injury of the carotid artery in normal and von Willebrand pigs. [Abstract no. 363.] *Circulation* **62**, III-98.

Getty, R. 1965 The gross and microscopic occurrence and distribution of spontaneous atherosclerosis in the arteries of swine. In *Comparative atherosclerosis: the morphology of spontaneous and induced atherosclerotic lesions in animals and its relation to human disease* (ed. J. C. Roberts, Jr & R. Straus, pp. 236–294. New York: Harper & Row.

Gimbrone, M. A., Jr, Aster, R. H., Cotran, R. S., Corkery, J., Jandl, J. H. & Folkman, J. 1969 Preservation of vascular integrity in organs perfused *in vitro* with a platelet-rich medium. *Nature, Lond.* **221**, 33–36.

Glagov, S. 1973 Mechanical stresses on vessels and the non-uniform distribution of atherosclerosis. *Med. Clins N. Am.* **58**, 63–77.

Harker, L. A., Ross, R., Slichter, S. J. & Scott, C. R. 1976 Homocystine-induced arteriosclerosis: the role of endothelial cell injury and platelet response in its genesis. *J. clin. Invest.* **58**, 731–741.

Hjart, P. F. 1964 Bleeding time and vascular factor in von Willebrand's disease. In *The hemophilias* (ed. K. M. Brinkhous), pp. 295–299.

Howard, M. A. & Firkin, B. 1971 Ristocetin – a new tool in the investigation of platelet aggregation. *Thromb. Diathes. haemorrh.* **26**, 362–369.

Howard, M. A., Montgomery, D. C. & Hardisty, R. M. 1974 Factor VIII-related antigen in platelets. *Thromb. Res.* **4**, 617–624.

Howard, M. A., Sawers, R. J. & Firkin, B. G. 1973 Ristocetin: a means of differentiating von Willebrand's disease into two groups. *Blood* **41**, 687–690.

Imai, H. & Thomas, W. A. 1968 Cerebral atherosclerosis in swine: role of necrosis in progression of diet-induced lesions from proliferative to atheromatous stage. *Expl molec. Path.* **8**, 330–357.

Jaffe, E. A., Hoyer, L. W. & Nachman, R. L. 1973 Synthesis of antihemophilic factor antigen by cultured human endothelial cells. *J. clin. Invest.* **52**, 2757–2764.

Jaffe, E. A., Hoyer, L. W. & Nachman, R. L. 1974 Synthesis of von Willebrand factor by cultured human endothelial cells. *Proc. natn. Acad. Sci. U.S.A.* **71**, 1906–1909.

Kimura, A., Bowie, E. J. W., Campbell, R. J. & Fass, D. N. 1979 Willebrand factor in hemostatis in the 'in vitro' bleeding time. *Blood* **54**, 1347–1357.

Larrieu, M. J., Caen, J. P., Meyer, D., Vanier, H., Sultan, Y. & Bernard, J. 1968 Congenital bleeding disorders with long bleeding time and normal platelet count. II. Von Willebrand's disease (report of 37 patients). *Am. J. Med.* **45**, 354–372.

Legrand, Y. J., Rodriguez-Zeballos, A., Kartalis, G., Fauvel, F. & Caen, J. P. 1978 Adsorption of factor VIII antigen-activity complex by collagen. *Thromb. Res.* **13**, 909–911.

Lewis, J. C. & Kottke, B. A. 1977 Endothelial damage and thrombocyte adhesion in pigeon atherosclerosis. *Science, N.Y.* **196**, 1007–1009.

Mannucci, P. M. 1977 Spectrum of von Willebrand's disease: a study of 100 cases. *Br. J. Haemat.* **35**, 101–112.

Mannucci, P. M., Pareti, F. I., Holmberg, L., Nilsson, I. M. & Ruggeri, Z. M. 1976 Studies on the prolonged bleeding time in von Willebrand's disease. *J. Lab. clin. Med.* **88**, 662–671.

Meyer, D. & Larrieu, M.-J. 1970 Von Willebrand factor and platelet adhesiveness. *J. clin. Path.* **23**, 228–231.

Meyer, D., Jenkins, C. S. P., Dreyfus, M. D., Fressinaud, E. & Larrieu, M.-J. 1974 Willebrand factor and ristocetin. II. Relationship between Willebrand factor, Willebrand antigen and factor VIII activity. *Br. J. Haemat.* **28**, 579–599.

Meyer, D., Larrieu, M.-J., Maroteaux, P. & Caen, J. P. 1967 Biological findings in von Willebrand's pedigrees: implications for inheritance. *J. clin. Path.* **20**, 190–194.

Moore, S., Friedman, R. J., Singal, D. P., Gauldie, J., Blajchman, M. A. & Roberts, R. S. 1976 Inhibition of injury-induced thromboatherosclerotic lesions by anti-platelet serum in rabbits. *Thromb. Haemostas.* **35**, 70–81.

Morawitz, P. & Jurgens, R. 1930 Gibt es eine Thrombasthenie? *Münch. med. Wschr.* **77**, 2001.

Mustard, J. F. 1975 Platelets, drugs and thrombosis, the problem. In *Platelets, drugs and thrombosis* (ed. J. Hirsh, J. F. Cade, A. S. Gallus &tE. Schonbaum), p. 322. Basel: S. Karger.

Nachman, R., Levine, R. & Jaffe, E. A. 1977 Synthesis of factor VIII antigen by cultured guinea pig mega-karyocytes. *J. clin. Invest.* **60**, 914–921.

Nilsson, I. M., Blombäck, M. & Blombäck, B. 1959 von Willebrand's disease in Sweden. Its pathogenesis and treatment. *Acta med. scand.* **164**, 263–278.

Nyman, D. 1980 Von Willebrand factor dependent platelet aggregation and adsorption of factor VIII-related antigen by collagen. *Thromb. Res.* **17**, 209–214.

Olson, J. D., Brockway, W. J., Fass, D. N., Magnuson, M. A. & Bowie, E. J. W. 1976 Evaluation of ristocetin–Willebrand factor assay and ristocetin-induced platelet aggregation. *Am. J. clin. Path.* **63**, 210–218.

Owen, C. A., Jr, Bowie, E. J. W., Zollman, P. E., Fass, D. N. & Gordon, H. 1974 Carrier of porcine von Wille-brand's disease. *Am. J. net. Res.* **35**, 245–248.

Perret, B. A., Furlan, M. & Beck, E. A. 1979 Studies on factor VIII-related protein. II. Estimation of molecular size difference between factor VIII oligomers. *Biochim. biophys. Acta* **578**, 164–174.

Pick, R., Chediak, J. & Glick, G. 1979 Aspirin inhibits development of coronary atherosclerosis in cynomolgus monkeys (Macaca fascicularis) fed an atherogenic diet. *J. clin. Invest.* **63**, 158–162.

Reidy, M. A. & Bowyer, D. E. 1977 Scanning electron microscopy of arteries: the morphology of aoertic endo-thelium in hemodynamically stressed areas associated with branches. *Atherosclerosis* **26**, 181–194.

Ross, R. & Harker, L. 1976 Hyperlipidemia and atherosclerosis: chronic hyperlipidemia initiates and maintains lesions by endothelial cell desquamation and lipid accumulation. *Science, N.Y.* **193**, 1094–1100.

Ross, R., Glomset, J., Kariya, N. & Harker, L. 1974 A platelet-dependent serum factor that stimulates the proliferation of arterial smooth muscle cells in vitro. *Proc. natn. Acad. Sci. U.S.A.* **71**, 1207–1210.

Ruggeri, Z. M. & Zimmerman, T. S. 1980 Variant von Willebrand disease. *J. clin. Invest.* **65**, 1318–1325.

Ruggeri, Z. M., Mannucci, P. M., Jeffcoate, S. L. & Ingram, G. I. C. 1976 Immunoradiometric assay of factor VIII-related antigen with observations in 32 patients with von Willebrand's disease. *Br. J. Haemat.* **33**, 221–232.

Sakariassen, K. S., Bolhuis, P. A. & Sixma, J. J. 1979 Human blood platelet adhesion to artery subendothelium is mediated by factor VIII-von Willebrand factor bound to the subendothelium. *Nature, Lond.* **279**, 636–638.

Salzman, E. W. 1963 Measurement of platelet adhesiveness: a simple *in vitro* technique demonstrating an abnorm-ality in von Willebrand's disease. *J. Lab. clin. Med.* **62**, 724–735.

Shiamoto, T., Yamashita, Y., Numano, F. & Sunaga, T. 1971 Scanning and transmission electron microscopic observation of endothelial cells in the normal condition and in initial stages of atherosclerosis. *Acta path. Japan* **21**, 93.

Silwer, J., Cronberg, S. & Nilsson, I. M. 1966 Occurrence of arteriosclerosis in von Willebrand's disease. *Acta med. scand.* **180**, 475–484.

Silwer, J. & Nilsson, I. M. 1964 On a Swedish family with 51 members affected by von Willebrand's disease. *Acta mea. scand.* **185**, 627–643.

Somer, J. B., Evans, G. & Schwartz, C. J. 1972 Influence of experimental aortic coarctation on the pattern of aortic Evans blue uptake in vivo. *Atherosclerosis* **16**, 127–133.

Stemerman, M. B. & Ross, R. 1972 Experimental arteriosclerosis. I. Fibrous plaque formation in primates, an electron microscope study. *J. exp. Med.* **136**, 769–789.

Texon, M. 1972 The hemodynamics basis of atherosclerosis: further observations: the ostial lesions. *Bull. N.Y. Acad. Med.* **48**, 733–740.

Tschopp, T. B., Weiss, H. J. & Baumgartner, H. R. 1974 Decreased adhesion of platelets to subendothelium in von Willebrand's disease. *J. Lab. clin. Med.* **83**, 296–300.

van Mourik, J. A., Bouma, B. N., laBruyere, W. T., deGraff, S. & Mochtar, I. A. 1974 Factor VIII, a series of homologous oligomers and a complex of two proteins. *Thromb. Res.* **4**, 155–164.

von Willebrand, E. A. 1926 Hereditär pseudohemofili. *Finska LäkSällsk. Handl.* **68**, 87.

von Willebrand, E. A., Jurgens, R. & Dahlberg, U. 1934 Konstitutionell trombopati, en ny arftlig blodarsjukdom. *Finska LäkSällsk. Handl.* **76**, 193.

Weinstein, M. & Deykin, D. 1979 Comparison of factor VIII-related von Willebrand factor proteins prepared from human cryoprecipitate and factor VIII concentrate. *Blood* **53**, 1095–1105.

Weiss, H. J. & Rogers, J. 1972 Correction of the platelet abnormality in von Willebrand's disease by cryo-precipitate. *Am. J. Med.* **53**, 734–738.

Weiss, H. J., Baumgartner, H. R., Tschopp, T. B. & Turitto, V. T. 1977 Interaction of platelets with subendo-thelium: a new method for identifying and classifying abnormalities of platelet function. *Ann. N.Y. Acad. Sci.* **283**, 293–309.

Weiss, H. J., Rogers, J. & Brand, H. 1973 Defective ristocetin-induced platelet aggregation in von Willebrand's disease and its correction by factor VIII. *J. clin. Invest.* **52**, 2697–2707.

Weiss, H. J., Tschopp, T. B. & Baumgartner, H. R. 1975 Impaired interaction (adhesion–aggregation) of platelets with the subendothelium in storage-pool disease and after aspirin ingestion: a comparison with von Willebrand's disease. *New Engl. J. Med.* **293**, 619–623.

Wesolowski, S. A., Fries, C. C., Sabnini, A. M. & Sawyer, P. N. 1965 The significance of turbulence in hemic systems and in the distribution of the atherosclerotic lesions. *Surgery* **57**, 155–162.

Wojcik, J. D., Van Horn, D. L., Webber, A. J. & Johnson, S. A. 1969 Mechanisms whereby platelets support the endothelium. *Transfusion* **9**, 324–335.

Zimmerman, T. S., Ratnofi, O. D. & Powell, A. E. 1971 Immunologic differentiation of classic hemophilia (factor VIII deficiency) and von Willebrand's disease. *J. clin. Invest.* **50**, 244–254.

Zimmerman, T. S., Roberts, J. & Edgington, T. S. 1975 Factor VIII-related antigen: multiple molecular forms in human plasma. *Proc. natn. Acad. Sci. U.S.A.* **72**, 5121–5125.

Zucker, M. B. 1963 *In vitro* abnormality of the blood in von Willebrand's disease correctable by normal plasma. *Nature Lond.* **197**, 601–602.

Discussion

J. McMichael, F.R.S. (2 *North Square, London, U.K.*) In rabbits, fibrous plaque produced by mechanical injury can form a lipid-rich lesion in the presence of low levels of cholesterol levels (Moore, 1973). Does Dr Bowie find it necessary to add cholesterol to get fatty plaques in his experimental atheroma in pigs?

Reference

Moore, S. 1973 *Lab. Invest.* **29**, 478.

E. J. W. Bowie. The atherosclerotic lesions discussed were induced by a 2 % cholesterol high-tallow diet. We do, however, see lipid in the spontaneously developing atherosclerotic lesions in animals that have a normal level of cholesterol.

C. R. W. Gray (*Thoracic Unit, Westminster Hospital, London, U.K.*). Dr Bowie's results show a dramatic difference in the distribution of fats in aortas from normal and von Willebrand pigs on a high-fat diet. Has he considered the possibility that the aortic fat deposits are derived from platelet lipids and not from plasma lipids?

E. J. W. Bowie. We have, of course, considered that possibility. We are currently studying the intimal, fatty depositions in the von Willebrand pigs.

Elspeth B. Smith (*Department of Chemical Pathology, University Medical Buildings, Foresterhill, Aberdeen, U.K.*). We have been measuring factor VIII-related antigen (VIII RA) in human aortic intima and lesions by using an immunoelectrophoretic assay, and have obtained very odd results. A large variety of plasma proteins in intima is invariably present in concentrations that are a function of their concentration in the patient's plasma and of their molecular mass; large molecules are retained to a much greater extent than small ones. However, factor VIII RA is an exception and is unpredictable; it was present in high concentration in some samples but in others that appeared morphologically similar we failed to recover any, despite normal concentrations in the patient's plasma. This variability was not confined to the endothelialized surfaces of intima; the concentration in the centres of plaques was actually twice the concentration in the caps but half appeared to contain no factor VIII RA at all, although all samples contained high concentrations of prothrombin.

I wonder if Dr Bowie has any explanation for this anomalous observation.

E. J. W. Bowie. I think that these results are very interesting, although I have no explanation for them. Factor VIII-related antigen exists in plasma as a series of polymers, the largest of which have extremely high relative molecular masses up to 20×10^6. Each polymer would diffuse at a different rate and this may account for the variability in the results. I certainly think that it is worth pursuing further.

Phil. Trans. R. Soc. Lond. B **294**, 281–290 (1981)

Printed in Great Britain

Inherited abnormalities of platelet glycoproteins

By J. P. Caen, A. T. Nurden and T. J. Kunicki†

Unité 150 INSERM, Hôpital Lariboisière, 6 rue Guy Patin,
75475 Paris Cedex 10, France

Glanzmann's thrombasthenia and the Bernard–Soulier syndrome are inherited blood disorders characterized by abnormalities in different aspects of platelet function during haemostasis. Platelets from patients with thrombasthenia do not aggregate in response to the normal physiological platelet aggregation inducing stimuli, while Bernard–Soulier platelets have a reduced capacity to adhere to exposed subendothelium. Deficiencies of different membrane glycoproteins have been located in the platelets of both disorders and suggest specific roles for membrane glycoproteins in different aspects of platelet function.

Introduction

When platelets aggregate, a stimulus received at a receptor within the platelet plasma membrane sets in motion a chain of events that results in the formation of bonds between adjacent cells. Similarly, when platelets adhere to subendothelial components exposed during vessel injury, the process is initiated by the interaction of specific stimuli with externally orientated membrane receptors and concluded with the formation of cohesive forces exposed at the platelet surface. Cell contact interactions in mammalian cell systems are often mediated by membrane glyco-proteins (Nicolson 1976), and glycoproteins have been shown to be major components of the normal human platelet surface (Phillips & Poh Agin 1977*a*). Evidence supporting a possible role for membrane glycoproteins in platelet surface contact interactions has come from studies performed on platelets isolated from patients with inherited disorders of platelet function.

Membrane glycoprotein composition of normal human platelets

Phillips (1972) and Nachman & Ferris (1972) initially described three glycoproteins after SDS–polyacrylamide gel electrophoresis of human platelet membranes solubilized by the detergent sodium dodecyl sulphate (SDS). These glycoproteins, in the molecular mass range $M_r = 150000$–90000, were located by staining for carbohydrate by using the periodate–Schiff reaction. Phillips (1972) termed the glycoproteins I, II and III and established the convention whereby the glycoprotein (GP) with the highest molecular mass was termed GPI, the next GPII and so on. Subsequently, it was shown by using lactoperoxidase-catalysed ^{125}I-labelled platelets that GPII contained two components that were denoted GPIIa and IIb (Phillips *et al.* 1975).

Thus the further convention was established that as heterogeneity within the major periodate–Schiff-staining bands became apparent, the newly resolved species within each molecular mass class were each given a different letter suffix. The glycoprotein composition of the platelet plasma membrane is now known to be complex (Phillips & Poh Agin 1977*a*; Clemetson *et al.*

† Current address: The Blood Center of Southeastern Wisconsin, 1701 West Wisconsin Avenue, Milwaukee, Wisconsin 53233, U.S.A.

19-2

1979), with the number of components observed depending largely on the sensitivity of the analytical approach used.

Some characteristics of the platelet membrane glycoproteins are illustrated in figure 1. Two different surface-labelling techniques have been used to incorporate a radioactive label into those molecules with part of their structure exposed at the human platelet surface. Lacto-peroxidase-catalysed iodination has been used as a method for incorporating ^{125}I into the tyrosine residues of polypeptide chains exposed at the platelet surface. Alternatively, washed

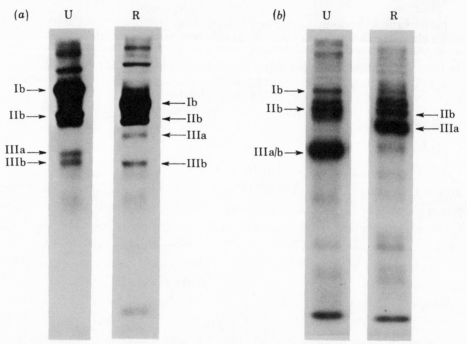

FIGURE 1. Identification of the surface-orientated membrane glycoproteins of normal human platelets after analysis by SDS–polyacrylamide gel electrophoresis of platelets whose surface proteins had been radiolabelled by two different surface labelling procedures. Washed human platelets were incubated (a) sequentially with neuraminidase, galactose oxidase and sodium [^{3}H]borohydride as described by McGregor et al. (1979), or (b) with lactoperoxidase and ^{125}I as described by Phillips & Poh Agin (1977a). The radiolabelled plate-lets were analysed by SDS–polyacrylamide gel electrophoresis on 7–12 % gradient acrylamide slab gels in the absence of (unreduced; U) or after (reduced; R) disulphide bond reduction as detailed by Nurden et al. (1981). Radiolabelled proteins were located by fluorography (^{3}H) or by radioautography (^{125}I).

platelets have been treated sequentially with neuraminidase, galactose oxidase and sodium [^{3}H]borohydride with the result that ^{3}H has been incorporated into galactose and N-acetyl-galactosamine residues of membrane glycoproteins. It may be noted that GPIb is labelled profusely with ^{3}H, probably as a result of its having a high carbohydrate content. In contrast, GPIIIa is weakly labelled with ^{3}H but strongly labelled with ^{125}I, suggesting that it has a lower sugar content and a large proportion of its protein structure exposed at the surface.

Also illustrated in figure 1 is the altered mobility of GPIb, IIb and IIIa following disulphide bond reduction. GPIb and IIb appear to be dimeric molecules, the subunits of which are linked by one or more disulphide bonds. Reduction results in the separation of a large, glyco-sylated polypeptide (α-chain) from a smaller polypeptide (β-chain) which may or may not be glycosylated (Phillips 1979). In contrast, GPIIIa appears to contain intramolecular disulphide bonds. Although the platelet plasma membrane contains many glycosylated components other than those labelled in figure 1, the four glycoproteins highlighted on this figure are those that have been best characterized to date; they will form the basis of this review. The surface orientation of the platelet membrane glycoproteins is confirmed by their rapid degradation when proteases are added to washed platelet suspensions (Nurden & Caen 1975; Kunicki & Aster 1979). Furthermore, the presence of a layer rich in bound carbohydrate at the outer surface of the platelet plasma membrane has been demonstrated by cytochemical procedures used in combination with electron microscopy (Behnke 1968).

GLANZMANN'S THROMBASTHENIA

A disease with an autosomal recessive inheritance, Glanzmann's thrombasthenia (G.t.) is characterized by the absence of platelet aggregation in response to ADP and all physiological aggregation-inducing agents (for a review see Hardisty 1977). As discussed elsewhere (Nurden & Caen 1979), the basic defect appears to lie in the inability of G.t. platelets to form the platelet–platelet cohesive forces that conclude the aggregation mechanism. The platelets of most patients are also unable to support clot retraction (Caen et al. 1966). Occasionally a modified clot retraction is observed, although the platelet aggregation defect remains unchanged. These patients have been described as type II thrombasthenia by Caen (1972).

Membrane fractions isolated from thrombasthenic platelets were first studied by Nurden & Caen (1974), who noted the presence of glycoprotein abnormalities. SDS–polyacrylamide gel electrophoresis followed by periodate–Schiff staining revealed marked reductions in the staining intensity normally observed in the GPII and III regions of the gel. Molecular differences in the surface composition of thrombasthenic platelets were confirmed by Phillips et al. (1975) with the use of the lactoperoxidase-catalysed procedure for labelling surface proteins with ^{125}I or [131]I.

Platelets from a larger number of thrombasthenic patients have now been examined by a number of different radiolabelling and SDS–polyacrylamide gel electrophoresis procedures (Phillips & Poh Agin 1977b; White et al. 1978; Hagen & Solum 1978; Kunicki & Aster 1978; Nurden & Caen 1979). Accumulated evidence from these studies suggests severe molecular deficiencies of GPIIb and IIIa as a specific membrane defect of thrombasthenic platelets. This finding is illustrated in figure 2.

Kunicki & Aster (1978) first showed that the platelet-specific alloantigen Pl[A1] (Zw[a]) was deleted from platelets in thrombasthenia; they then proved (Kunicki & Aster 1979) that the Pl[A1] antigenic marker was associated with GPIIIa on normal human platelets. Further support for this conclusion was provided by Van Leeuwen et al. (1979), who showed that the allelic counterpart of Pl[A1], Pl[A2] (Zw[b]), was also missing from G.t. platelets.

Triton X-100 solubilized normal human and thrombasthenic platelet proteins were studied by crossed immunoelectrophoresis (c.i.e.) by using a polyspecific rabbit antiserum against normal human platelets (Hagen et al. 1980). The treatment with the non-ionic detergent resulted in the solubilization of 90% of the total platelet protein. Two immunoprecipitates were observed to be missing from the patterns obtained by using G.t. platelets. In terms of the nomenclature used, these were denoted bands 16 and 24. Band 24 was identified as being given by platelet fibrinogen. Band 16 was shown to be heavily labelled with ^{125}I when normal human platelets whose surface proteins had been labelled with ^{125}I were analysed. Elution of band 16 from unstained agarose gels was followed by SDS–polyacrylamide gel electrophoresis.

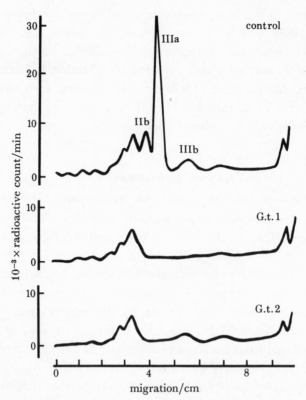

FIGURE 2. The abnormal surface structure of platelets isolated from patients with Glanzmann's thrombasthenia. The surface proteins of normal human platelets and those isolated from two patients with G.t. were labelled with ^{125}I by the lactoperoxidase-catalysed procedure. The radiolabelled platelets were analysed by SDS–polyacrylamide gel electrophoresis in 6 % acrylamide tube gels after disulphide bond reduction as detailed by Nurden *et al.* (1981). After electrophoresis the gels were cut into 1 mm segments and the radioactivity contained in each segment measured in a γ-ray counter.

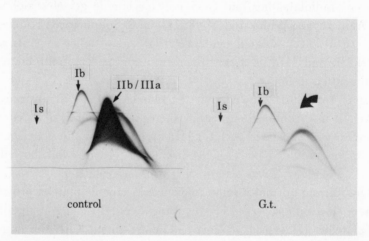

FIGURE 3. Analysis of the membrane glycoprotein composition of thrombasthenic platelets by crossed immuno-electrophoresis. The surface proteins of normal human platelets and those isolated from a patient with G.t. were labelled with ^{125}I by the lactoperoxidase-catalysed procedure. The platelets were solubilized in the presence of 1 % Triton X-100 and c.i.e. performed according to the procedures detailed by Hagen *et al.* (1980). The immunoglobulin fraction of a multispecific rabbit antiserum prepared against washed, normal human platelets was incorporated into the agarose gel for the second dimension of electrophoresis. The immunoprecipitates containing radiolabelled antigens were located by radioautography.

In this way GP IIb and IIIa were identified as the platelet antigens contained within the band 16 precipitate (Hagen *et al.* 1980). Their uniform distribution throughout the immunoprecipitation line suggested the presence of a membrane complex containing these antigens. Figure 3 illustrates the absence of band 16 from a radioautograph obtained after the analysis of radiolabelled G.t. platelets by c.i.e. Recent studies have shown the presence of intermediate levels of GP IIb/IIIa, $53 \pm 5 \%$ (mean $\pm$ s.d.), in several kindred patients, with thrombasthenia (Kunicki *et al.* 1981 *a*). The presence of intermediate levels of GP IIb/IIIa in the platelets of presumed heterozygotes for the thrombasthenia trait suggests a direct link between the inheritance of the disorder and the glycoprotein defect.

The above results all refer to thrombasthenic platelets that lack the ability to support either platelet aggregation or clot retraction. When platelets from a patient with type II thrombasthenia were analysed by c.i.e., band 24 (fibrinogen) was detected as normal, while band 16 (IIb/IIIa) was reduced to approximately 13 % of the normal size (Hagen *et al.* 1980). Both functional and biochemical heterogeneity is exhibited in thrombasthenia.

BERNARD–SOULIER SYNDROME

The Bernard–Soulier (B.–S.) syndrome is a second platelet disorder with an autosomal recessive inheritance. This syndrome is characterized by a moderate to severe thrombocytopenia (low circulating platelet count), the presence of unusually large platelets on blood smears and a number of platelet function abnormalities (see Hardisty 1977). The primary haemostatic defect appears to be the inability of B.–S. platelets to adhere to the exposed subendothelial surface (Caen *et al.* 1976). Recent studies suggest that this is due to a defect in the interaction between the B.–S. platelet and microfibrils in the subendothelium (Legrand *et al.* 1980). As discussed elsewhere (Nurden & Caen 1979), the abnormality is probably related to the absence of agglutination of B.–S. platelets by ristocetin in the presence of normal human plasma, which in turn strongly suggests a defective interaction between the von Willebrand protein and its platelet receptor. Platelet aggregation rapidly follows platelet stimulation by ADP or collagen in the B.–S. syndrome; however, a decreased aggregation response to thrombin has been reported and characterized (Jamieson & Okumura 1978).

A specific glycoprotein abnormality in B.–S. platelets was first described by Nurden & Caen (1975), who observed a much decreased carbohydrate staining intensity of GP I after the analysis of isolated B.–S. platelet membranes by SDS–polyacrylamide gel electrophoresis. A greater resolution of the platelet surface components has been achieved in subsequent studies, which suggest a specific abnormality primarily affecting GP Ib (Nurden & Caen 1979; Nurden *et al.* 1981). This finding is illustrated in figure 4. Here, SDS–solubilized normal human and B.–S. platelet glycoproteins have been analysed by SDS–polyacrylamide gel electrophoresis in the absence of disulphide bond reduction. As shown earlier (figure 1), GP Ib is well separated from the other major carbohydrate-containing membrane glycoproteins when electrophoresis is performed without disulphide bond reduction.

The protein content of B.–S. platelets is increased twofold to fourfold (Nurden *et al.* 1981); however, analysis of their protein composition by using 7–12 % acrylamide gradient gels showed normal polypeptide profiles. The increased protein content of B.–S. platelets is probably related to their increased granule content (Rendu *et al.* 1981) and to their increased size (see Hardisty 1977). When the surface composition of B.–S. platelets was studied by lactoperoxidase-catalysed iodination, ^{125}I was found to be incorporated into all of the normally labelled surface components with the exception of GPIb (Nurden *et al.* 1981). That B.–S. platelets were deficient in GPIb was further suggested by the studies of Hagen *et al.* (1980), who showed that a specific immunoprecipitate (band 13) was missing when B.–S. platelets were studied by c.i.e. Subsequent studies have clearly identified band 13 as being given by GPIb (T. Kunicki, unpublished observations).

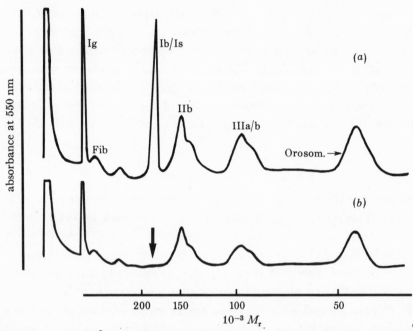

Figure 4. The abnormal membrane glycoprotein composition of Bernard–Soulier platelets. Washed normal human platelets (*a*) and those isolated from a patient with the B.–S. syndrome (*b*) were analysed by SDS–polyacrylamide gel electrophoresis on 7 % acrylamide tube gels as detailed by Nurden *et al.* (1981) and in the absence of disulphide bond reduction. Glycoproteins were located by staining for carbohydrate with the periodate–Schiff reaction after electrophoresis. Densitometric profiles of the stained gels are illustrated.

The position of the immunoprecipitate given by GPIb is clearly shown on figure 3. Glyco-calicin or GPIs are the names given to a glycopeptide of high molecular mass, derived from GPIb through the action of a protease that is active in platelet homogenates in the presence of divalent cations (Solum *et al.* 1980). GPIs is often clearly observed after c.i.e. as a fast migrating component giving an immunoprecipitate with a line of identity with GPIb. This precipitate may also be observed on figure 3. An antiserum prepared against purified glyco-calicin has been used in previously reported c.i.e. studies (Hagen *et al.* 1980), where it was concluded that both GPIs and its precursor membrane glycoprotein were absent from the platelets of B.–S. patients. These, and our previous results (Nurden & Caen 1979), strongly suggest that the precursor of glycocalicin is GPIb.

In an earlier study, Kunicki *et al.* (1978) showed that B.–S. platelets, while possessing the Pl[A1] antigen, lacked the receptor for quinine- or quinidine-dependent antibodies that was present on the platelets of all normal subjects tested. This receptor was subsequently shown to be associated with membrane GPIb or a structural analogue of this glycoprotein as isolated by chromatography on wheatgerm lectin affinity columns (Kunicki *et al.* 1981 *b*). The absence of this receptor appears to be a specific characteristic of the B.–S. platelet surface.

CURRENT THOUGHTS ON THE POSSIBLE ROLES OF MEMBRANE GLYCOPROTEINS
IN NORMAL HUMAN PLATELET FUNCTION

The crucial question to be answered is whether the observed functional defects of thrombasthenic and Bernard–Soulier platelets are a direct result of glycoprotein deficiencies. Fibrinogen has long been known as an essential cofactor for platelet aggregation. Recent studies have shown that specific receptor sites for fibrinogen are exposed on the platelet surface after stimulation with ADP, adrenalin (Plow & Marguerie 1980) and probably other aggregation inducers. No such receptor sites are exposed on thrombasthenic platelets after stimulation (Mustard *et al.* 1979) despite the normal binding of [^{14}C]ADP (Legrand & Caen 1976) to the thrombasthenic platelet membrane. Thus one possible explanation for the absence of aggregation in thrombasthenia is that the fibrinogen bridge, which may link one platelet to another in the aggregate, is unable to form.

The IgG L... is an alloantibody isolated from the serum of a thrombasthenic patient; it induces a 'thrombasthenia-like' functional state on normal human platelets (Levy-Toledano *et al.* 1978). When the antibody was used in crossed immunoelectrophoresis it precipitated GPIIb/IIIa (Hagen *et al.* 1980), which appear to be present as a divalent cation dependent complex in Triton X-100 extracts of normal human platelets (Kunicki *et al.* 1981 c). Recent studies have shown that IgG L... inhibits the ADP-dependent binding of fibrinogen to the normal human platelet surface (Lee *et al.* 1981). As Ca^{2+} ions are an essential cofactor for platelet aggregation (Born & Cross 1964), a tempting hypothesis is that GPIIb/IIIa may contribute structurally to the fibrinogen receptor that mediates platelet aggregation. Alternatively, in the absence of GPIIb/IIIa it is possible that the fibrinogen receptor does not become exposed after platelet stimulation with ADP or other aggregating agents.

Platelet adhesion to microfibrils present within the subendothelial tissues exposed during vessel injury appears to depend on the presence of plasma von Willebrand factor (v.W.f.) (Legrand *et al.* 1980). Ristocetin-induced platelet agglutination appears to be mediated by the binding of v.W.f. to the platelet surface (Kao *et al.* 1979). Both ristocetin-induced platelet agglutination and adhesion of normal human platelets to subendothelium were inhibited by an antibody that developed in a patient with the Bernard–Soulier syndrome who had received multiple transfusions of normal human platelet concentrates to arrest an episode of bleeding (Tobelem *et al.* 1976). Indirect immunoprecipitation tests with the use of this antibody (IgGP...) and Nonidet P40-extracted surface antigens of normal human platelets showed that it interacted with an antigen of apparent relative molecular mass 150000 (Degos *et al.* 1977). The antigen was absent from B.–S. platelets and appeared to be GPIb. The effect of the IgGP... was specific; it did not inhibit ADP- or collagen-induced platelet aggregation. Recent studies have shown that B.–S. platelets lack the ristocetin-induced v.W.f. binding receptor on the platelet surface (Moake *et al.* 1980). A tempting hypothesis, therefore, is that GPIb may contribute structurally to the v.W.f. receptor that appears to mediate platelet adhesion to microfibrils. Alternatively, it is possible that in the absence of GPIb this receptor does not become exposed after platelet stimulation.

Conclusions

Blood platelets provide the initial response to injury in normal vessels by forming a platelet plug to prevent bleeding and to promote vessel healing. Since most platelet functions are mediated through cell surface interactions, the study of platelet membrane glycoproteins has been an important area of research. Progress has been made in defining the functional roles of some of the surface constituents. Our approach has been to investigate the membrane defects present in the platelets of patients with inherited abnormalities of platelet function, and to examine the effects on platelet function of antisera monospecific for different membrane antigens. Such studies have suggested specific roles for different membrane glycoproteins in platelet aggregation and adhesion. It is not yet known whether membrane glycoproteins directly mediate these processes or that their absence in abnormal membranes prevents the exposure of receptors for protein cofactors that mediate the platelet response after platelet activation. Studies are continuing to identify those molecules responsible for platelet 'stickiness', both after normal platelet activation and in platelet pathology.

References (Caen *et al.*)

Behnke, O. 1968 Electron microscopical observations on the surface coating of human blood platelets. *J. ultrastruct. Res.* **24**, 51–69.

Born, G. V. R. & Cross, M. J. 1964 Effects of inorganic ions and of plasma proteins on the aggregation of blood platelets by adenosine diphosphate. *J. Physiol., Lond.* **170**, 397–414.

Caen, J. P. 1972 Glanzmann's thrombasthenia. *Clinics Haemat.* **1**, 383–392.

Caen, J. P., Castaldi, P. A., Leclerc, J. C., Inceman, S., Larrieu, M. J., Probst, M. & Bernard, J. 1966 Congenital bleeding disorders with long bleeding time and normal platelet count. 1. Glanzmann's thrombasthenia (report of fifteen patients). *Am. J. Med.* **41**, 4–26.

Caen, J. P., Nurden, A. T., Jeanneau, C., Michel, H., Tobelem, G., Levy-Toledano, S., Sultan, Y., Valensi, F. & Bernard, J. 1976 Bernard–Soulier syndrome: a new platelet glycoprotein abnormality. Its relationship with platelet adhesion to subendothelium and with the factor VIII von Willebrand protein. *J. Lab. clin. Med.* **87**, 586–596.

Clemetson, K. J., Capitanio, A. & Luscher, E. F. 1979 High resolution two-dimensional gel electrophoresis of the proteins and glycoproteins of human blood platelets. *Biochim. biophys. Acta* **553**, 11–24.

Degos, L., Tobelem, G., Lethielleux, P., Levy-Toledano, S., Caen, J. & Colombani, P. 1977 Molecular defects in platelets from patients with Bernard–Soulier syndrome. *Blood* **50**, 899–903.

Hagen, I. & Solum, N. O. 1978 Further studies on the protein composition and surface structure of normal platelets and platelets from patients with Glanzmann's thrombasthenia and Bernard–Soulier syndrome. *Thromb. Res.* **38**, 914–923.

Hagen, I., Nurden, A., Bjerrum, O. J., Solum, N. O. & Caen, J. 1980 Immunochemical evidence for protein abnormalities in platelets from patients with Glanzmann's thrombasthenia and Bernard–Soulier syndrome. *J. clin. Invest.* **65**, 722–731.

Hardisty, R. H. 1977 Disorders of platelet function. *Br. med. Bull.* **33**, 207–212.

Jamieson, G. A. & Okumura, T. 1978 Reduced thrombin binding and aggregation in Bernard–Soulier platelets. *J. clin. Invest.* **61**, 861–864.

Kao, K.-J., Pizzo, S. V. & McKee, P. A. 1979 Platelet receptors for human factor VIII/von Willebrand protein: functional correlation of receptor occupancy and ristocetin-induced platelet aggregation. *Proc. natn. Acad. Sci. U.S.A.* **76**, 5317–5320.

Kunicki, T. J. & Aster, R. H. 1978 Deletion of the platelet-specific alloantigen Pl^{A1} from platelets in Glanzmann's thrombasthenia. *J. clin. Invest.* **61**, 1225–1231.

Kunicki, T. J. & Aster, R. H. 1979 Isolation and immunologic characterisation of the human platelet alloantigen Pl^{A1}. *Molec. Immunol.* **16**, 353–360.

Kunicki, T., Johnson, M. M. & Aster, R. H. 1978 Absence of the platelet receptor for drug-dependent antibodies in the Bernard–Soulier syndrome. *J. clin. Invest.* **62**, 716–719.

Kunicki, T. J., Pidard, D., Cazenave, J.-P., Nurden, A. T. & Caen, J. P. 1981a Inheritance of the human platelet alloantigen, Pl^{A1}, in type 1 Glanzmann's thrombasthenia. *J. clin. Invest.* **67**, 717–725.

Kunicki, T. J., Pidard, D., Rosa, J.-P. & Nurden, A. T. 1981c The formation of Ca^{++}-dependent complexes of platelet membrane glycoproteins IIb and IIIa in solution as determined by crossed immunoelectrophoresis. *Blood.* (In the press.)

Kunicki, T. J., Russell, N. R., Nurden, A. T., Aster, R. H. & Caen, J. P. 1981 b Further studies of the human platelet receptor for quinine- and quinidine-dependent antibodies. *J. Immunol.* **126**, 398–406.

Lee, H., Nurden, A. T., Thomaidis, A. & Caen, J. P. 1981 Fibrinogen binding to type I and type II thrombasthenic platelets and to normal platelets in the presence of an acquired IgG-antibody from a thrombasthenic patient. *Br. J. Haemat.* (In the press.)

Legrand, C. & Caen, J. P. 1976 Binding of ¹⁴C-ADP by thrombasthenic platelet membranes. *Haemostasis* **5**, 231–238.

Legrand, Y., Fauvel, F., Gutman, N., Muh, J. P., Tobelem, G., Souchon, H., Karniguian, A. & Caen, J. P. 1980 Microfibrils (MF) platelet interaction: requirement of von Willebrand factor. *Thromb. Res.* **19**, 737–739.

Levy-Toledano, S., Tobelem, G., Legrand, C., Bredoux, R., Degos, L., Nurden, A. T. & Caen, J. P. 1978 An acquired IgG antibody occurring in a thrombasthenic patient: its effect on normal human platelet function. *Blood* **51**, 1065–1071.

McGregor, J. L., Clemetson, K. J., James, E. & Dechavanne, M. 1979 A comparison of techniques used to study externally orientated proteins and glycoproteins of human blood platelets. *Thromb. Res.* **16**, 437–452.

Moake, J. L., Olson, J. D., Troll, J. H., Tang, S. S., Funicella, T. & Peterson, D. M. 1980 Binding of radioiodinated human von Willebrand factor to Bernard–Soulier, thrombasthenic and von Willebrand's disease platelets. *Thromb. Res.* **19**, 21–27.

Mustard, J. F., Kinlough-Rathbone, R. L., Packham, M. A., Perry, D. W., Harfenist, E. J. & Pai, K. R. M. 1979 Comparison of fibrinogen association with normal and thrombasthenic platelets on exposure to ADP or chymotrypsin. *Blood* **54**, 987–993.

Nachman, R. L. & Ferris, B. 1972 Studies on the proteins of human platelet membranes. *J. biol. Chem.* **247**, 4468–4475.

Nicolson, G. L. 1976 Transmembrane control of the receptors on normal and tumor cells. I. Cytoplasmic influence over cell surface components. *Biochim. biophys. Acta* **457**, 57–108.

Nurden, A. T. & Caen, J. P. 1974 An abnormal platelet glycoprotein pattern in three cases of Glanzmann's thrombasthenia. *Br. J. Haemat.* **28**, 253–260.

Nurden, A. T. & Caen, J. P. 1975 Specific roles for platelet surface glycoproteins in platelet function. *Nature, Lond.* **255**, 720–722.

Nurden, A. T. & Caen, J. P. 1979 The different glycoprotein abnormalities in thrombasthenic and Bernard–Soulier platelets. *Semin. Hemat.* **16**, 234–250.

Nurden, A. T., Dupuis, D., Kunicki, T. J. & Caen, J. P. 1981 Analysis of the glycoprotein and protein composition of Bernard–Soulier platelets by single and two-dimensional SDS–polyacrylamide gel electrophoresis. *J. clin. Invest.* (In the press.)

Phillips, D. R. 1972 Effect of trypsin on the exposed polypeptides and glycoproteins in the human platelet membrane. *Biochemistry, Wash.* **11**, 4582–4588.

Phillips, D. R. 1979 Surface labelling as a tool to determine structure–function relationships of platelet plasma membrane glycoproteins. *Thromb. Haemostas.* **42**, 1638–1651.

Phillips, D. R. & Poh Agin, P. 1977 a Platelet plasma membrane glycoproteins. Evidence for the presence of nonequivalent disulfide bonds using nonreduced–reduced two-dimensional gel electrophoresis. *J. biol. Chem.* **252**, 2120–2126.

Phillips, D. R. & Poh Agin, P. 1977 b Platelet membrane defects in Glanzmann's thrombasthenia. Evidence for decreased amounts of two major glycoproteins. *J. clin. Invest.* **60**, 535–545.

Phillips, D. R., Jenkins, C. S. P., Lüscher, E. F. & Larrieu, M.-J. 1975 Molecular differences of exposed surface proteins on thrombasthenic platelet plasma membranes. *Nature, Lond.* **257**, 599–600.

Plow, E. F. & Marguerie, G. A. 1980 Induction of the fibrinogen receptor on human platelets by epinephrine and the combination of epinephrine and ADP. *J. biol. Chem.* **255**, 10971–10977.

Rendu, F., Nurden, A. T., Lebret, M. & Caen, J. P. 1981 Further investigations on Bernard–Soulier platelet abnormalities: A study of 5-HT uptake and mepacrine fluorescence. *J. Lab. clin. Med.* (In the press.)

Solum, N. O., Hagen, I. & Sletback, T. 1980 Further evidence for glycocalicin being derived from a larger amphiphilic platelet membrane glycoprotein. *Thromb. Res.* **18**, 773–785.

Tobelem, G., Levy-Toledano, S., Bredoux, R., Michel, H., Nurden, A., Caen, J. P. & Degos, L. 1976 New approach to determination of specific functions of platelet membrane sites. *Nature, Lond.* **263**, 427–429.

Van Leeuwen, E. F., Zonnevels, G. T. E., Von Riesz, L. E., Jenkins, C. S. P., Van Mourik, J. A. & Von dem Borne, A. E. G., Jr 1979 Absence of the complete platelet-specific alloantigens Zw (Pl^A1) on platelets in Glanzmann's thrombasthenia and the effect of anti-Zw^a antibody on platelet function [abstract]. *Thromb. Haemostas.* **42**, 422.

White, G. C., Workman, E. F. & Lundblad, R. L. 1978 Thrombin binding to thrombasthenic platelets. *J. Lab. clin. Med.* **91**, 76–82.

Discussion

J. R. O'BRIEN (*Central Laboratory, St Mary's Hospital, Portsmouth, U.K.*). Professor Caen's two types of thrombasthenia seem quite distinct. Has he examined patients with a bleeding diathesis in whom aggregation is diminished but not absent? We have two such families and so I wonder if there may be other variants.

J. P. CAEN. There are two types of thrombasthenia without any aggregation, but outside these two groups there is also a group of mild thrombasthenia to which the family Dr O'Brien mentions probably belongs.

It would be very interesting to look at the fibrinogen binding and at the glycoprotein content of those platelets.

Phil. Trans. R. Soc. Lond. B **294**, 291–303 (1981)

Printed in Great Britain

Overview of drugs in arterial thrombosis

By T. W. Meade

*M.R.C. Epidemiology and Medical Care Unit, Northwick Park Hospital,
Watford Road, Harrow, Middlesex HA1 3UJ, U.K.*

The recent history of randomized controlled trials in the prevention of ischaemic heart disease (i.h.d.) is considered. In 1970, it seemed that little could be done to prevent recurrence of the disease and there was almost no information on the potential for preventing its onset. Over the past decade, this rather pessimistic view has changed to one of guarded optimism. Yet there are still no drug régimes that command general support. One reason for the inconclusive results of recent trials may have been the assumption that myocardial infarction and sudden death share the same pathology. Another reason is the diversity of pathogenetic mechanisms and prognoses in i.h.d. Many patients probably stand little chance of benefiting from a particular drug either because it affects mechanisms other than those responsible for their disease or because their prognosis, excellent or hopeless, is unlikely to be influenced whatever treatment they receive. It is consequently difficult to ensure reasonable chances of demonstrating benefits in those who may really stand to gain. A tendency for pharmacological information to become available during or after a large trial, rather than beforehand, has added to the difficulties. Despite all their problems, randomized controlled trials remain the only way of testing drugs for the prevention of arterial disease. Suggestions are made for increasing the chances of clear results in future trials and of reaching the stage of benefit demonstrated sufficiently convincingly to form a basis for clinical practice. These suggestions include the use of factorial designs enabling the evaluation of more than one drug in a particular trial and the development of methods for selecting homogeneous groups of patients.

1. Introduction

In 1970, it seemed that little could be done to prevent the recurrence (secondary prevention) of ischaemic heart disease (i.h.d.). Dietary intervention aimed at lowering blood cholesterol levels had proved ineffective (Medical Research Council 1968; Leren 1970). Several trials of anti-coagulants had collectively suggested some benefit (International Anticoagulant Review Group 1970) though no trial on its own had done so convincingly. The uncertainty that followed these trials, together with the risks of bleeding and the need for continuous laboratory control of treatment, led to the abandonment of anticoagulants for routine management. The verdict on anticoagulants, however, was 'not proven' rather than 'proven of no value'; the question remains open and is considered again later in this paper.

Now, 10 years later, several other agents have been tested in secondary prevention trials and experience from primary prevention trials is also beginning to accumulate. By contrast with the situation a decade ago, many now believe that the prevention of i.h.d. by pharmacological means is possible. Yet there are still no specific drugs which command general support. Why is this?

This contribution reviews the developments that have changed the outlook for i.h.d. prevention from one of considerable pessimism to one of guarded optimism. It identifies some of the difficulties that will have to be overcome in reaching the next stage – that of benefit demonstrated sufficiently clearly to form a basis for clinical practice. The paper cites several trials to exemplify different points, but it is not a comprehensive review of these trials. The main emphasis is on i.h.d., though the prevention of cerebrovascular disease is also considered.

2. Ischaemic heart disease:
heterogeneity of manifestations, mechanisms and prognosis
(a) Manifestations

Terms such as ischaemic or coronary heart disease have for many years been used to include different clinical manifestations: sudden death, myocardial infarction and angina pectoris. At autopsy, advanced vessel wall disease is seen in most of those who die suddenly or after the established clinical features of myocardial infarction. But evidence of recent thrombosis and cardiac necrosis is found less often after sudden death than after myocardial infarction (Mitchell 1978). The interpretation of this observation is not straightforward (Meade 1981). The very intense fibrinolytic activity associated with sudden death could be enough to lyse thrombi responsible for a swift and catastrophic arrhythmic event. Platelet microthrombi may be responsible for sudden death (Haerem 1978). Explanations such as these – largely though not entirely conjectural – are compatible with a thrombotic explanation for sudden death as well as for myocardial infarction. But the two presentations should not be assumed to share exactly the same pathology. Besides morbid anatomical differences, there are differences in the apparent effects of drugs and of dietary changes on the occurrence of sudden death and myocardial infarction. The secondary prevention trials of aspirin have indicated a possible benefit against reinfarction. This contrasts with a less convincing effect against fatal events (mostly 'sudden') (*Lancet* 1980). The same contrast has been reported in a dietary trial (Turpeinen *et al.* 1979) and in the W.H.O. primary prevention trial of clofibrate (Committee of Principal Investigators 1978).

(b) Mechanisms

Table 1 summarizes the intended drug effects of the main i.h.d. trials so far reported.

The first five approaches are intended to prevent or diminish possible pathogenetic changes in the coronary circulation. The sixth deals with electrical and myocardial abnormalities. A feature of most of the secondary prevention trials has been their tendency to favour the active treatments (assuming that the drugs do indeed exert their benefits via the intended effects, a point considered again later). Although their results are far from conclusive, this tendency, together with evidence from other sources, suggests that all the mechanisms summarized in table 1 are involved in the pathogenesis of recurrent i.h.d. The same applies to the onset of first episodes of i.h.d., studied in primary prevention trials. Clofibrate reduced the incidence of non-fatal myocardial infarction by 25 % (Committee of Principal Investigators 1978), though it had no effect on the incidence of fatal heart attacks or angina pectoris. A later report (Committee of Principal Investigators 1980) described the 25 % higher mortality from all causes in the clofibrate treated group. The widespread use of clofibrate for the primary prevention of i.h.d. is thus contra-indicated. The beneficial effect of clofibrate on non-fatal infarction is, however, a valuable observation in terms of understanding the pathogenesis of this manifestation of i.h.d. Two primary prevention trials (referred to again in §5) have demonstrated reductions in the incidence of cardiovascular disease after the detection and treatment of hypertension (Hypertension Detection and Follow-up Program 1979; Australian Therapeutic Trial 1980). (Results of primary prevention trials of aspirin are awaited.)

Thus, quite apart from their clinical implications, the trials have emphasized the limitations of thinking of i.h.d. and its prevention in terms of single processes. There must be some people in whom one disorder is the leading cause of a first or recurrent clinical episode of i.h.d. But this disorder may be in lipid metabolism, in blood pressure control, in 'hypercoagulability' or in platelet sensitivity. In other people, combinations of disorders are probably responsible for subsequent events. There is, therefore, almost certainly a considerable diversity of pathogenetic mechanisms in i.h.d.

TABLE 1. PREVENTION OF ARTERIAL DISEASE, ESPECIALLY I.H.D.: INTENDED DRUG EFFECTS ON PATHOGENETIC MECHANISMS

1. Prevention of fibrin formation
2. Enhancement of fibrin dissolution
3. Prevention of platelet aggregation
4. Lowering of blood lipids
5. Lowering of blood pressure (principally for stroke prevention)
6. Prevention of arrhythmias

1. Secondary prevention	International Anticoagulant Review Group (1970)
	Sixty Plus Reinfarction Study (1980)
2. Secondary prevention	European Collaborative Study (1975)
	European Co-operative Study Group (1979)
3. Secondary prevention	Elwood et al. (1974)
	Elwood & Sweetnam (1979)
	Coronary Drug Project Research Group (1976)
	Anturane Reinfarction Trial (1978, 1980)
	Aspirin Myocardial Infarction Study Research Group (1980)
	Persantine–Aspirin Reinfarction Study Research Group (1980)
4. Primary prevention	Committee of Principal Investigators (1978, 1980)
Secondary prevention	Dewar & Oliver (1971) (and accompanying reports)
	Coronary Drug Project Research Group (1975)
	Rosenhamer & Carlson (1980)
5. Primary prevention (principally)	Veterans Administration (1967, 1970)
	Hypertension Detection and Follow-up Program (1979)
	Australian Therapeutic Trial (1980)
6. Secondary prevention	Wilhelmson et al. (1974)
	Multicentre International Study (1975, 1977)
	Baber et al. (1980)

The references are illustrative rather than comprehensive, especially for 1, 2 and 6.

(c) Prognosis

Many patients die soon after a myocardial infarct, whatever treatment they are given. On the other hand, many make a rapid recovery, also probably uninfluenced by treatment. There remains a proportion, of unknown size, in whom treatment may be able to alter the prognosis.

(d) Implications

The combined effects of differences in the manifestations, mechanisms and prognosis of i.h.d. mean that participants in preventive trials are likely to be heterogeneous in a number of important respects. But a drug with a specific action may only be capable of influencing one type of outcome (e.g. sudden death) in a relatively small proportion of patients. Thus i.h.d. prevention trials are subject to a low ratio of 'signal' to 'noise'.

The consequences of the heterogeneity of participants in trials vary according to whether these are of secondary or primary prevention.

Patients become eligible for secondary prevention trials because they have survived a myocardial infarction and not, other than exceptionally, because they can be shown to have had a particular disorder, such as hyperlipidaemia. Even on blood pressure, systematic pre-morbid information will usually be lacking. In addition, the infarct will itself lead to wide-ranging changes – in blood lipids (Dodds & Mills 1959), clotting factors (Meade 1981) and blood pressure – thus making it almost impossible retrospectively to assess the contribution of different processes to the event. Secondary prevention trials are therefore particularly susceptible to the consequences of the diversity of pathogenetic mechanisms in i.h.d. Entering patients into such a trial because they have had infarcts is rather like entering patients into a leukaemia chemotherapy trial without knowing the cell type. In either case, some of the patients stand to benefit. Many, however, do not, and their effect is to increase the difficulty of demonstrating benefit in those for whom the drug may indeed be useful.

Secondary prevention trials are also especially affected by the differences in prognosis referred to earlier. The number of patients required could be reduced, perhaps appreciably, if it were possible to exclude those likely to do very well or very badly, regardless of treatment. Some progress in this direction might be made through the prognostic value of electrocardiographic (e.c.g.) excercise testing shortly before discharge from hospital. Thus, the 1 year mortality in patients without S–T changes during exercise was 2.1%, compared with 27% in those with S–T segment depression (Théroux et al. 1979). This approach would mean screening large numbers of patients and would also preclude very early entry into a trial. On the other hand, those with a hopeless prognosis would have died by the time exercise testing was feasible. The test would then identify those at high risk but among whom treatment might make a substantial impact. Clinical e.c.g. details, blood pressure readings and chest X-ray findings were among measures used to predict outcome in the placebo group of the Coronary Drug Project (1974). In a 3 year follow-up period, 30.7% of the deaths took place in the 10% of patients at greatest risk. (Over 90% of the deaths were cardiovascular; 81.6% were due to i.h.d.) It is surprising that more use has not hitherto been made of readily available clinical information which might be used to select high-risk groups for secondary prevention trials.

From a statistical point of view, the higher mortality and recurrence rates in secondary than in primary prevention trials are, of course, an advantage, though even in secondary trials the magnitude of these rates is not enough to avoid the need for hundreds or even thousands of patients.

Primary prevention trials are carried out in participants who can often be selected according to the characteristic to be modified, for example blood cholesterol levels in the W.H.O. trial of clofibrate or blood pressure in the trials of anti-hypertensive agents. Thus, in theory at least, the existence of several different pathogenetic mechanisms does not present as great a problem as for secondary prevention trials. But the opportunity of focusing on one mechanism depends on having a valid and biologically plausible measure of risk, such as the blood cholesterol level, which has been shown to be associated with the later occurrence of the disease. There is no such measure of platelet function. The primary prevention trials of aspirin in progress or being planned make use of participants in whom no particular attempt has been made to select those at high risk or in whom risk is assessed on 'conventional' risk factors such as blood cholesterol or smoking habit, and which may or may not reflect platelet activity. This is unsatisfactory, particularly as, in statistical terms, the incidence of first i.h.d. events in an unselected group is low so that trials require very large numbers of participants. Platelet function depends not only on intrinsic properties of the platelets themselves but on plasma, vessel wall and haemodynamic influences as well. Difficult and time-consuming though it may prove, tests that reflect these features and are predictive of i.h.d. must be a high research priority if basic knowledge on platelets is to bear full fruit in practical terms.

In both primary and secondary prevention trials, sudden death and myocardial infarction can and probably should be regarded as separate endpoints, for reasons discussed earlier. This means that the number of participants required will have to be based on separate mortality and incidence rates rather than on the rate for both combined.

3. EARLY ENTRY

Many believe that future secondary prevention trials should be based on very early, if not immediate, entry after infarction. In the second South Wales aspirin trial (Elwood & Sweetnam 1979), half the patients were admitted within 7 days. The interval in the Anturane Reinfarction Trial (1980) was 25–35 days. Otherwise, entry into recent trials (i.e. excluding the anti-coagulant trials) has been between about 6 weeks and several years after infarction. The optimum interval may vary for different drugs, but the general principle of entry within days or a few weeks, rather than months or years, is sound. However, early entry trials raise two major problems.

One difficulty is that very early entry may result in the inclusion of patients who do not stand to benefit, either because it is eventually clear that they have not had myocardial infarcts or because their prognosis is hopeless, whatever treatment they receive. This difficulty can be allowed for by delaying entry for 2 or 3 days. By that time, it will be possible to exclude most of those who have not had infarcts and many of those who have had very serious episodes will have died. Any requirement for exercise testing (suggested earlier) will delay entry still further. It is a matter for judgement whether the possible advantages of such a test outweigh the disadvantages of the delay.

The second difficulty is that drugs other than those tested in the trial will almost certainly have to be administered. A particular example is the likely use of β-blocking agents in perhaps a quarter of those recruited to an early entry trial of aspirin or sulphinpyrazone. This difficulty raises pharmacological questions about possible interactions (§4). It also raises the precise objectives of i.h.d. trials, primary as well as secondary. Are these trials intended (a) to test the policy of using a particular drug ('pragmatic') or (b) to give a precise assessment of the clinical effectiveness of the drug under ideal conditions ('explicative')? An argument for the pragmatic approach is that it reflects the realities of clinical practice, where several drugs may be used simultaneously and there is no certainty that all the patients will actually take a particular drug in accordance with instructions. Another reason for the pragmatic approach arises from the recurring question of whether to include the results from patients who deviate from the treatment schedule or who default from follow-up. These patients have to be excluded from an explicative trial, to ensure that the results are based only on patients known to have adhered to their allocated treatment régime for most if not all of the trial. But the greater the number of patients omitted from the analysis, the greater the risk becomes of biases affecting the comparison of outcome in treated and control groups. This problem is avoided by the 'intention to treat' attitude of pragmatic trials. Analysis is based on all the patients entered, according to the régime to which they were originally allocated, whether or not they adhere to this régime and, as far as possible, even if they default from follow-up. Although the pragmatic approach will probably reduce the power of a trial, a result suggesting a beneficial effect also implies a beneficial effect in explicative terms. This is exemplified by the recent Dutch trial of stopping anticoagulants in those aged 60 years or more. The adverse effect of discontinuing anticoagulants on recurrent myocardial infarction was quite clear on a pragmatic as well as an explicative analysis (Sixty Plus Reinfarction Study 1980). The effect on mortality was suggestive though not significant at a conventional level on the pragmatic analysis; it was highly significant on the explicative. Although stopping anticoagulants is not the same as starting the treatment, the Dutch trial is a reminder that the issue of anticoagulants after infarction has never been satisfactorily resolved.

4. Pharmacological considerations

Further attention to a number of pharmacological topics might increase the value of preventive trials in i.h.d.

(a) Mode of action

A major stimulus to a clinical trial is knowledge of the action of a drug on some process involved in pathogenesis. But trials demonstrate the clinical benefit (or otherwise) of the drug in question: they do not prove that the drug necessarily confers the benefit by the process that formed the basis for its use in the trial. Thus, clofibrate probably lowers the plasma fibrinogen level (Dormandy et al. 1974) as well as that of blood cholesterol. Although the original reason for testing sulphinpyrazone (Anturane Reinfarction Trial 1980) was its effects on platelet function, it has been suggested that it acts as an anti-arrhythmic drug or that it modifies myocardial function (Forfar et al. 1980). Increasingly precise information on modes of action is clearly required, to take full advantage of the possibility of selecting patients for trials according to the pathogenetic mechanisms predominantly responsible for their disease or predisposition to it.

(b) Dose–response

Even for hypotensive agents, dose–response data are far from complete. Most clofibrate trials have used doses that resulted in only modest cholesterol-lowering effects. The early and encouraging results of a Swedish trial of clofibrate and nicotinic acid (Rosenhamer & Carlson 1980) may be due to the relatively large fall in cholesterol levels that it has achieved. (For the reasons discussed in §2b, the widespread use of clofibrate is now contra-indicated. But the dose–response effects of the clofibrate trials are nevertheless valid illustrations.) One reason for the uncertain benefits of anticoagulants in the early trials may have been the failure to achieve and then maintain optimal levels of anticoagulation. The clear-cut results of the Dutch trial of stopping anticoagulants probably owe much to the particular attention paid to this point.

(c) Interactions

It has already been pointed out that in early entry secondary prevention trials, participants will often be exposed to non-trial as well as trial drugs, which may interact. Trial drugs (if more than one are used in combination) may also interact with one another. The theoretical possibility of harmful interactions has been a reason for deciding not to proceed with trials which on other grounds seem justified. It is therefore important to try to distinguish between interactions that have a high chance of actually occurring and of being clinically harmful and those that are less likely to occur or, if they do, unlikely to be of any consequence. Interactions between drugs and the characteristics of those who take them, such as their sex or age, may be of a greater relevance than interactions between drugs themselves.

(d) Side-effects

Trials are an excellent source of information about the adverse as well as the beneficial effects of drugs. Yet common adverse effects could be detected in controlled comparisons involving far smaller numbers than those needed to demonstrate benefits in terms of mortality and reinfarction. These smaller comparisons would not, it is true, detect rare but serious harmful effects such as those of clofibrate on mortality from all causes (Committee of Principal Investigators 1980) or those of practolol. But less serious effects such as lethargy or impotence could be detected, with greater confidence than hitherto, before rather than during or after a major clinical trial. Information thus obtained would be useful in making choices between what may be an increasingly large number of possible drugs. It may be that sulphinpyrazone impairs renal function (Wilcox et al. 1980), the evidence to this effect having only become available, however, well after the completion of the Anturane Reinfarction Trial (1980).

(e) Compliance

Side effects at therapeutic levels and other factors will affect compliance with trial régimes. Again, this is a feature that should be established with some certainty before rather than after the main trial.

In summary, the scale, planning and conduct of clinical trials will benefit from the availability, beforehand rather than afterwards, of increasingly precise and comprehensive pharmacological information.

5. HYPERTENSION AND ARTERIAL DISEASE

The main stimulus to the detection and treatment of hypertension has been the predominance of raised blood pressure as a determinant of cerebrovascular disease (Gordon & Kannel 1972). This association is much more striking than the relation between raised blood pressure and i.h.d., though raised pressure is also associated with an increased risk of i.h.d. (Gordon & Kannel 1972). There were thus expectations that the treatment of high blood pressure might reduce the incidence of i.h.d. as well as of stroke. In contrast to clear reductions in stroke incidence, however, early trials suggested little or no benefit in terms of i.h.d. (Veterans Administration 1967, 1970). These trials have been followed by others concerned with milder degrees of hypertension. Both the American Hypertension Detection and Follow-up Program (1979) and the Australian Therapeutic Trial (1980) showed significant reductions in mortality from all causes, these reductions being mainly accounted for by cardiovascular disease. It is not clear whether the beneficial effect in the trial in the U.S.A. was due specifically to antihypertensive treatment or to the higher level of general medical care received by those in the more actively treated group. Both trials suggested possible benefits for i.h.d. as well as more obvious benefits for stroke. However, neither of these trials included β-blocking agents as a primary treatment. Whether these agents are more effective in preventing i.h.d. than those so far studied remains to be seen. Propranolol is one of the primary treatments in the Medical Research Council's mild hypertension trial (Medical Research Council 1977).

6. OTHER PREVENTIVE MEASURES

This review is concerned specifically with prevention by drugs. The primary prevention of i.h.d. by modifications of life-style is, however, widely advocated. These modifications form part of trials (see, for example, Rose *et al.* 1980) whose main results are awaited. Giving up cigarette smoking is an effective method of secondary prevention though this view is largely based on the results of non-randomized comparisons. The growing use of coronary artery surgery as a means of managing angina should also be borne in mind (Second Interim Report 1980).

7. FUTURE DIRECTIONS

For the time being, it has to be accepted that the combination of the low signal/noise ratio and the statistically low event rates mean that secondary prevention i.h.d. trials testing active treatments against inactive placebos will often need 2000 participants, or more. If and when interest shifts to secondary trials of a new agent against an older one of established value the numbers needed may be even larger. Primary prevention trials may call for over 10000 participants, particularly if the latter cannot be selected by a test related to the pathogenetic mechanism to be modified. With the uncertain clinical implications of past trials in mind there are signs of resistance to further i.h.d. trials. This might be justified if it appeared that the prevention of i.h.d. would follow some basic advance in pathogenesis or treatment so fundamental that further large-scale trials were unnecessary. This seems improbable. It is hard to envisage any development – even the discovery of thromboxane and prostacyclin – that would overturn the view of i.h.d. as a condition of many disordered processes, making it unnecessary to test new drugs and to identify patients likely to benefit from them. An alternative to further clinical trials is trial by pharmacological theory, exemplified by predictions of drug interactions in early entry trials or trials using more than one drug, and by much of the controversy surrounding the question of aspirin dose. An almost certain consequence of abandoning clinical trials is that the use of drugs for i.h.d. prevention would be determined by the promotional expertise of the pharmaceutical industry. More and more drugs would join the list of those of uncertain benefit: anticoagulants, aspirin, sulphinpyrazone.

To these rather negative reasons for further trials there is the more positive reason referred to earlier. Although they were inconclusive, secondary prevention trials that have been reported (table 1) have nearly all suggested benefits attributable to the drugs in question. The reductions in event rates characteristic of many of the trials – 20 % or so – are often described as marginal. But reductions of this magnitude would be of considerable value in a disease as common as i.h.d. Reductions might be much larger than 20 % in groups of patients of otherwise poor prognosis taking drugs that modify the particular pathogenetic mechanism(s) responsible for their disease. It has been suggested that one of the reasons for the unconvincing results of the aspirin trials is that doses were too large, thus inhibiting prostacyclin as well as thromboxane production. But it is at least as likely that the results were a reflection of low signal/noise ratios. On these grounds there are good reasons for further trials, as the need and opportunity arise and recognizing that these trials will continue to be large, difficult and expensive for the foreseeable future. There are, however, some measures that can be taken to maximize the chances of useful information.

8. Some solutions

Most of the steps to be taken follow from what has already been said. They include the reconfirmation of some aspects of trial design and analysis that have recently been questioned. The suggestions that follow are not intended to be a summary of trial design and analysis but mostly arise from the particular problems of trials of drugs in arterial disease. Some of the suggestions may enable trials to be smaller than hitherto. Some have the opposite effect. But they should all, if practicable, increase the chances of clear results.

(a) Measures for immediate implementation

(i) Randomization

It has recently been suggested that 'historical controls' can be used as a basis for comparison with treated patients (Cranberg 1979). This approach, using as it does some retrospective data, has the superficial appeal of ease and economy. It is liable to be utterly misleading, particularly in just such situations as the secondary prevention of i.h.d. The biases that can arise from not randomizing may result in an apparent but spurious difference in outcome between treated and control groups of the same magnitude as any true difference (Doll & Peto 1980). Is the difference then due to treatment or to bias? Alternatives to randomization or modifications of it have been suggested (Weinstein 1974; Machin 1979; Zelen 1979) but have not been adopted. At present, and probably indefinitely, there is no acceptable substitute for classical random allocation.

(ii) Adequate numbers

It is not only pointless but unethical (Altman 1980) to initiate trials with numbers too small for a reasonable chance of clear results. Failure to demonstrate a drug's benefit in too small a trial does not provide any useful evidence that it is without effect, either. Trials of this sort merely add to existing uncertainty. The economy of numbers suggested by combining sudden death and infarction as outcomes cannot be made if they are considered separately. Another factor tending to increase required numbers is growing concern at the effects of multiple statistical inspections of trial data, as they accumulate. On the other hand, increasing awareness by statisticians of the requirements of clinicians and vice versa is gradually leading to an improved mutual understanding of what can sometimes be achieved with numbers that are less than ideal.

There is no easy solution to the problem of large sample sizes in arterial disease trials but this is not, in itself, an argument against further trials.

(iii) Factorial designs

The use of two drugs, either separately or in combination, may have statistical as well as clinical advantages (Armitage 1980). There will be four groups in a two-drug factorial trial: patients on one drug alone, those on the other alone, those on both and those on neither. It may be possible to assess the independent value of the two drugs in a trial no larger than a trial to assess a single drug. In addition, clinicians need information on the benefits of drugs used in combination. The main disadvantage of factorial trials lies in the possibility of drug interactions. If these are marked, that is if the two drugs used together have markedly greater or smaller effects than the sum of their separate effects, the effect of either drug on its own can only be assessed on half the data, with a consequent reduction in the power of the trial. This highlights the need for as much information as possible, before rather than during or after the trial, on interactions of clinical significance. The use of factorial designs deserves wider consideration than it has so far received. The Canadian trial of aspirin and sulphinpyrazone in cerebrovascular disease suggested a benefit attributable to aspirin, but not to sulphinpyrazone or to both drugs together (Canadian Co-operative Study Group 1978). The benefit was confined to men.

(iv) *Pragmatic analyses*

The reasons for these have already been discussed.

(v) *Distinction between different endpoints*

The reasons for distinguishing between sudden death and infarction have been discussed.

(vi) *Record of all patients*

Records should be kept of all the patients considered for a trial, even if they are not included in it. This simple procedure, rarely carried out, enables some assessment of the extent to which trial patients are or are not representative of all patients with the diagnosis in question. The Anturane Re-infarction Trial (1978, 1980) extrapolated its findings to myocardial infarction patients as a whole, but because of the very high proportion of patients excluded from the trial it is doubtful whether this was justified.

(b) *Possible measures for the medium term*

Some measures might have an effect on trials in the medium term, depending on the initiation and outcome of future research.

(i) *Selection by prognosis*

Attention has already been drawn to the considerable advantages of secondary prevention trials that exclude patients likely to do very well or very badly whatever treatment they are given.

(ii) *Pharmacological precision*

It is clear that some important pharmacological questions only arise as a result of large-scale trials. Others arise quite independently while trials are in progress: the implications of prostacyclin, for example. These questions cannot be foreseen. However, some of the features discussed earlier can to some extent be anticipated. If so, the increasingly precise and comprehensive information that may emerge before rather than after future trials can only be of value.

(c) *A possible measure for the longer term*

A measure which might, in the longer term, improve trial design and conduct is selection by pathogenesis.

It is hard to imagine much progress towards the selection of patients for secondary prevention trials according to the processes mainly responsible for their first event. Selection by prognosis (§b(i) above) may eventually be possible. Participants in primary prevention trials can (and have) been selected according to their blood pressure and blood lipid levels. It may eventually be possible to select according to clotting factor levels (Meade *et al.* 1980). A major deficiency, however, is any test of platelet function, as defined in §2d, that is predictive of subsequent i.h.d. If and when such a test becomes available, the rationale and conduct of trials of agents that modify platelet function are likely to be improved.

9. CONCLUSION

Implementing some of these suggestions implies the need for priorities in the field of research on arterial disease and some coordination of ensuing research programmes. This is a controversial topic. There must, though, be some reasonable compromise between the extremes of having no guidelines other than the personal interests of workers in the field and of attempting to override these interests altogether.

The simultaneous frustrations and the potential of trials of drugs in arterial disease are considerable. In a paraphrase of Churchill's description of democracy as a form of government, these trials seem to be the worst way of going about the problem – except for all the other ways that have been tried from time to time.

Note added in proof (23 April 1981). Particularly encouraging results have recently been reported from the Norwegian secondary prevention trial of the β-blocking agent timolol. (Norwegian Multicentre Study Group 1981 Timolol-induced reduction in mortality and reinfarction in patients surviving acute myocardial infarction. *New Engl. J. Med.* **304**, 801–807.)

REFERENCES (Meade)

Altman, D. G. 1980 Statistics and ethics in medical research. *Br. med. J.* **281**, 1182–1184.
Anturane Reinfarction Trial Research Group 1978 Sulphinpyrazone in the prevention of cardiac death after myocardial infarction. *New Engl. J. Med.* **298**, 289–295; 333–334.
Anturane Reinfarction Trial Research Group 1980 Sulphinpyrazone in the prevention of sudden death after myocardial infarction. *New Engl. J. Med.* **302**, 250–256.
Armitage, P. 1980 Clinical trials in the secondary prevention of myocardial infarction and stroke. *Thromb. Haemostas.* **43**, 90–94.
Aspirin Myocardial Infarction Study Research Group 1980 A randomized controlled trial of aspirin in persons recovered from myocardial infarction. *J. Am. med. Ass.* **243**, 661–669.
Australian Therapeutic Trial Management Committee 1980 The Australian Therapeutic Trial in Mild Hypertension. *Lancet* i, 1261–1267.
Baber, N. S., Wainwright Evans, D., Howitt, G., Thomas, M., Wilson, C., Lewis, J. A., Dawes, P. M., Handler, K. & Tuson, R. 1980 Multicentre postinfarction trial of propranolol in 49 hospitals in the United Kingdom, Italy and Yugoslavia. *Br. Heart J.* **44**, 96–100.
Canadian Co-operative Study Group 1978 A randomized trial of aspirin and sulphinpyrazone in threatened stroke. *New Engl. J. Med.* **299**, 53–59.
Committee of Principal Investigators 1978 A co-operative trial in the primary prevention of ischaemic heart disease using clofibrate. *Br. Heart J.* **40**, 1069–1118.
Committee of Principal Investigators 1980 WHO cooperative trial on primary prevention of ischaemic heart disease using clofibrate to lower serum cholesterol: mortality follow-up. *Lancet* ii, 379–385.
Coronary Drug Project Research Group 1974 Factors influencing long-term prognosis after recovery from myocardial infarction – three-year findings of the coronary drug project. *J. chron. Dis.* **27**, 267–285.
Coronary Drug Project Research Group 1975 Clofibrate and niacin in coronary heart disease. *J. Am. med. Ass.* **231**, 360–381.
Coronary Drug Project Research Group 1976 Aspirin in coronary heart disease. *J. chron. Dis.* **29**, 625–642.
Cranberg, L. 1979 Do retrospective controls make clinical trials 'inherently fallacious?' *Br. med. J.* ii, 1265–1266.
Dewar, H. A. & Oliver, M. F. 1971 Secondary prevention trials using clofibrate: a joint commentary on the Newcastle and Scottish trials. *Br. med. J.* iv, 784–786.

Dodds, C. & Mills, G. L. 1959 Influence of myocardial infarction on plasma-lipoprotein. *Lancet* i, 1160–1163.

Doll, R. & Peto, R. 1980 Randomized controlled trials and retrospective controls. *Br. med. J.* **280**, 44.

Dormandy, J. A., Gutteridge, J. M. C., Hoare, E. & Dormandy, T. L. 1974 Effect of clofibrate on blood viscosity in intermittent claudication. *Br. med. J.* iv, 259–262.

Elwood, P. C. & Sweetnam, P. M. 1979 Aspirin and secondary mortality after myocardial infarction. *Lancet* ii, 1313–1315.

Elwood, P. C., Cochrane, A. L., Burr, M. L., Sweetnam, P. M., Williams, G., Welsby, E., Hughes, S. J. & Renton, R. 1974 A randomized controlled trial of acetyl salicylic acid in the secondary prevention of mortality from myocardial infarction. *Br. med. J.* i, 436–440.

European Collaborative Study 1975 Controlled trial of urokinase in myocardial infarction. *Lancet* ii, 624–630.

European Co-operative Study Group 1979 Streptokinase in acute myocardial infarction. *New Engl. J. Med.* **301**, 797–802.

Forfar, J. C., Russell, D. C. & Oliver, M. F. 1980 Haemodynamic effects of sulphinpyrazone on exercise responses in normal subjects. *Lancet* ii, 718–720.

Gordon, T. & Kannel, W. B. 1972 Predisposition to atherosclerosis in the head, heart and legs. The Framingham Study. *J. Am. med. Ass.* **221**, 661–666.

Haerem, J. W. 1978 Sudden, unexpected coronary death. *Acta path. microbiol. scand.*, Sect. A, Suppl. no. 265.

Hypertension Detection and Follow-up Program Cooperative Group 1979 Five-year findings of the hypertension detection and follow-up program. *J. Am. med. Ass.* **242**, 2562–2571, 2572–2577.

International Anticoagulant Review Group 1970 Collaborative analysis of long-term anticoagulant administration after acute myocardial infarction. *Lancet* i, 203–209.

Lancet 1980 Aspirin after myocardial infarction. *Lancet* i, 1172–1173.

Leren, P. 1970 The Oslo diet heart study; eleven year report. *Circulation* **42**, 935–942.

Machin, D. 1979 On the possibility of incorporating patients from non-randomising centres into a randomised clinical trial. *J. chron. Dis.* **32**, 347–353.

Meade, T. W. 1981 The epidemiology of atheroma and thrombosis. In *Haemostasis and thrombosis*. Edinburgh: Churchill Livingstone. (In the press.)

Meade, T. W., Chakrabarti, R., Haines, A. P., North, W. R. S., Stirling, Y. Thompson, S. G. & Brozović, M. 1980 Haemostatic function and cardiovascular death: early results of a prospective study. *Lancet* i, 1050–1054.

Medical Research Council 1968 Report of the Research Committee: controlled trial of soya-bean oil in myocardial infarction. *Lancet* ii, 693–700.

Medical Research Council 1977 Report of Medical Research Council Working Party on Mild to Moderate Hypertension. *Br. med. J.* i, 1437–1440.

Mitchell, J. R. A. 1978 Clinical events resulting from thrombus formation, *Br. med. Bull.* **34**, 103–106.

Multicentre International Study 1975 Improvement in prognosis of myocardial infarction by long-term beta-adrenoreceptor blockade using practolol. *Br. med. J.* iii, 735–740.

Multicentre International Study 1977 Reduction in mortality after myocardial infarction with long-term beta-adrenoreceptor blockade. *Br. med. J.* ii, 419–421.

Persantine–Aspirin Reinfarction Study Research Group 1980 Persantine and aspirin in coronary heart disease. *Circulation* **62**, 449–461.

Rose, G., Heller, R. F., Tunstall Pedoe, H. & Christie, D. G. S. 1980 Heart disease prevention project: randomised controlled trial in industry. *Br. med. J.* **280**, 747–751.

Rosenhamer, G. & Carlson, L. A. 1980 Effect of combined clofibrate–nicotinic acid treatment in ischaemic heart disease. *Atherosclerosis* **37**, 129–38.

Second Interim Report by the European Coronary Surgery Study Group 1980 Prospective randomised study of coronary artery bypass surgery in stable angina pectoris. *Lancet* ii, 491–495.

Sixty Plus Reinfarction Study Research Group 1980 A double-blind trial to assess long-term oral anticoagulant therapy in elderly patients after myocardial infarction. *Lancet* ii, 989–994.

Théroux, P., Waters, D. D., Halphen, C., Debaisieux, J.-C. & Mizgala, H. F. 1979 Prognostic value of exercise testing soon after myocardial infarction. *New Engl. J. Med.* **301**, 341–345.

Turpeinen, O., Karvonen, M. J., Pekkarinen, M., Miettinen, M., Elosuo, R. & Paavilainen, E. 1979 Dietary prevention of coronary heart disease: the Finnish mental hospital study. *Int. J. Epidemiol.* **8**, 99–118.

Veterans Administration Cooperative Study Group on Antihypertensive Agents 1967 Effects of treatment on morbidity in hypertension. *J. Am. med. Ass.* **202**, 1028–1034.

Veterans Administration Cooperative Study Group on Antihypertensive Agents 1970 Effects of treatment on morbidity in hypertension. *J. Am. med. Ass.* **213**, 1143–1152.

Weinstein, M. C. 1974 Allocation of subjects in medical experiments. *New Engl. J. Med.* **291**, 1278–1285.

Wilcox, R. G., Richardson, D., Hampton, J. R., Mitchell, J. R. A. & Banks, D. C. 1980 Sulphinpyrazone in acute myocardial infarction: studies on cardiac rhythm and renal function. *Br. med. J.* **281**, 531–534.

Wilhelmsson, C., Wilhelmsen, L., Vedin, J. A. & Tibblin, G. 1974 Reduction of sudden deaths after myocardial infarction by treatment with alprenolol. Preliminary results. *Lancet* ii, 1157–1164.

Zelen, M. 1979 A new design for randomized clinical trials. *New Engl. J. Med.* **300**, 1242–1245.

Discussion

J. McMICHAEL, F.R.S. (2 *North Square, London, NW*11 7*AA, U.K.*). The best-matched secondary trial of polyunsaturated fats was under the M.R.C. (*Lancet* ii, 693 (1968)). It produced no benefit. Massive inter-centre trials are often vitiated by diagnostic differences and interpretations. France has notoriously been under-recording coronary deaths since the war. Experimental viral infections (*Lancet* ii, 821 (1978)) can produce the disease and so, possibly, can other infections. We cannot take rational steps towards prevention until we know more about causes from direct observation and experiment.

T. W. MEADE. Clinical trials can provide information on causes and mechanisms as well as on prevention.

Phil. Trans. R. Soc. Lond. B **294**, 305–329 (1981)

Printed in Great Britain

Prostacyclin: its biosynthesis, actions and clinical potential

By S. Moncada and J. R. Vane, F.R.S.

Wellcome Research Laboratories, Langley Court, Beckenham, Kent BR3 3BS, U.K.

Prostacyclin (PGI_2) is the product of arachidonic acid metabolism generated by the vessel wall of all mammalian species studied, including man. Prostacyclin is a potent vasodilator and the most potent inhibitor of platelet aggregation so far described. Prostacyclin inhibits aggregation through stimulation of platelet adenyl cyclase leading to an increase in platelet cyclic AMP. In the vessel wall, the enzyme that synthesizes prostacyclin is concentrated in the endothelial layer. Prostacyclin can also be a circulating hormone released from the pulmonary circulation. Based on these observations we proposed that platelet aggregability *in vivo* is controlled via a prostacyclin mechanism.

The discovery of prostacyclin has given a new insight into arachidonic acid metabolism and has led to a new hypothesis about mechanisms of haemostasis. Reductions in prostacyclin production in several diseases, including atherosclerosis and diabetes, have been described and implicated in the pathophysiology of these diseases. Additionally, since prostacyclin powerfully inhibits platelet aggregation and promotes their disaggregation, this agent could have an important use in the therapy of conditions in which increased platelet aggregation takes place and in which, perhaps, a prostacyclin deficiency exists.

Prostacyclin has been used beneficially in humans during extracorporeal circulation procedures such as cardiopulmonary bypass, charcoal haemoperfusion and haemodialysis. Its possible use in other conditions such as peripheral vascular disease or transplant surgery is at present being investigated.

During 1975, Moncada and coworkers began to look for biosynthesis of thromboxane A_2 (TXA_2) by various tissues other than platelets. Vascular tissues did not generate TXA_2, but the cascade bioassay technique (Vane 1964) showed that microsomal fractions of blood vessels converted the endoperoxide precursor enzymically into an unknown product that was labile and relaxed the coeliac and mesenteric arteries of the rabbit (Moncada *et al.* 1976*a*). They called this substance PGX, and showed also that it inhibited platelet aggregation; in fact it was the most potent inhibitor of platelet aggregation known, being 30–40 times more potent than PGE_1 (Moncada & Vane 1978). In later work PGX was characterized further; it potently relaxed coronary (Dusting *et al.* 1977*a*) as well as splanchnic vascular strips *in vitro* (Bunting *et al.* 1976), dilated vascular beds *in vivo* (Armstrong *et al.* 1977, 1978; Dusting *et al.* 1978*c*) and had strong antithrombotic activity *in vivo* (Higgs *et al.* 1977; Ubatuba *et al.* 1979). Furthermore, it was the major metabolite of arachidonic acid in vascular tissues (Johnson *et al.* 1976; Salmon *et al.* 1978). PGX was the unstable intermediate in the formation of 6-oxo-$PGF_{1\alpha}$, a compound described by Pace-Asciak (1976) as a product of prostaglandin (PG) endoperoxides in the rat stomach. The work that led to the elucidation of the structure of PGX was carried out as a collaborative effort between scientists from the Wellcome Research Laboratories and from the Upjohn Company (Johnson *et al.* 1976). PGX was then renamed prostacyclin with the abbreviation of PGI_2. It has now been given the approved name of epoprostenol, but the trivial name of prostacyclin will be used throughout this review.

The discovery of prostacyclin, together with the isolation and characterization of the prosta-glandin endoperoxides and TXA_2 which preceded it (Hamberg & Samuelsson 1973; Hamberg et al. 1974, 1975; Nugteren & Hazelhof 1973), have added substantially to our understanding of platelet – vessel wall interactions, and opened new lines of research in haemostasis and thrombosis. Another consequence that is also gathering momentum is a better understanding of the basis of some diseases. In this chapter we shall deal mainly with the way in which the balance between aggregatory and anti-aggregatory metabolites of arachidonic acid affects the processes of haemostasis and thrombosis. We shall discuss the regulation and pharmacological manipulation of prostacyclin biosynthesis as well as disturbances in its biosynthesis in some pathological conditions. The therapeutic potential of prostacyclin as an antithrombotic agent will be addressed in the last section.

The ability of the vessel wall to synthesize prostacyclin is greatest at the intimal surface and progressively decreases towards the adventitia (Moncada et al. 1977). Cultures of cells from vessel walls also show that endothelial cells are the most active producers of prostacyclin (MacIntyre et al. 1978; Weksler et al. 1977 b); moreover, this production persists after numerous subcultures in vitro (Christofinis et al. 1979).

Initially it was demonstrated that vessel microsomes in the absence of cofactors could utilize prostaglandin endoperoxides, but not arachidonic acid, to synthesize prostacyclin (Moncada et al. 1976 a). Later it was shown that fresh vascular tissue could utilize both precursors, although the endoperoxides were much better substrates (Bunting et al. 1976). Moreover, vessel micro-somes, fresh vascular rings or endothelial cells treated with indomethacin could, when incubated with platelets, generate a prostacyclin-like anti-aggregating activity (Bunting et al. 1976, 1977; Gryglewski et al. 1976). The release of this substance was inhibited by 15-hydroperoxyarachi-donic acid (15-HPAA) and other fatty acid hydroperoxides known to be selective inhibitors of prostacyclin formation (Gryglewski et al. 1976; Moncada et al. 1976 b; Salmon et al. 1978). From all these data we concluded that the vessel wall can synthesize prostacyclin from its own endogenous precursors, but also that it can utilize prostaglandin endoperoxides released by the platelets, thus suggesting a biochemical cooperation between platelet and vessel wall (Moncada & Vane 1978, 1979 b).

This hypothesis was challenged by Needleman et al. (1978), who demonstrated that while arachidonic acid was rapidly converted to prostacyclin by perfused rabbit hearts and kidneys, PGH_2 was not readily transformed. They concluded that some degree of vascular damage is necessary for the endoperoxide to be utilized by prostacyclin synthetase. On the other hand, incubation of platelet-rich plasma (p.r.p.) with fresh, indomethacin-treated arterial tissue leads to an increase in platelet cyclic AMP (cAMP) (Best et al. 1977) that parallels the inhibition of the aggregation and can be abolished by previous treatment of the vascular tissue with tranyl-cypromine, a less active inhibitor of prostacyclin formation (Gryglewski et al. 1976). Further-more, Tansik et al. (1978) showed that lysed aortic smooth muscle cells could be supplied with prostaglandin endoperoxides by lysed human platelets to form prostacyclin. Finally, un-disturbed endothelial cell monolayers readily transform PGH_2 to prostacyclin (Marcus et al. 1978).

Needleman et al. (1979) and Hornstra et al. (1979), using vessel microsomes or fresh vascular tissue, concluded that endoperoxides from platelets cannot be utilized by other cells under their experimental conditions. However, more recently, Marcus et al. (1979; see also Marcus et al., this symposium) showed that feeding of endoperoxides to endothelial cells suspended in p.r.p.

takes place *in vitro*, but only when the platelet number is around normal blood levels. Too high a platelet concentration induces a platelet–platelet interaction that limits the platelet – endothelial cell reaction. It should be stressed, however, that the possibility of platelet-released endoperoxides being utilized by endothelial cells has not yet been tested *in vivo*. Adherence of the platelet to the vessel wall could well provide the proximity that would be needed for such 'cooperation'.

It is also possible that formed elements of blood such as the white cells, which produce endoperoxides and TXA_2 (Davison *et al.* 1978; Goldstein *et al.* 1977; Higgs *et al.* 1976) could interact with the vessel wall to promote formation of prostacyclin. Moreover, leucocytes themselves generate prostacyclin in whole blood, especially in the presence of thromboxane synthetase inhibitors (Flower & Cardinal 1979). Thus, prostacyclin might regulate white cell behaviour (Higgs *et al.* 1978*b*; Weksler *et al.* 1977*a*), and help to control white cell activity during the inflammatory response. Interestingly, an artificial surface, when exposed to blood *in vivo*, initially becomes coated with platelets, but this coat is slowly replaced by a pavement of white cells. The white cell pavement is then unattractive to platelets, and this could be due to prostacyclin generation by the leucocytes.

Bradykinin and angiotensin release prostaglandins from the kidney (Aiken & Vane 1973; McGiff *et al.* 1970, 1972), lungs (Vane & Ferreira 1976) and other organs *in vivo* (Ferreira *et al.* 1973). Before the discovery of prostacyclin, Gimbrone & Alexander (1975) had demonstrated that angiotensin II stimulated the generation of an immunoreactive, PGE-like substance by human umbilical endothelial cells in culture. Needleman and coworkers (Blumberg *et al.* 1977; Needleman 1976; Needleman *et al.* 1975) had also described the release by angiotensin and bradykinin of a PGE-like substance from rabbits' isolated perfused hearts and mesenteric vessels. The PGE-like substance was characterized by bioassay on gastrointestinal tissues and chromatographic mobility on thin-layer plates. It is now clear that these techniques do not readily distinguish between prostacyclin (or 6-oxo-PGF_{1a}) and PGE_2 (Moncada & Vane 1978; Omini *et al.* 1977), and Needleman *et al.* (1978) have now shown that bradykinin or angiotensin II release a prostacyclin-like substance from Langendorff-perfused hearts of rabbits. Moreover, Dusting and coworkers (Dusting & Mullins 1980; Dusting *et al.* 1981) demonstrated that angiotensins I and II release much more prostacyclin than PGE_2 from perfused isolated mesenteric vasculature of rats, and prostacyclin was identified as the major prostacyclin released from the pulmonary circulation of the dog *in vivo* by antiotensin I or II (Mullane & Moncada 1980*b*). In contrast, the isolated perfused kidney of the rabbit converts exogenous arachidonate predominately into prostacyclin, but PGE_2 is the main prostanoid released by bradykinin and angiotensin II into the venous effluent (Needleman *et al.* 1978). However, perfusion of isolated kidneys with albumin-free Krebs's solution produces a large increase in glomerular filtration rate so that medullary perfusion is enhanced. Since PGE_2 is prevalent in the medulla and the effluent assayed is a mixture of venous and urinary outflow, this technique could account for the large quantities of PGE_2. In the canine kidney *in vivo*, prostacyclin and not PGE_2 was identified as the main prostaglandin released into renal venous blood by angiotensin and bradykinin (Mullane & Moncada 1980*b*). Small quantities of PGE_2 (approximately 10 % of those of prostacyclin) were observed in some experiments by these workers. These findings have renewed interest in the concept proposed by Vane & McGiff (1975) that prostaglandins released by angiotensin and bradykinin may modulate or partly mediate the renal and vascular actions of these peptides.

The pulmonary circulation has long been recognized for its ability to transform arachidonic acid rapidly into more polar products. Indeed most known metabolites of arachidonic acid have at one time or another been proposed as major products generated by the lungs. Isolated perfused lungs of guinea pigs, rats and rabbits release prostaglandins E_2 and $F_{2\alpha}$, TXA_2, lipoxygenase metabolites of arachidonic acid, prostacyclin and metabolites of all these substances when they are challenged with histamine, bradykinin, 5-hydroxytryptamine, arachidonic acid or anaphylactic shock. These products are also generated when pulmonary tissue is subjected to mechanical trauma. Gryglewski (1979) has recently reviewed evidence that isolated perfused lungs of cats, rats, rabbits and guinea-pigs release spontaneously a prostacyclin-like substance, and little other arachidonate-derived material, when perfused through the pulmonary artery with Krebs's solution. Prostacyclin has been identified in the pulmonary effluent by relaxation of bovine coronary artery strips, by disaggregation of platelet clumps, and by mass spectrometric quantification of the stable degradation product of prostacyclin, 6-oxo-$PGF_{1\alpha}$. The output of prostacyclin is blocked by cyclo-oxygenase inhibitors and is stimulated by low concentrations of arachidonic acid (100 ng/ml), angiotensin I, angiotension II or bradykinin.

The release of prostacyclin induced by angiotensin I is blocked by the converting enzyme inhibitor, captopril, in isolated guinea pig lungs, rat mesenteric vasculature (Dusting & Mullins 1980; Dusting et al. 1981; Grodzinska & Gryglewski 1980; Gryglewski 1979) and the pulmonary and renal circulation of anaesthetized dogs in vivo (Mullane & Moncada 1980a). Prostacyclin release induced by angiotensin I or II is also abolished by the receptor antagonists saralasin or [Sar¹–Ala⁸]-angiotensin II in both the rat and the dog (Dusting 1981a; Dusting et al. 1981; Gryglewski 1979). Thus, prostacyclin is released by activation of an angiotensin II receptor, and is not released directly by angiotensin I. Activation of the angiotensin II receptor appears to be linked to a phospholipase, since angiotensin II-stimulated prostacyclin release can be abolished by dexamethasone or mepacrine (Dusting 1981a).

Other peptides or amines tested do not release prostacyclin from perfused lungs (Gryglewski 1979). Noradrenalin and vasopressin do not release prostacyclin from rat mesenteric vessels, despite their potent vasoconstrictor effects (Dusting & Mullins 1980; Dusting et al. 1981). Moreover prostacyclin release into the circulation of the dog was not observed after injections of adrenalin, noradrenalin or 5-hydroxytryptamine (Mullane & Moncada 1980b), despite changes in systemic blood pressure.

Therefore, the release of prostacyclin induced by angiotensin and bradykinin does not appear to be a simple consequence of the mechanical events associated with alterations in vessel diameter. These observations, together with the finding that low concentrations of prostacyclin are released from the lungs in vivo, prompted the proposal that the pulmonary endothelium may be regarded as an endocrine organ regulating platelet behaviour (Gryglewski et al. 1978a, b; Moncada et al. 1978).

In rats and dogs, prostacyclin is a much more powerful vasodepressor agent than PGE_2, but only when the two substances are given intravenously, and not if they are given into the aorta (Armstrong et al. 1977, 1978). Using dogs, we showed by direct bioassay in circulating blood that prostacyclin escapes the pulmonary inactivation process (Dusting et al. 1977b), which normally removes 95 % or more of PGE_2 or $PGF_{2\alpha}$ in a single circulation in vivo. Thus, prostacyclin can recirculate (Dusting et al. 1978b). Furthermore, infused arachidonic acid is converted into prostacyclin in passage across the lung circulation in vivo (Dusting et al. 1978a; Mullane et al. 1979). Therefore, prostacyclin generated in the lung or elsewhere would not be confined to a local site of action, and is potentially a circulating hormone.

Gryglewski *et al.* (1978 *a*) developed a technique for continuously measuring platelet aggregation in circulating blood of anaesthetized cats, and showed that arterial blood contained higher concentrations of an anti-aggregatory substance than mixed venous blood. They concluded that the arterial–venous difference was due to prostacyclin released from the lungs since the difference was abolished by aspirin or by incubating the blood at 37 °C for 10 min, during which time prostacyclin activity disappears (Dusting *et al.* 1977 *b*, 1978 *b*). Moncada *et al.* (1978) applied this technique to anaesthetized rabbits, and came to the same conclusion, since the greater disaggregatory activity present in arterial blood was abolished by an antibody raised against 5,6-dihydro prostacyclin (6β-PGI_1), which cross-reacts with prostacyclin. Moreover, the prostacyclin-like, disaggregatory substance in arterial blood is increased during hyperventilation of the lungs, or after pulmonary embolism by intravenous injection of air (Gryglewski 1979). In a recent study, 6-oxo-$PGF_{1\alpha}$, measured by mass spectrometry, was at a higher concentration in the arterial than in the venous side of the circulation of five patients undergoing cardiac catheterization (Hensby *et al.* 1979 *a*). Thus, the lungs may constantly release small amounts of prostacyclin into the passing blood. This, combined with 50 % overall inactivation in one circulation through peripheral tissues (Dusting *et al.* 1978 *b*), would account for higher levels in arterial than in venous blood.

Three reservations about these results should be mentioned. First, in the studies with anaesthetized cats and rabbits, blood was drawn through an extracorporal circuit with a peristaltic pump. Under such conditions, the circulating blood volume would be slightly reduced and this may lead to a stimulation of the renin–angiotensin system, which in turn could stimulate prostacyclin release (see below). In addition, it is now well recognized that surgical procedures in anaesthetized small animals can exaggerate the contribution of prostaglandins to renal homoeostasis (Terragno *et al.* 1977), and by analogy, the same may be true for the lungs. Secondly, in these extracorporeal experiments platelet emboli dislodged from the collagen strips return to the animal in the venous blood. The trapping of platelet emboli in the lungs may be an additional stimulus for generation of prostacyclin under these conditions (Aiken 1979). Platelet emboli are also generated, and returned to the animal in other extracorporeal systems, particularly when venous blood is reoxygenated for bioassay on a cascade of smooth muscle strips. Thirdly, the biotransformation of prostacyclin in the human circulation is not yet fully understood, and the assumption that 6-oxo-$PGF_{1\alpha}$ determined in blood samples is a reliable index of concentrations of active prostacyclin in circulating blood may not be valid. Recent studies of human platelet aggregation performed within 3 min of withdrawal of arterial or venous blood (Steer *et al.* 1980) led to the conclusion that circulating levels of prostacyclin in resting man were too low to influence aggregability of platelets, but again it is important to note that these tests were performed *in vitro*. Studies in which levels of prostacyclin or its metabolites have been determined in man have failed to clarify the situation. Prostacyclin-like activity was detectable in human venous blood used to superfuse various tissues sensitive to prostacyclin (Neri Serneri *et al.* 1980). The level rose by several nanograms per millilitre with relief of ischaemia, and was reduced by pretreatment with indomethacin. However, in a study in which 6-oxo-$PGF_{1\alpha}$ in human blood samples was measured by mass spectrometry, levels of 80 pg/ml in venous blood and approximately double that in arterial blood were obtained (Hensby *et al.* 1979 *a*). Although these levels are lower than those achieved by bioassay, they are still much higher than those obtained by measuring the daily turnover in urine of a metabolite of prostacyclin (Oates *et al.* 1980). Further work is necessary to establish clearly the routes of catabolism of both prostacyclin and 6-oxo-PGF$_{1\alpha}$ in the human circulation, to determine whether there is an effective level of circulating prostacyclin in normal man at rest or during exercise.

Prostacyclin is the most potent endogenous inhibitor of platelet aggregation yet discovered. It is 30–40 times more potent than PGE$_1$ (Moncada & Vane 1977). and more than 1000 times more active than adenosine (Born 1962). *In vivo*, prostacyclin applied locally in low concentrations inhibits thrombus formation due to ADP in the microcirculation of the hamster cheek pouch (Higgs *et al.* 1977) and given systemically to the rabbit it prevents electrically induced thrombus formation in the carotid artery and increases bleeding time (Ubatuba *et al.* 1979). The duration of these effects *in vivo* in short: they disappear within 30 min of administration. Prostacyclin disaggregates platelets *in vitro* (Moncada *et al.* 1976 *b*; Ubatuba *et al.* 1979), in extracorporeal circuits where platelet clumps have formed on collagen strips (Gryglewski *et al.* 1978 *a*, *c*), and in the circulation of man (Szczeklik *et al.* 1978 *b*). Moreover, it inhibits thrombus formation in a coronary artery model in the dog when given locally or systemically (Aiken *et al.* 1979) and protects against sudden death (thought to be due to platelet aggregation) induced by intravenous arachidonic acid in rabbits (Bayer *et al.* 1979).

Prostacyclin is unstable and its activity disappears within 15 s on boiling or within 10 min at 22 °C at neutral pH. In blood at 37 °C, the activity of prostacyclin (as measured by bioassay on vascular smooth muscle) has a half-life of 2–3 min (Dusting *et al.* 1977 *b*, 1978 *b*). It has been reported that prostacyclin has an extended stability in plasma or blood (Gimeno *et al.* 1980; Wynalda & Fitzpatrick 1980) and that this may be associated with binding to albumin or with metabolism to 6-oxo-PGE$_1$ (Blasko *et al.* 1980). The relevance of these observations to the actual biological activity remains unclear. Alkaline pH increases the stability of prostacyclin (Cho & Allen 1978; Johnson *et al.* 1976) so that at pH 10.5 at 25 °C, it has a half-life of 100 h. It can be stabilized as a pharmaceutical preparation by freeze-drying and can be reconstituted in an alkaline glycine buffer for use in man.

The generation of prostacyclin is an active mechanism by which the vessel wall could be protected from deposition of platelet aggregates. Prostacyclin formation thus provides an explanation of the long recognized fact that contact with healthy vascular endothelium is not a stimulus for platelet clumping. An imbalance between formation of prostacyclin and TXA$_2$ could be of dramatic consequence.

Vascular damage leads to platelet adhesion but not necessarily to thrombus formation. When the injury is minor, platelet thrombi are formed which break away from the vessel wall and are washed away by the circulation. The degree of injury is an important determinant, and there is general agreement that for the development of thrombosis, severe damage or physical detachment of the endothelium must occur. All these observations are in accord with the differential distribution of prostacyclin synthetase across the vessel wall, decreasing in concentration from the intima to the adventitia (Moncada *et al.* 1977). Moreover, the proaggregating elements increase from the subendothelium to the adventitia. These two opposing tendencies render the endothelial lining anti-aggregatory and the outer layers of the vessel wall thrombogenic (Moncada *et al.* 1977).

The ability of the vascular wall actively to prevent aggregation has been postulated before (Saba & Mason 1974). For instance, the presence of an ADPase in the vessel wall has led to the suggestion that this enzyme, by breaking down ADP, limits platelet aggregation (Heyns *et al.* 1974; Lieberman *et al.* 1977). We have confirmed the presence of an ADPase in the vessel wall.

However, the anti-aggregating activity is mainly related to the release of prostacyclin, for 15-HPAA or 13-hydroperoxylinoleic acid (13-HPLA), two inhibitors of prostacyclin formation that have no activity on ADPase, abolish most if not all of the anti-aggregatory activity of vascular endothelial cells (Bunting et al. 1977). Similar results have been obtained with an antiserum which cross-reacts with and neutralizes prostacyclin in vitro (Bunting et al. 1978). Endothelial cells pretreated with this antiserum can no longer inhibit ADP-induced aggregation (Bunting et al. 1978; Christofinis et al. 1979).

It is not yet clear whether prostacyclin is responsible for all the thromboresistant properties of the vascular endothelium and it would be unusual for an important biological principle to rely on a single mechanism. However, Czervionke et al. (1979), using endothelial cell cultures, have demonstrated that platelet adherence in the presence of thrombin increases from 4 % to 44 % after treatment with 1 mM aspirin. This increase was accompanied by a decrease in 6-oxo-PGF$_{1\alpha}$ formation from 107 nM to less than 3 nM and could be reversed by addition of 25 nM endogenous prostacyclin. This suggests that prostacyclin, although not responsible for all the thromboresistant properties of vascular endothelium, plays an important role in the control of platelet aggregability.

Prostacyclin inhibits platelet aggregation (platelet–platelet interaction) at much lower concentrations than those needed to inhibit adhesion (platelet–collagen interaction) (Higgs et al. 1978a). This suggests that prostacyclin can allow platelets to stick to vascular tissue and to interact with it, while at the same time preventing or limiting thrombus formation. Certainly, platelets adhering to a site where prostacyclin synthetase is present could well feed the enzyme with endoperoxide, thereby producing prostacyclin and preventing other platelets from clumping onto the adhering platelets, limiting the cells to a monolayer. Weiss & Turitto (1979) have observed some degree of inhibition of platelet–endothelium interactions with low concentrations of prostacyclin at high shear rates, but at none of the concentrations used could they observe total inhibition of platelet adhesion.

Prostacyclin inhibits platelet aggregation by stimulating adenylate cyclase, leading to an increase in cAMP levels in the platelets (Gorman et al. 1977; Tateson et al. 1977). In this respect prostacyclin is much more potent than either PGE$_1$ or PGD$_2$ (Tateson et al. 1977). 6-Oxo-PGF$_{1\alpha}$ has relatively weak antiaggregatory activity and is almost devoid of activity on platelet cAMP (Tateson et al. 1977).

Prostacyclin is not only more potent than PGE$_1$ in elevating cAMP but the elevation persists longer. The elevation induced by PGE$_1$ in platelets in vitro starts falling after 30 s, while prostacyclin stimulation is not maximal until after 30 s. It is then maintained for 2 min after which it gradually wanes over 30 min (Gorman et al. 1977). Prostacyclin also strongly stimulates adenylate cyclase in isolated membrane preparations (Gorman et al. 1977).

Prostacyclin, PGE$_1$ and PGD$_2$ stimulate adenylate cyclase by acting on two distinct receptors on the platelet membrane (Miller & Gorman 1979; Whittle et al. 1978). PGE$_1$ and prostacyclin act on one, whereas PGD$_2$ acts on another. This is shown by differences in activity in different species (Whittle et al. 1978), and by the use of a prostaglandin antagonist (Eakins et al. 1976) that selectively prevents the inhibition of platelet aggregation induced by PGD$_2$ but not that induced by prostacyclin or PGE$_1$ (Whittle et al. 1978). Moreover, studies of agonist-specific sensitization of cAMP accumulation in platelets show that PGE$_1$ or PGE$_2$ can desensitize for subsequent PGE$_1$ or prostacyclin activation, and that subthreshold concentrations of prostacyclin desensitize for PGE$_1$ stimulation. PGD$_2$, however, desensitizes to a further dose of PGD$_2$ but not to PGE$_1$ or prostacyclin. These results suggest (Miller & Gorman 1979; Whittle *et al.* 1978) that the receptor in platelets previously described as a PGE$_1$ receptor (MacDonald & Stuart 1974) is, in fact, a prostacyclin receptor.

There have not been many detailed studies of the mechanism of action of prostacyclin. In contrast to TXA$_2$, it enhances Ca^{2+} sequestration (Kazer-Glanzman *et al.* 1977). Moreover, inhibitory effects on platelet phospholipase (Lapetina *et al.* 1977; Minkes *et al.* 1977) and platelet cyclo-oxygenase have been described (Malmsten *et al.* 1976). All these activities are related to its ability to increase cAMP levels in platelets. Moreover, prostacyclin inhibits endoperoxide-induced aggregation, which suggests additional sites of action still undefined but dependent on the cAMP effect (Minkes *et al.* 1977). These observations have extended and given important biological significance to the original observation of Vargaftig & Chignard (1975), who demonstrated that substances such as PGE$_1$ that increase cAMP in platelets inhibit the release of TXA$_2$ (measured as rabbit aorta contracting activity) in platelets. Prostacyclin, by inhibiting several steps in the activation of the arachidonic acid cascade, exerts an overall control of platelet aggregability *in vivo*.

The fact that prostacyclin increases cAMP levels in cells other than platelets (Gorman *et al.* 1979; Hopkins *et al.* 1978) and the possibility that in those cells an interaction with the thromboxane system could lead to a similar control of cell behaviour to that observed in platelets, suggests that the prostacyclin–thromboxane A$_2$ system has wider biological significance in cell regulation.

Prostacyclin relaxes *in vitro* most vascular strips, including rabbit coeliac and mesenteric arteries (Bunting *et al.* 1976), bovine coronary arteries (Dusting *et al.* 1977*a*; Needleman *et al.* 1978), human and baboon cerebral arteries (Boullin *et al.* 1979), and lamb ductus arteriosus (Coceani *et al.* 1978). Exceptions to this include the porcine coronary arteries (Dusting *et al.* 1977*c*), some strips of rat venous tissue, and isolated human saphenous vein (Levy 1978), which are weakly contracted by prostacyclin. Whether these same effects are induced in the corresponding circulations in the intact animals or man has not been studied. In the human umbilical arterial strip, prostacyclin induces a dose-dependent relaxation at low concentrations (less than 1 μM) and a dose-dependent contraction at higher concentrations (more than 10 μM) (Pomerantz *et al.* 1978). As mentioned earlier, prostacyclin, and not PGE$_2$, is the main metabolite of arachidonic acid in isolated vascular tissue, and this has led to an intense reassessment of the effects and role of arachidonic acid and its metabolites in vascular tissue and the cardiovascular system (for review see Dusting *et al.* 1979).

In their early experiments, Gryglewski *et al.* (1976) observed that a fatty acid peroxide, 15-hydroperoxyarachidonic acid, strongly and selectively inhibited prostacyclin synthetase, the enzyme responsible for the formation of prostacyclin from endoperoxides in vessel microsomes (i.c.$_{50}$ = 0.5 μg/ml). Other fatty acid hydroperoxides and their methyl esters also inhibit this enzyme (Moncada & Vane 1978; Salmon *et al.* 1978). Tranylcypromine, which is a well known inhibitor of enzymes not related to the metabolic pathway of arachidonic acid, is a somewhat weaker inhibitor of prostacyclin synthetase (i.c.$_{50}$ = 160 μg/ml) than are the fatty acid hydroperoxides (Gryglewski *et al.* 1976). Unfortunately, hydroperoxides of fatty acids are not useful tools for examining the role of endogenous prostacyclin biosynthesis *in vivo* (Dusting *et al.* 1978*c*), probably because they are rapidly reduced by enzymes such as glutathione peroxidase (Christopherson 1968). Other substances that inhibit prostacyclin synthetase in blood vessel microsomes include an analogue of prostaglandin endoperoxide (9,11-diaza- and 9,11-epoxyimino-prosta-5,12-dienoic acid) (Fitzpatrick *et al.* 1978), and a hydroperoxy derivative of indole (Terashita *et al.* 1979).

Prostaglandin endoperoxides are at the crossroads of arachidonic acid metabolism, for they are precursors of substances with opposing biological properties. On the one hand, TXA_2 produced by the platelets contracts large blood vessels and induces platelet aggregation; on the other prostacyclin produced by the vessel wall is a strong vasodilator and the most potent inhibitor of platelet aggregation known. Each substance has opposing effects on cAMP concentrations in platelets (Moncada & Vane 1979 *b*), thereby giving a balanced control mechanism which will therefore affect thrombus and haemostatic plug formation. Selective inhibition of the formation of TXA_2 should lead to an increased bleeding time and inhibition of thrombus formation, whereas inhibition of prostacyclin formation should be propitious for a 'prothrombotic state'. The amount of control exerted by this system can be tested, for selective inhibitors of each pathway have been described (see above and Moncada & Vane (1978) and Nijkamp *et al.* (1977)).

The use of aspirin as a pharmacological tool to investigate the interaction between these two substances has been fruitful. Aspirin is active against platelet cyclo-oxygenase *in vivo* and *in vitro*. Moreover, this effect is long lasting because aspirin acetylates the active site of the enzyme leading to irreversible inhibition (Roth & Majerus 1975; Roth & Siok 1978). Because platelets are unable to synthesize new protein (Marcus 1978), they cannot replace the cyclo-oxygenase. The inhibition will therefore only be overcome by new platelets coming into the circulation after the block of cyclo-oxygenase in megakaryocytes has worn off (Burch *et al.* 1978). Interestingly, the cyclo-oxygenase of vessel walls seems less sensitive to aspirin than that of platelets (Baenziger *et al.* 1977). Indeed, it has been suggested that indomethacin as well as aspirin may have restricted access to the cyclo-oxygenase that generates prostacyclin in the lung during stimulation by angiotensin (Dusting 1981 *a*, *b*). Thus, the secretion of prostacyclin into the circulation may be partly resistant to inhibition after single doses of these anti-inflammatory drugs.

Studies in rabbits and cats also suggest that administration of low doses of aspirin reduce the formation of TXA_2 more than that of prostacyclin (Amezcua *et al.* 1978; Korbut & Moncada 1978). Infusions of arachidonic acid in untreated animals had an antithrombotic effect and increased bleeding time. These effects were potentiated by small doses of aspirin (up to 10 mg/kg) and blocked by larger doses (20–200 mg/kg), which presumably inhibit formation of both prostacyclin and TXA_2.

Endothelial cells recover from aspirin inhibition more rapidly than do platelets in rabbits and rats (Kelton *et al.* 1978; Villa *et al.* 1979). Endothelial cells probably recover their ability to synthesize prostacyclin by regeneration of cyclo-oxygenase (Czervionke *et al.* 1978; Kelton *et al.* 1978), because recovery can be prevented by the protein synthesis inhibitor cycloheximide (Czervionke *et al.* 1979).

Until the discovery of prostacyclin, the use of aspirin as an antithrombotic agent based on its effects on platelets seemed logical (Majerus 1976), although the results of clinical trials were inconclusive (Verstraete 1976). Now, however, the situation needs further clarification, especially with respect to the optimal dose of aspirin. Aspirin in large doses (200 mg/kg) increases thrombus formation in a model of venous thrombosis in the rabbit (Kelton *et al.* 1978), and *in vitro* treatment of endothelial cells with aspirin enhances thrombin-induced platelet adherence to them (Czervionke *et al.* 1978). In addition, there is an inverse correlation between the amount of prostacyclin produced by the tissue on the one hand, and platelet adhesion or aggregation on the other. Moreover, aspirin treatment of arterial tissue *in vitro* increases its thrombogenicity (Baumgartner & Tschopp 1979).

In man, O'Grady & Moncada (1978) showed that a small single dose of aspirin (0.3 g) increased bleeding time 2 h after ingestion, whereas a large dose (3.9 g) had no effect. Some workers have confirmed these results (Rajah *et al.* 1978), but others have been unable to do so (Godal *et al.* 1979). The variability might be linked to the differences in methodology or to the age of the subjects. Indeed, Jorgensen *et al.* (1979, 1980) showed that the cutaneous bleeding time in man decreases with age and the response to aspirin varies according to the age, being prolonged in young male volunteers and not in older subject. Moreover, platelet aggregation and TXA_2 formation are blocked 2 h after a single dose of aspirin (3.9 g). The bleeding time is unchanged at that time, but 24 and 72 h after aspirin it is increased and slowly recovers towards pretreatment levels over a period of 168 h, in a manner that mirrors the recovery of TXA_2 formation and platelet aggregability (Amezcua *et al.* 1979). An extension of the concept comes from the demonstration that tranylcypromine, an inhibitor of prostacyclin formation, enhances platelet aggregation in an experimental model of thrombosis in the microcirculation of the brain of the mouse (Rosenblum & El-Sabban 1978).

All these results show that the prostacyclin–thromboxane balance is an important mechanism of control of platelet aggregability *in vivo*. Clearly, manipulation of this control mechanism might lead to prothrombotic or antithrombotic states of clinical relevance. In this context it is interesting that Mustard's group has shown that hydrocortisone treatment of normal or thrombocytopenic rats blocks prostacyclin formation in the vessel wall and decreases the bleeding time (Blajchman *et al.* 1979), a result that would be expected because steroids prevent activation of phospholipase (Flower 1978), and should thereby inhibit the vascular release of prostacyclin induced by substances that release endogenous arachidonic acid, such as angiotension.

Attempts to measure, in man, TXB_2 and prostacyclin or 6-oxo-$PGF_{1\alpha}$ after different aspirin dose schedules have confirmed the higher sensitivity of platelet cyclo-oxygenase to aspirin. Masotti *et al.* (1979) found that aspirin at 3.0–3.5 mg/kg gave, in a sample removed 2 h later, a 50 % inhibition of *ex vivo* platelet aggregation by several agents, while 5.0 mg/kg was needed for 50 % inhibition of prostacyclin formation as measured by cascade superfusion bioassay. It has also recently been demonstrated that a single daily dose of aspirin (160 mg) reduced significantly (by 40 %) the incidence of thrombosis over a 5 month observation period in artificial arterio-venous shunts in patients (Harter *et al.* 1979).

From all these results it is clear that a selective inhibitor of thromboxane formation should now be tested for antithrombotic efficacy (Moncada & Vane 1977, 1978), because theoretically this provides an advantage over aspirin in allowing prostacyclin formation by vessel walls or other cells either from their own endoperoxides or from those released by platelets. This should be the main criterion for determining a 'superior' mechanism of action over a small dose of aspirin. Studies *in vivo* are not yet available, but Needleman *et al.* (1979) made the observation that when platelets were treated with a thromboxane synthetase inhibitor *in vitro*, endoperoxides were available for utilization by the vessel wall. Interestingly, in the presence of a thromboxane synthetase inhibitor, arachidonic acid or collagen added to blood *in vitro* lead to the formation of 6-oxo-$PGF_{1\alpha}$ rather than TXB_2. Platelets cannot synthesize prostacyclin, so some other cell in the blood must have done so (Blackwell *et al.* 1978; Flower & Cardinal 1979).

These results support our suggestion that thromboxane synthetase inhibitors might have a superior antithrombotic effect to simple cyclo-oxygenase inhibitors (Moncada & Vane 1977, 1978). It is important to realize at this stage, however, that all these observations have been made *in vitro*, and that *in vivo* experiments are necessary to clarify further the nature of the interaction between platelets and normal or damaged vessel walls.

Whether other drugs exert their antithrombotic effect by acting on the prostacyclin–thromboxane system is not yet known, but studies with the use of sulphinpyrazone in cultured endothelial cells (Gordon & Pearson 1978) and ticlopidine given orally to rats (Ashida & Abiko 1978) suggest that these compounds have little or no effect on prostacyclin formation at concentrations at which they affect platelet behaviour. A compound that might stimulate prostacyclin formation in humans after oral ingestion has also been described (Vermylen *et al.* 1979).

Selective inhibition of prostacyclin formation by lipid peroxides could also lead to a condition in which platelet aggregation is increased; this could play a role in the development of atherosclerosis. Indeed, lipid peroxidation takes place as a non-enzymic reaction (Harman & Piette 1966), and it is known to occur in certain pathological conditions (Slater 1972). Hence, lipid peroxides present in these conditions could be shifting the balance of the system in favour of TXA_2 and predisposing to thrombus formation.

The role of lipid peroxides in the development of atherosclerosis has been debated for almost 30 years, since Glavind *et al.* (1952) described the presence of lipid peroxides in human atherosclerotic aortae. They found the peroxide content in diseased arteries to be directly proportional to the severity of the atherosclerosis. Subsequent investigations by Woodford *et al.* (1965) suggested that Glavind's findings were based on artefacts, ascribing the presence of lipid peroxides to their formation during the preparative procedure. Despite this, the presence of conjugated diene hydroperoxides in lipids of human atheroma has again been reported (Fukazumi 1965; Fukazumi & Iwata 1963), and lipid peroxides have been found in atherosclerotic rabbit aortae (Iwakami 1965) subjected to an extraction procedure that avoids lipid peroxidation *in vitro*. Some authors (Brooks *et al.* 1971; Harland *et al.* 1971) favour the suggestion that lipid peroxides do accumulate in atherosclerotic plaques, whether or not these peroxides act by inhibiting prostacyclin formation and as a consequence reduce the arteries' defence mechanism. This theory is of interest especially since other substances related to atherosclerosis such as the cholesterol carriers, the low-density lipoproteins (LDLs), also inhibit prostacyclin formation in endothelial cell cultures (Nordoy *et al.* 1978).

Gryglewski and coworkers (Dembinska *et al.* 1977) have found that there is a substantial reduction in prostacyclin formation in the vascular tissue of rabbits made atherosclerotic, and more recently there has been a report that human tissue obtained from atherosclerotic plaque does not produce prostacyclin, whereas tissue obtained from a normal vessel does (D'Angelo *et al.* 1978). Sinzinger *et al.* (1979) have also shown that different types of atherosclerotic lesions ranging from fatty streaks to complicated lesions all produced much less prostacyclin than normal arteries. Nordoy *et al.* (1978) have shown that low-density lipoproteins inhibit prostacyclin formation. Gryglewski *et al.* (unpublished observations) have recently confirmed this link by their finding that LDLs contain high concentrations of lipid peroxides. High-density lipoproteins (HDLs), on the other hand, prevent the inhibitory effect of LDLs on prostacyclin formation. From epidemiological studies there is a positive correlation between the plasma concentration of LDLs and the risk of developing clinical coronary heart disease (Medalie *et al.* 1973), but a stronger, inverse relation has recently been demonstrated between HDL–cholesterol levels and coronary heart disease (Havel 1979). Since the mechanisms relating changes in plasma lipoproteins to increased tendency for thrombosis have not yet been adequately defined, the interaction of lipoproteins with prostacyclin biosynthesis promises to be an exciting area for further study.

Before the discovery of prostacyclin, it was suggested that the use of dietary dihomo-γ-linolenic acid, the precursor of the monoenoic series of prostaglandins, could be an approach to the prevention of thrombosis, because PGG_1 and TXA_1 are not proaggregating and PGE_1 is anti-aggregating (Willis *et al.* 1974). Other reports tend to agree with this proposal (Sim & McCraw 1977), but there is some doubt, because feeding rabbits with dihomo-γ-linolenic acid leads to an increase in the tissue content of this acid without change in platelet responsiveness, at least to ADP (Oelz *et al.* 1976). The main criticism of all this work, including that of human platelets (Kernoff *et al.* 1977), is that the conclusions are based on studies performed *in vitro* in which platelets are studied as isolated cells without contact with vessel walls.

It is now evident that the use of dihomo-γ-linolenic acid in an attempt to direct the synthetic machinery of the platelets is not the most rational approach for the prevention of thrombosis. This is because the endoperoxides PGG_1 and PGH_1 are not substrates for prostacyclin synthetase; indeed, they or their precursor might adversely affect the prostacyclin protective mechanism. Eicosapentaenoic acid (C20:5ω3), the precursor of the trienoic prostaglandins, could, however, act as a precursor for an antiaggregating agent, $\Delta\text{-}^{17}$prostacyclin (PGI_3), and it is known that C20:5ω3 is itself a weak anti-aggregating agent. TXA_3, if generated, is a weaker proaggregating agent than TXA_2 (Gryglewski *et al.* 1979). Thus, the use of this fatty acid could afford a dietary protection against thrombosis. Indeed, it has been suggested that the low incidence of myocardial infarction in Eskimos and their increased tendency to bleed could be due to the high eicosapentaenoic acid and low arachidonate content of their diet and consequently of their tissue lipid (Dyerberg *et al.* 1978). In Greenland Eskimos, there is an elevated content of C20:5ω3 (compared with Danes) in the platelet lipids and a prolonged bleeding time. Furthermore, their platelets are resistant to aggregation (Dyerberg & Bang 1979). In a recent study in which thrombosis and subsequent infarction were induced in dogs, dietary supplementation with fish oil resulted in a more normal electrocardiogram pattern and a reduced infarction size compared with the control group (Culp *et al.* 1980). The understanding of the role of fatty acids and their oxidized products in thrombosis and/or atherosclerosis is, however, at an early stage, and much experimental and clinical work is needed before the full picture emerges (see also Dyerberg, this symposium).

β-Thromboglobulin is a small protein related to platelet factor IV and is stored in the α-granules of platelets and released with other granular constituents during aggregation or adherence of the platelets to a damaged vessel wall (Moore *et al.* 1975). Hope *et al.* (1979) demonstrated that β-thromboglobulin inhibits formation of prostacyclin by bovine aortic endothelial cells in culture, at concentrations that are exceeded locally during platelet aggregation and release. Platelet factor IV does not have this action (Hope *et al.* 1979). This phenomenon may be an important component of the process of thrombosis, but the precise mechanism of inhibition has not been determined.

MacIntyre *et al.* (1978) have found in cell-free plasma a factor that stimulates prostacyclin production by pig aortic endothelial cells. Thrombin, trypsin and a calcium ionophore have also been shown to stimulate prostacyclin formation in human endothelial cells (Weksler *et al.* 1978). The mechanism of action and significance of these factors in regulating prostacyclin biosynthesis has yet to be established. Finally, unidentified factors that inhibit prostacyclin formation have been found in renal cortex (Terragno *et al.* 1978) and in a microsomal fraction of rat placenta (Harrowing & Williams 1979). Both these inhibitors appear to act at the cyclo-oxygenase level and they may be related to a similar endogenous cyclo-oxygenase inhibitor found in plasma (Saeed *et al.* 1977). More work is necessary to define the significance and function of these factors.

Increased production of prostaglandin endoperoxides or TXB_2 *in vitro* by platelets has been found in blood from patients with arterial thrombosis, deep venous thrombosis or recurrent thrombosis; these conditions are associated with a shortened platelet survival time (Lagarde & Dechavanne 1977). In addition, increased sensitivity of platelets to aggregating agents and increased release of TXB_2 has been described in rabbits made atherosclerotic by diet (Shimamoto *et al.* 1978) and in patients who survived myocardial infarction (Szczeklik *et al.* 1978 a). An increased level of TXB_2 in blood has been observed in patients with Prinzmetal's angina (Lewy *et al.* 1979). Moreover, platelets from rats made diabetic release more TXB_2 than platelets from normal rats (Harrison *et al.* 1978; Johnson *et al.* 1978).

Changes in prostacyclin production associated with disease have also been postulated. An increased production in uraemic patients has been suggested to explain their haemostatic defect (Remuzzi *et al.* 1977). On the other hand, a lack of prostacyclin production has been suggested in patients with idiopathic thrombocytopaenic purpura (Remuzzi *et al.* 1978), and a recent report suggests the absence of detectable levels of 6-oxo-$PGF_{1\alpha}$ in humans suffering from this condition (Hensby *et al.* 1979 b). Both diseases may be linked by the accumulation during uraemia or the lack of production during idiopathic thrombocytopaenic purpura of a 'plasma factor' that stimulates prostacyclin synthesis (MacIntyre *et al.* 1978). A lower release of prostacyclin by the blood vessels of rats made diabetic has also been described (Harrison *et al.* 1978; Johnson *et al.* 1978): this decreased production can be corrected by chronic insulin treatment (Harrison *et al.* 1978). Prostacyclin production by blood vessels from patients with diabetes is also lower than normal (Johnson *et al.* 1979), and circulating levels of 6-oxo-$PGF_{1\alpha}$ are reduced in diabetic patients with proliferative retinopathy (Dollery *et al.* 1979).

Pace-Asciak *et al.* (1978) demonstrated that aortae from spontaneously hypertensive rats of the Japanese strain generate more prostacyclin than aortae from normotensive rats when incubated with exogenous arachidonic acid *in vitro*. Furthermore, Armstrong *et al.* (1976) found that prostaglandin endoperoxide (PGH_2) has a greater hypotensive effect in genetically hypotensive rats of the New Zealand strain than in normotensive controls, whereas PGE_2 had a similar hypotensive action in the two strains. These results indicate that PGH_2 may be more readily converted to prostacyclin in hypertensive rats, and it has been suggested that the greater formation of prostacyclin in blood vessels represents an adaptive mechanism to the elevated arterial pressure (Pace-Asciak *et al.* 1978). However, chronic treatment with indomethacin or aspirin does not alter arterial pressure in spontaneously hypertensive rats (Antonaccio *et al.* 1979; DiNicolantonio *et al.* 1981), although it does markedly reduce the vasodepressor action of intravenous arachidonic acid (DiNicolantonio *et al.* 1981).

It is interesting that plasma exchange in patients suffering from hypertension as a complication of haemolytic uraemic syndrome restored a 'prostacyclin stimulating factor', and led to improved control of blood pressure (Remuzzi *et al.* 1978). Moreover, others have reported that plasma exchange has an antihypertensive effect in patients with glomerulonephritis and essential hypertension (Whitworth *et al.* 1978). These observations suggest that essential hypertension in man may be associated with impairment, rather than enhancement, of prostacyclin formation in the vasculature. Clearly, more work is necessary to define any role of prostacyclin in the experimental models of hypertension in the rat, and to substantiate the relevance of development of hypertension in the rat to essential hypertension in man.

Intra-arterial thrombus formation and haemostatic plug formation have been described in general terms as equivalent phenomena (Mustard & Packham 1975). It is, however, possible that the relative importance of prostacyclin and TXA_2 in these conditions is different, because prostacyclin, at least under some conditions, is an unstable circulating hormone (Gryglewski *et al.* 1978*a*; Moncada *et al.* 1978) as well as a locally generated one. Its role in controlling intra-arterial thrombus formation might be more important than that of TXA_2, which seems to be generated only after strong interaction between aggregating platelets or by their interaction with vessel wall materials.

As far as aspirin is concerned, more information is needed on the rate of recovery of the endothelial cyclo-oxygenase *in vivo* after single doses of aspirin. Equally important is the assessment of any cumulative effect of a multiple-dose régime on platelet and endothelial cyclo-oxygenase, to establish the optimal interval of administration. The demonstration of the ability of aspirin to prevent thromboembolism in some circumstances but not in others (Jobin 1978; Verstraete 1976) may suggest a qualitative or quantitative difference in the underlying pathophysiology. Further clinical trials should be conducted in which aspirin is given at low doses either alone or combined with phosphodiesterase inhibitors such as dipyridamole. Ideally, a selective inhibitor of thromboxane synthetase should be developed to be used alone or in combination with phosphodiesterase inhibitors (Moncada & Vane 1978).

A more direct approach to antithrombotic therapy, however, would be to control platelet cAMP; increasing platelet cAMP inhibits most forms of aggregation whether or not they are dependent on arachidonic acid metabolic products. Since prostacyclin is the most powerful substance known in both preventing aggregation and increasing platelet cAMP (Gorman *et al.* 1977; Tateson *et al.* 1977), prostacyclin or an analogue, alone or in combination with a phosphodiesterase inhibitor, should be a more comprehensive approach to the control of platelet aggregation *in vivo*. Alternatively, drugs that stimulate endogenous prostacyclin production (Vermylen *et al.* 1979) could be developed. Several of these possibilities are at present being explored.

Prostacyclin or chemical analogues may find a use as a 'hormone replacement' therapy in conditions such as atherosclerosis, acute myocardial infarction or 'crescendo angina' and other states in which excessive platelet aggregation may take place in the circulation or in specific areas such as in organ transplants. Moreover, we have suggested its use in extracorporeal circulations such as cardiopulmonary bypass and renal dialysis (Moncada & Vane 1979*a*). In these systems the main problems are platelet loss with the formation of micro-aggregates which, when returning to the patient in bypass, are responsible for the cerebral and renal impairment observed after operation (Abel *et al.* 1976; Branthwaite 1972). In addition, there are side effects associated with the chronic use of heparin, especially the development of osteoporosis (Griffith *et al.* 1965).

Several anti-platelet drugs have been proposed to deal with these two problems and some have been used with moderate success. PGE_1 has been reported to be beneficial during cardiopulmonary bypass in dogs (Balanowski *et al.* 1977). However, prostaglandins of the E type induce diarrhoea (Main & Whittle 1975), an effect not shared by prostacyclin (Robert *et al.* 1979; Ubatuba *et al.* 1979). Therefore, prostacyclin is not only more potent but more specific in achieving platelet protection. Prostacyclin has proved beneficial in several systems of extra-corporeal circulation in experimental animals, including renal dialysis, cardiopulmonary by-pass and charcoal haemoperfusion (Bunting *et al.* 1979; Coppe *et al.* 1979; Longmore *et al.* 1979; Woods *et al.* 1978). In one of these systems (renal dialysis), prostacyclin can replace heparin altogether (Woods *et al.* 1978). In charcoal haemoperfusion, heparin is also necessary since charcoal seems to activate the clotting cascade directly (Bunting *et al.* 1979).

Prostacyclin has potent effects on platelets and on the cardiovascular system in man (Szczeklik *et al.* 1978 *b*). During infusion of prostacyclin in healthy volunteers for 60 min at rates ranging from 2 to 16 ng kg^{-1} min^{-1} there was a dose-related inhibition of platelet aggregation measured in platelet-rich plasma and in whole blood (O'Grady *et al.* 1979). Similar inhibition of platelet aggregation was seen when the responses were measured 15 or 45 min after starting the infusion. At infusions of 8 ng kg^{-1} min^{-1}, partial inhibition of aggregation was demonstrable for up to 105 min after the end of infusion, and this persistence of effect on platelets has recently been confirmed (Chierchia *et al.* 1979). Template bleeding time was not significantly increased though Szczeklik *et al.* (1978 *b*) found an approximate doubling of bleeding time in response to prostacyclin at 20 ng kg^{-1} min^{-1}.

Prostacyclin disperses circulating platelet aggregates (Szczeklik *et al.* 1978 *b*). Significant inhibition of platelet aggregation induced by ADP was seen (FitzGerald *et al.* 1979) when prostacyclin was administered under blind conditions at rates of 4 and 8 ng kg^{-1} min^{-1}. Other haematological variables such as platelet count, platelet factor 3 concentration, accelerated partial thromboplastin time, prothrombin time, euglobin clot lysis time, concentration of fibrinogen degradation products and blood glucose were not affected by prostacyclin (O'Grady *et al.* 1979; Szczeklik *et al.* 1978 *b*).

It was originally suggested (Szczeklik *et al.* 1978 *b*) that prostacyclin had direct positive chronotropic and inotropic effects in man. However, in a double blind controlled study with the use of prostacyclin up to 4 ng kg^{-1} min^{-1} an increase in heart rate accompanied by decrease in diastolic blood pressure, pre-ejection period and QS_2 index was observed (Warrington & O'Grady 1980). Systolic blood pressure, left ventricular ejection time index and the normalized first derivative of the apex cardiogram were unaltered by prostacyclin. These findings were consistent with an arteriolar vasodilator effect of prostacyclin, which would be expected to lower diastolic and mean blood pressure and thus reflexly increase heart rate and contractility.

When heart rate was increased by more than 10 % over control values during prostacyclin infusion, peripheral temperature measured at the great toe increased by 1–6 K (O'Grady *et al.* 1979). Increases in skin temperature as well as facial flushing were also observed at rates of 2–5 ng kg^{-1} min^{-1} (Szczeklik *et al.* 1978 *b*). Facial flushing invariably occurs at doses above 4 ng kg^{-1} min^{-1} when an increase in heart rate of more than 10 % is recorded (O'Grady *et al.* 1979). This flushing limits the extent to which double blind studies with prostacyclin can be performed.

The cardiovascular effects of prostacyclin are shorter-lived than those on platelets and dis-appear within 15 min of the end of infusion (O'Grady *et al.* 1979). Plasma renin activity rises significantly during prostacyclin infusion but plasma noradrenalin and plasma aldosterone levels did not change significantly (FitzGerald *et al.* 1979).

Renal blood flow measured by using ^{125}I-hippuran increased in response to an infusion of prostacyclin (6 ng kg^{-1} min^{-1}) that caused a small reduction in diastolic blood pressure, while the glomerular filtration rate measured by using ^{51}Cr-EDTA remained unchanged (J. Henry & J. O'Grady, unpublished).

Headache has been reported when doses greater than 8 ng kg^{-1} min^{-1} are administered (FitzGerald et al. 1979; O'Grady et al. 1979; Szczeklik et al. 1978b). Colicky central abdominal discomfort has been less frequently experienced but was reproducible in one subject (O'Grady et al. 1979). The precise mechanism of these gastrointestinal effects is unclear. It may be that they reflect the contraction of human gastrointestinal smooth muscle by prostacyclin; they may also be vagally mediated or represent secondary effects of prostacyclin or of its metabolic products.

Ill-defined sensations of unease and restlessness have been experienced by subjects receiving higher infusion rates of prostacyclin (Chierchia et al. 1979; O'Grady et al. 1979; Szczeklik et al. 1978b). In two subjects, the administration of prostacyclin at the rate of 50 ng kg^{-1} min^{-1} (Szczeklik et al. 1978b) caused sudden weakness with pallor and nausea, a fall in systolic and diastolic blood pressure and bradycardia. It is possible that this effect is mediated by a vagal reflex, which has been observed in dogs (Chapple et al. 1978a, b).

Following reports that PGE$_1$ has been used successfully in the treatment of peripheral vascular disease (Carlson & Olsson 1976), prostacyclin has been shown to have a similar effect, producing a long-lasting increase in muscle blood flow, disappearance of ischaemic pain and healing of trophic ulcers after an intra-arterial infusion to the affected limb for 3 days (Szczeklik et al. 1979). In a subsequent trial in 30 patients, symptoms were alleviated in 22 patients; this improvement was sustained for up to 15 months in 12 of them (Szczeklik et al. 1980; see also Gryglewski et al., this symposium).

Recently, the first report (Gimson et al. 1980) on the use of prostacyclin during charcoal haemoperfusion in humans has demonstrated that there is a protection against platelet loss and activation (assessed by the prevention of the release into the plasma of β-thromboglobulin). These are basically the results obtained in clinical trials with prostacyclin in cardiopulmonary bypass operations (Bunting et al. 1981; Walker et al. 1980; see also Longmore, this symposium). Many other uses of prostacyclin are yet to be explored in clinical conditions. One of them is its use in transplant surgery, where in animals, prostacyclin added to the washing solution normally used to flush the donor kidney before transplant improved the efficacy (Munday et al. 1981). Prostacyclin also protected against hyperacute kidney rejection in a dog model (Munday et al. 1980). Results in these and other areas will certainly be produced in the near future.

REFERENCES (Moncada & Vane)

Abel, R. M., Buckley, M. J., Austen, W. G., Barnett, G. O., Beck, C. H. & Fischer, J. E. 1976 Etiology, incidence and prognosis of a prospective analysis of 500 consecutive patients. J. thorac. cardiovasc. Surg. 71, 323–333.

Aiken, J. W. 1979 See Discussion following 'Is the lung an endocrine organ that secretes prostacyclin?', by R. J. Gryglewski. In Prostacyclin (ed. J. R. Vane & S. Bergström), p. 287. New York: Raven Press.

Aiken, J. W., Gorman, R. R. & Shebuski, R. J. 1979 Prevention of blockage of partially obstructed coronary arteries with prostacyclin correlates with inhibition of platelet aggregation. Prostaglandins 17, 483–494.

Aiken, J. W. & Vane, J. R. 1973 Intrarenal prostaglandin release attenuates the renal vasoconstrictor activity of angiotensin. J. Pharmac. exp. Ther. 184, 678–687.

Amezcua, J.-L., O'Grady, J., Salmon, J. A. & Moncada, S. 1979 Prolonged paradoxical effect of aspirin on platelet behaviour and bleeding time in man. Thromb. Res. 16, 69–79.

Amezcua, J.-L., Parsons, M. & Moncada, S. 1978 Unstable metabolites of arachidonic acid, aspirin and the formation of the haemostatic plug. Thromb. Res. 13, 477–488.

Antonaccio, M. J., Harris, D., Goldenberg, H., High, J. P. & Rubin, B. 1979 The effects of captopril, propranolol and indomethacin on blood pressure and plasma renin activity in spontaneously hypertensive and normotensive rats. *Proc. Soc. exp. Biol. Med.* **162**, 429–433.

Armstrong, J. M., Boura, A. L. A., Hamberg, M. & Samuelsson, B. 1976 A comparison of the vasodepressor effects of the cyclic endoperoxides PGG_2 and PGH_2 with those of PGD_2 and PGE_2 in hypertensive and normotensive rats. *Eur. J. Pharmac.* **39**, 251–258.

Armstrong, J. M., Chapple, D. J., Dusting, G. J., Hughes, R., Moncada, S. & Vane, J. R. 1977 Cardiovascular actions of prostacyclin (PGI_2) in chloralose anaesthetized dogs. *Br. J. Pharmac.* **61**, 136P.

Armstrong, J. M., Lattimer, N., Moncada, S. & Vane, J. R. 1978 Comparison of the vasodepressor effects of prostacyclin and 6-oxo-prostaglandin $F_{1\alpha}$ with those of prostaglandin E_2 in rats and rabbits. *Br. J. Pharmac.* **62**, 125–130.

Ashida, S.-I. & Abiko, Y. 1978 Effect of ticlopidine and acetylsalicylic acid on generation of prostaglandin I_2-like substance in rat arterial tissue. *Thromb. Res.* **13**, 901–908.

Baenziger, N. L., Dillender, M. J. & Majerus, P. 1977 Cultured human skin fibroblasts and arterial cells produce a labile platelet-inhibitory prostaglandin. *Biochem. biophys. Res. Commun.* **78**, 294–301.

Balanowski, P. J. P., Bauer, J., Machiedo, G. & Neville, W. E. 1977 Prostaglandin influence on pulmonary intravascular leukocytic aggregation during cardiopulmonary bypass. *J. thorac. cardiovasc. Surg.* **73**, 221–224.

Baumgartner, H. R. & Tschopp, Th.B. 1979 Platelet interaction with aortic sub-endothelium (S.E.) in vitro. Locally produced PGI_2 inhibits adhesion and formation of mural thrombi in flowing blood. In *Thrombosis and haemostasis abstracts* (VII Int. Congress on Thrombosis and Haemostasis), p. 6.

Bayer, B. L., Blass, K. E. & Förster, W. 1979 Antiaggregatory effect of prostacyclin (PGI_2) *in vivo. Br. J. Pharmac.* **66**, 10–12.

Best, L. C., Martin, T. J., Russell, R. G. G. & Preston, F. E. 1977 Prostacyclin increases cyclic AMP levels and adenylate cyclase activity in platelets. *Nature, Lond.* **267**, 850–851.

Blackwell, G. J., Flower, R. J., Russell-Smith, N., Salmon, J. A., Thorogood, P. B. & Vane, J. R. 1978 I-*n*-Butylimidazole: a potent and selective inhibitor of 'thromboxane synthetase'. *Br. J. Pharmac.* **64**, 436P.

Blajchman, M.A., Senyi, A. F., Hirsh, J., Surya, Y., Buchanan, M. & Mustard, J. F. 1979 Shortening of the bleeding time in rabbits by hydrocortisone caused by inhibition of prostacyclin generation by the vessel wall. *J. clin. Invest.* **63**, 1026–1035.

Blasko, G., Nemesanszky, E., Szabo, G., Stadier, I. & Palos, L. A. 1980. The effects of PGI_2 and PGI_2 analogues with increased stability on platelet cAMP and aggregation. *Thromb. Res.* **17**, 673–681.

Blumberg, A. L., Denny, S. E., Marshall, G. R. & Needleman, P. 1977 Blood vessel hormone interactions: angiotensin, bradykinin and prostaglandins. *Am. J. Physiol.* **232**, H303–310.

Born, G. V. R. 1962 Aggregation of blood platelets by adenosine diphosphate and its reversal. *Nature, Lond.* **194**, 927–929.

Boullin, D. J., Bunting, S., Blaso, W. P., Hunt, T. M. & Moncada, S. 1979 Response of human and baboon arteries to prostaglandin endoperoxides and biologically generated and synthetic prostacyclin: their relevance to cerebral arterial spasm in man. *Br. J. clin. Pharmac.* **7**, 139–147.

Branthwaite, M. A. 1972 Neurological damage related to open heart surgery. *Thorax* **27**, 748–753.

Brooks, C. J. W., Steel, G., Gilbert, J. D. & Harland, W. A. 1971 Lipids of human atheroma. 4. Characteristics of a new group of polar sterol esters from human atherosclerotic plaques. *Atherosclerosis* **13**, 223–237.

Bunting, S., Gryglewski, R., Moncada, S. & Vane, J. R. 1976 Arterial walls generate from prostaglandin endoperoxides a substance (prostaglandin X) which relaxes strips of mesenteric and coeliac arteries and inhibits platelet aggregation. *Prostaglandins* **12**, 897–913.

Bunting, S., Moncada, S., Reed, P., Salmon, J. A. & Vane, J. R. 1978 An antiserum to 5,6-dihydro prostacyclin (PGI_1) which also binds prostacyclin. *Prostaglandins* **15**, 565–574.

Bunting, S., Moncada, S. & Vane, J. R. 1977 Antithrombotic properties of vascular endothelium. *Lancet* ii, 1075–1076.

Bunting, S., Moncada, S., Vane, J. R., Woods, H. F. & Weston, M. J. 1979 Prostacyclin improves hemocompatability during charcoal hemoperfusion. In *Prostacyclin* (ed. J. R. Vane & S. Bergström), pp. 361–369. New York: Raven Press.

Bunting, S., O'Grady, J., Moncada, S., Vane, J. R., Fabiani, J. N., Terrier, E. & Dubost, C. 1981 The use of prostacyclin in cardiopulmonary bypass. (In preparation.)

Burch, J. W., Stanford, N. & Majerus, P. W. 1978 Inhibition of platelet prostaglandin synthetase by oral aspirin. *J. clin. Invest.* **61**, 314–319.

Carlson, L. A. & Olsson, A. G. 1976 Intravenous prostaglandin E_1 in severe peripheral vascular disease. *Lancet* ii, p. 810.

Chapple, D. J., Dusting, G. J., Hughes, R. & Vane, J. R. 1978*a* A vagal reflex contributes to the hypotensive effect of prostacyclin in anaesthetized dogs. *J. Physiol., Lond.* **281**, 43–44P.

Chapple, D. J., Dusting, G. J., Hughes, R. & Vane, J. R. 1978*b* Some direct and reflex cardiovascular actions of prostacyclin (PGI_2) and PGE_2 in anaesthetized dogs. *Br. J. Pharmac.* **68**, 437–447.

Chierchia, S., Ciabattoni, G., Cinotti, G., Maseri, A., Patrono, C., Pulgiese, F., Distante, A., Simonetti, I. & Bernini, W. 1979 Haemodynamic and antiaggregatory effects of prostacyclin (PGI_2) in the healthy man. *Circulation* **59-60**, suppl. II, p. 83.

Cho, M. J. & Allen, M. A. 1978 Chemical stability of prostacyclin (PGI₂) in aqueous solutions. *Prostaglandins* **25**, 943–954.

Christofinis, G. J., Moncada, S., Bunting, S. & Vane, J. R. 1979 Prostacyclin (PGI₂) release by rabbit aorta and human umbilical vein endothelial cells after prolonged subculture. In *Prostacyclin* (ed. J. R. Vane & S. Bergström), pp. 77–84. New York: Raven Press.

Christopherson, B. O. 1968 Formation of monohydroxypolenic fatty acids from lipid peroxides by a glutathione peroxidase. *Biochim. biophys. Acta* **164**, 35.

Coceani, F., Bishai, I., White, E., Bodach, E. & Olley, P. M. 1978 Action of prostaglandins, endoperoxides and thromboxanes on the lamb ductus arteriosus. *Am. J. Physiol.* **234**, H117–H122.

Coppe, D., Wonders, T., Snider, M. & Salzman, E. W. 1979 Preservation of platelet number and function during extracorporeal membrane oxygenation (ECMO) by regional infusion of prostacyclin. In *Prostacyclin* (ed. J. R. Vane & S. Bergström), pp. 371–383. New York: Raven Press.

Culp, B. R., Lands, W. E. M., Lucchesi, B. R., Pitt, B. & Romson, J. 1980 The effect of dietary supplementation of fish oil on experimental myocardial infarction. *Prostaglandins* **20**, 1021–1031.

Czervionke, R. L., Hoak, J. C. & Fry, G. L. 1978 Effect of aspirin on thrombin-induced adherence of platelets to cultured cells from the blood vessel walls. *J. clin. Invest.* **62**, 847–857.

Czervionke, R. L., Smith, J. B., Fry, G. L. & Hoak, J. C. 1979 Inhibition of prostacyclin by treatment of endothelium with aspirin. *J. clin. Invest.* **63**, 1089–1092.

D'Angelo, V., Villa, S., Myslieviec, M., Donati, M. B. & De Gaetano, G. 1978 Defective fibrinolytic and prostacyclin-like activity in human atheromatous plaques. *Thromb. Haemostas.* **39**, 535–536.

Davison, E. M., Ford-Hutchinson, A. W., Smith, M. J. H. & Walker, J. R. 1978 The release of thromboxane B₂ by rabbit peritoneal polymorphonuclear leukocytes. *Br. J. Pharmac.* **63**, 407P.

Dembinska-Kiec, A., Gryglewska, T., Zmuda, A. & Gryglewski, R. J. 1977 The generation of prostacyclin by arteries and by the coronary vascular bed is reduced in experimental atherosclerosis in rabbit. *Prostaglandins* **14**, 1025–1034.

DiNicolantonio, R., Dusting, G. J., Hutchinson, J. S. & Mendelsohn, F. A. O. 1981 Failure of aspirin to modify the hypotensive action of captopril in spontaneously hypertensive rats. *Clin. exp. Pharmac. Physiol.* (Submitted for publication.)

Dollery, C. T., Friedman, L. A., Hensby, C. N., Kohner, E., Lewis, P. J., Porta, M. & Webster, J. 1979 Circulating prostacyclin may be reduced in diabetes. *Lancet* ii, 1365.

Dusting, G. J. 1981a Prostacyclin released by angiotensins from lungs and isolated vascular tissue. In *Proceedings of the 28th International Congress of Physiological Sciences*. Budapest: Publishing House of the Hungarian Academy of Sciences. (In the press.)

Dusting, G. J. 1981b On angiotensin-induced release of a prostacyclin (PGI₂)-like substance from the lung. *J. Cardiovasc. Pharmac.* (In the press.)

Dusting, G. J., Moncada, S., Mullane, K. M. & Vane, J. R. 1978a Implications of prostacyclin (PGI₂) generation for modulation of vascular tone. *Clin. Sci. molec. Med.* **55**, 195s–198s.

Dusting, G. J., Moncada, S. & Vane, J. R. 1977a Prostacyclin (PGX) is the endogenous metabolite responsible for relaxation of coronary arteries by arachidonic acid. *Prostaglandins* **13**, 3–15.

Dusting, G. J., Moncada, S. & Vane, J. R. 1977b Disappearance of prostacyclin in the circulation of the dog. *Br. J. Pharmac.* **62**, 414–514P.

Dusting, G. J., Moncada, S. & Vane, J. R. 1977c Prostacyclin is a weak contractor of coronary arteries in the pig. *Eur. J. Pharmac.* **45**, 301–304.

Dusting, G. J., Moncada, S. & Vane, J. R. 1978b Recirculation of prostacyclin (PGI₂) in the dog. *Br. J. Pharmac.* **64**, 315–320.

Dusting, G. J., Moncada, S. & Vane, J. R. 1978c Vascular actions of arachidonic acid and its metabolites in perfused mesenteric and femoral beds of the dog. *Eur. J. Pharmac.* **49**, 65–72.

Dusting, G. J., Moncada, S. & Vane, J. R. 1979 Prostaglandins, their intermediates and precursors: cardiovascular roles and regulatory mechanisms in normal and abnormal circulatory systems. *Proc. Cardiovasc. Dis.* **21**, 405–430.

Dusting, G. J. & Mullins, E. M. 1980 Stimulation by angiotensin of prostacyclin biosynthesis in rats and dogs. *Clin. exp. Pharmac. Physiol.* **7**, 545–550.

Dusting, G. J., Mullins, E. M. & Nolan, R. D. 1981 Prostacyclin release accompanying angiotensin conversion in rat mesenteric vasculature. (Submitted for publication.)

Dyerberg, J. & Bang, H. O. 1979 Haemostatic function and platelet polyunsaturated fatty acids in Eskimos. *Lancet* ii, 433–435.

Dyerberg, J., Bang, H. O., Stofferson, E., Moncada, S. & Vane, J. R. 1978 Eicosapentaenoic acid and prevention of thrombosis and atherosclerosis? *Lancet* ii, 117–119.

Eakins, K. E., Rajadhyaksha, V. & Schroer, R. 1976 Prostaglandin antagonism by sodium *p*-benzyl-4-(1-oxo-2(4-chlorobenzyl)-3-phenylpropyl)phenyl phosphonate (N-0164). *Br. J. Pharmac.* **58**, 333–339.

Ferreira, S. H., Moncada, S. & Vane, J. R. 1973 Prostaglandins and the mechanism of analgesia produced by aspirin-like drugs. *Br. J. Pharmac.* **49**, 86–97.

FitzGerald, G. A., Friedman, L. A., Miyamori, I., O'Grady, J. & Lewis, P. J. 1979 A double blind placebo controlled crossover study of prostacyclin in man. *Life Sci.* **25**, 665–672.

Fitzpatrick, F. A., Bundy, G. L., Gorman, R. R. & Honohan, T. 1978 9,11-Epoxyiminoprosta-5,13-dienoic acid is a thromboxane A_2 antagonist in human platelets. *Nature, Lond.* **275**, 764–766.

Flower, R. J. 1978 Steroidal anti-inflammatory drugs as inhibitors of phospholipase A_2. In *Advances in prostaglandin and thromboxane research* (ed. R. Paoletti & B. Samuelsson), pp. 105–112. New York: Academic Press.

Flower, R. J. & Cardinal, D. C. 1979 Use of a novel platelet aggregometer to study the generation by, and actions of prostacyclin in whole blood. In *Prostacyclin* (ed. J. R. Vane & S. Bergström), pp. 211–220. New York: Raven Press.

Fukazumi, K. 1965 Lipids of the atherosclerotic artery. III. A hypothesis on the cause of atherosclerosis from the viewpoint of fat chemistry. *J. pharm. Soc. Japan* **14**, 119–122.

Fukazumi, K. & Iwata, Y. 1963 Lipids of atherosclerotic artery. II. Dialysis of lipids of abdominal aorta and lipids in lipid protein complexes existing in the aorta. *J. pharm. Soc. Japan* **12**, 93–97.

Gimbrone, M. A. & Alexander, R. W. 1975 Angiotensin II stimulation of prostaglandin production in cultured human vascular endothelium. *Science, N.Y.* **189**, 219–220.

Gimeno, M. F., Sterin-Borda, L., Borda, E. S., Lazzari, M. A. & Gimeno, A. L. 1980 Human plasma transforms prostacyclin (PGI_2) into a platelet antiaggregatory substance which contracts isolated bovine coronary arteries. *Prostaglandins* **19**, 907–916.

Gimson, A. E. S., Hughes, R. D., Mellon, P. J., Woods, H. F., Langley, P. G., Canalese, J., Williams, R. & Weston, M. J. 1980 Prostacyclin to prevent platelet activation during charcoal haemoperfusion in fulminant hepatic failure. *Lancet* i, 173–175.

Glavind, J., Hartmann, S., Clemmesen, J., Jessen, K. E. & Dam, H. 1952 Studies on the role of lipoperoxides in human pathology. II. The presence of peroxidized lipids in the atherosclerotic aorta. *Acta path. microbiol. scand.* **30**, 1.

Godal, H. C., Eika, C., Dybdahl, J. H., Daae, L. & Larsen, S. 1979 Aspirin and bleeding time. *Lancet* i, 1236.

Goldstein, I. M., Malmsten, C. L., Kaplan, Kindahl, H., Samuelsson, B. & Weissman, G. 1977 Thromboxane generation by stimulated human granulocytes: inhibition by glucocorticoids and superoxide dismutase. *Clin. Res.* **25**, 518A.

Gordon, J. L. & Pearson, J. D. 1978 Effects of sulphinpyrazone and aspirin on prostaglandin I_2 (prostacyclin) synthesis by endothelial cells. *Br. J. Pharmac.* **64**, 481–483.

Gorman, R. R., Bunting, S. & Miller, O. V. 1977 Modulation of human platelet adenylate cyclase by prostacyclin (PGX). *Prostaglandins* **13**, 377–388.

Gorman, R. R., Hamilton, R. D. & Hopkins, N. K. 1979 Stimulation of human foreskin fibroblast adenosine 3′5′-cyclic monophosphate levels by prostacyclin (prostaglandin I_2). *J. biol. Chem.* **254**, 1671–1676.

Griffith, G. C., Nichols, G., Asher, J. D. & Flanagan, B. 1965 Heparin osteoporosis. *J. Am. med. Ass.* **193**, 91–94.

Grodzinska, L. & Gryglewski, R. J. 1980 Angiotensin-induced release of prostacyclin from perfused organs. *Pharmac. Res. Commun.* **12**, 339–347.

Gryglewski, R. J. 1979 Prostacyclin is a circulatory hormone. *Biochem. Pharmac.* **28**, 3161–3166.

Gryglewski, R. J., Bunting, S., Moncada, S., Flower, R. J. & Vane, J. R. 1976 Arterial walls are protected against deposition of platelet thrombi by a substance (prostaglandin X) which they make from prostaglandin endoperoxides. *Prostaglandins* **12**, 685–714.

Gryglewski, R. J., Korbut, R. & Ocetkiewicz, A. C. 1978a Generation of prostacyclin by lungs in vivo and its release into the arterial circulation. *Nature, Lond.* **273**, 765–767.

Gryglewski, R. J., Korbut, R., Ocetkiewicz, A., Splawinski, J., Wojtaszek, B. & Swiens, J. 1978b Lungs as a generator of prostacyclin. Hypothesis on physiological significance. *Naunyn Schmiedebergs Arch. Pharmac.* **304**, 45–50.

Gryglewski, R. J., Korbut, R., Ocetkiewicz, A. C. & Stachwa, T. 1978c In vivo method for quantitation of antiplatelet potency of drugs. *Naunyn Schmiedebergs Arch. Pharmac.* **302**, 25–30.

Gryglewski, R. J., Salmon, J. A., Ubatuba, F. B., Weatherley, B. C., Moncada. S. & Vane, J. R. 1979 Effects of all cis-5,8,11,14,17-eicosapentaenoic acid and PGH_3 on platelet aggregation. *Prostaglandins* **18**, 453–478.

Hamberg, M. & Samuelsson, B. 1973 Detection and isolation of an endoperoxide intermediate in prostaglandin biosynthesis. *Proc. natn. Acad. Sci. U.S.A.* **70**, 899–903.

Hamberg, M., Svensson, J. & Samuelsson, B. 1975 Thromboxanes: a new group of biologically active compounds derived from prostaglandin endoperoxides. *Proc. natn. Acad. Sci. U.S.A.* **72**, 2994–2998.

Hamberg, M., Svensson, J., Wakabayashi, T. & Samuelsson, B. 1974 Isolation and structure of two prostaglandin endoperoxides that cause platelet aggregation. *Proc. natn. Acad. Sci. U.S.A.* **71**, 345–349.

Harland, W. A., Gilbert, J. D., Steel, G. & Brooks, C. J. W. 1971 Lipids of human atheroma. 5. The occurrence of a new group of polar sterol esters in various stages of human atherosclerosis. *Atherosclerosis* **13**, 239–246.

Harman, D. & Piette, L. H. 1966 Free radical theory of aging: free radical reaction in serum. *J. Geront.* **21**, 560–565.

Harrison, H. E., Reece, A. H. & Johnson, M. 1978 Decreased vascular prostacyclin in experimental diabetes. *Life Sci.* **23**, 351–356.

Harrowing, P. D. & Williams, K. I. 1979 Homogenates of rat placenta contain a factor(s) which inhibits uterine arachidonic acid metabolism. *Br. J. Pharmac.* **67**, 428P.

Harter, H. R., Burch, J. W., Majerus, P. W., Standford, N., Pelmes, J. A., Anderson, C. B. & Weerts, C. A. 1979 Prevention of thromboembolism in patients of haemodialysis by low dose aspirin. *New Engl. J. Med.* **301**, 577–579.

Havel, R. J. 1979 High density lipoproteins, cholesterol transport and coronary heart disease. *Circulation* **60**, 1–3.

Hensby, C. N., Barnes, P. J., Dollery, C. T. & Dargie, H. 1979a Production of 6-oxo-PGF$_{1\alpha}$ by human lung *in vivo. Lancet* ii, 1162–1163.

Hensby, C. N., Lewis, P. J., Hilgard, P., Mufti, G. J., Hows, J. & Webster, J. 1979b Prostacyclin deficiency in thrombotic thrombocytopenic purpura. *Lancet* ii, 748.

Heyns, A. du P., van den Berg, D. J., Potgieter, G. M. & Retief, F. P. 1974 The inhibition of platelet aggregation by an aorta intima extract. *Thromb. Diathes. haemorrh.* **32**, 417–431.

Higgs, E. A., Moncada, S., Vane, J. R., Caen, J. P., Michel, H. & Tobelem, G. 1978a Effect of prostacyclin (PGI$_2$) on platelet adhesion to rabbit arterial subendothelium. *Prostaglandins* **16**, 17–22.

Higgs, G. A., Bunting, S., Moncada, S. & Vane, J. R. 1976 Polymorphonuclear leukocytes produce thromboxane A$_2$-like activity during phagocytosis. *Prostaglandins* **12**, 749–757.

Higgs, G. A., Moncada, S. & Vane, J. R. 1977 Prostacyclin (PGI$_2$) inhibits the formation of platelet thrombi induced by adenosine diphosphate (ADP) *in vivo. Br. J. Pharmac.* **61**, 137P.

Higgs, G. A., Moncada, S. & Vane, J. R. 1978b Prostacyclin reduces the number of 'slow moving' leucocytes in hamster pouch cheek venules. *J. Physiol., Lond.* **280**, 55P–56P.

Hope, W., Martin, T. J., Chesterman, C. N. & Morgan, F. J. 1979 Human β-thromboglobulin inhibits PGI$_2$ production and binds to a specific site in bovine aortic endothelial cells. *Nature, Lond.* **228**, 210–212.

Hopkins, N. K., Sun, F. F. & Gorman, R. R. 1978 Thromboxane A$_2$ biosynthesis in human lung fibroblasts, WI 38. *Biochem. biophys. Res. Commun.* **85**, 827–836.

Hornstra, G., Haddeman, E. & Don, J. A. 1979 Blood platelets do not provide endoperoxides for vascular prostacyclin production. *Nature, Lond.* **279**, 66–68.

Iwakami, M. 1965 Peroxidase as a factor of atherosclerosis. *Nagoya J. med. Sci.* **28**, 50–66.

Jobin, F. 1978 *Semin. Thromb. Haemostas.* **4**, 199–240.

Johnson, M., Harrison, H. E., Raftery, A. T. & Elder, J. B. 1979 Vascular prostacyclin may be reduced in diabetes in man. *Lancet* i, 325–326.

Johnson, M., Reece, A. H. & Harrison, H. E. 1978 Decreased vascular prostacyclin in experimental diabetes. In *Abstracts of 7th International Congress of Pharmacology*, Paris, p. 342. Oxford: Pergamon Press.

Johnson, R. A., Morton, D. R., Kinner, J. H., Gorman, R. R., McGuire, J. C., Sun, F. F., Whittaker, N., Bunting, S., Salmon, J., Moncada, S. & Vane, J. R. 1976 The chemical structure of prostaglandin X (prostacyclin). *Prostaglandins* **12**, 915–928.

Jorgensen, K. A., Dyerberg, J., Olesen, A. S. & Stoffersen, E. 1980 Acetylsalicylic acid, bleeding time and age. *Thromb. Res.* **19**, 799–805.

Jorgensen, K. A., Olesen, A. S., Dyerberg, J. & Stoffersen, E. 1979 Aspirin and bleeding time: dependency of age. *Lancet* ii, 302.

Kazer-Glanzman, R., Jakabova, M., George, J. & Luscher, E. 1977 Stimulation of calcium uptake in platelet membrane vesicles by adenosine 3',5'-cyclic monophosphate and protein kinase. *Biochim. biophys. Acta* **446**, 429–440.

Kelton, J. G., Hirsch, J., Carter, C. J. & Buchanan, M. R. 1978 Thrombogenic effect of high dose aspirin in rabbits: relationship to inhibition of vessel wall synthesis of prostaglandin I$_2$-like activity. *J. clin. Invest.* **62**, 892–895.

Kernoff, P. B. A., Willis, A. L., Stone, R. J., Davies, J. A. & McNicol, G. P. 1977 Antithrombotic potential of dihomo-γ-linolenic acid in man. *Br. med. J.* ii, 1441–1444.

Korbut, R. & Moncada, S. 1978 Prostacyclin (PGI$_2$) and thromboxane A$_2$ interaction *in vivo*. Regulation by aspirin and relationship with antithrombotic therapy. *Thromb. Res.* **13**, 489–500.

Lagarde, M. & Dechavanne, M. 1977 Increase of platelet prostaglandin cyclic endoperoxides in thrombosis. *Lancet* i, 88.

Lapetina, E. G., Schmitges, G. J., Chandrabose, K. & Cuatrecasas, P. 1977 Cyclic adenosine 3',5'-monophosphate and prostacyclin inhibit membrane phospholipase activity in platelets. *Biochem. biophys. Res. Commun.* **76**, 828–835.

Levy, S. V. 1978 Contractile responses to prostacyclin (PGI$_2$) of isolated human saphenous and rat venous tissue. *Prostaglandins* **16**, 93–97.

Lewy, R. I., Smith, J. B., Silver, M. J., Wiener, L. & Walinsky, P. 1979 Detection of thromboxane A$_2$ in peripheral blood of patients with Prinzmetal's angina. *Prostaglandins Med.* **2**, 243–248.

Lieberman, G. E., Lewis, G. P. & Peters, T. J. 1977 A membrane-bound enzyme in rabbit aorta capable of inhibiting adenosine-diphosphate-induced platelet aggregation. *Lancet* ii, 330–332.

Longmore, D. B., Bennett, G., Gueirrara, S., Smith, M., Bunting, S., Reed, P., Moncada, S., Read, N. G. & Vane, J. R. 1979 Prostacyclin: a solution to some problems of extracorporeal circulation. *Lancet* i, 1001–1005.

MacDonald, J. W. D. & Stuart, R. K. 1974 Interactions of prostaglandins E_1 and E_2 in regulation of cyclic AMP and aggregation in human platelets: evidence for a common prostaglandin receptor. *J. Lab. clin. Med.* **84**, 111–121.

MacIntyre, D. E., Pearson, J. D. & Gordon, J. L. 1978 Localisation and stimulation of prostacyclin production in vascular cells. *Nature, Lond.* **271**, 549–551.

Main, I. H. M. & Whittle, B. J. R. 1975 Potency and selectivity of methyl analogues of prostaglandin E_2 on rat gastrointestinal function. *Br. J. Pharmacol.* **54**, 309–317.

Majerus, P. W. 1976 Why apirin? *Circulation* **54**, 357–359.

Malmsten, C., Granstrom, E. & Samuelsson, B. 1976 Cyclic AMP inhibits synthesis of prostaglandin endoperoxide (PGG_2) in human platelets. *Biochem. biophys. Res. Commun.* **68**, 569–576.

Marcus, A. J. 1978 The role of lipids in platelet function with particular reference to the arachidonic acid pathway. *J. Lipid Res.* **19**, 793–826.

Marcus, A. J., Weksler, B. B. & Jaffe, E. A. 1978 Enzymatic conversion of prostaglandin endoperoxide H_2 and arachidonic acid to prostacyclin by cultured human endothelial cells. *J. biol. Chem.* **253**, 7138–7141.

Marcus, A. J., Weksler, B. B., Jaffe, E. A. & Broekman, M. J. 1979 Synthesis of prostacyclin (PGI_2) from platelet-derived endoperoxides by cultured human endothelial cells. *Blood*, **54**, suppl. 1, abstr. 803, p. 290 a.

Masotti, G., Galanti, G., Pogessi, L., Abbate, R. & Neri Serneri, G. G. 1979 Differential inhibition of prostacyclin production and platelet aggregation by aspirin. *Lancet* ii, 1213–1216.

McGiff, J. C., Crowshaw, K., Terragno, N. A. & Lonigro, A. J. 1970 Release of a prostaglandin E-like substance into renal venous blood in response to angiotensin II. *Circuln Res.* **26–27**, suppl. 1, I-121–I-130.

McGiff, J. C., Terragno, N. A., Malik, K. U. & Lonigro, A. J. 1972 Release of a prostaglandin E-like substance from canine kidney by bradykinin. Comparison with eledoisin. *Circuln Res.* **31**, 36–43.

Medalie, J. H., Kahn, H. A., Naufeld, H. N., Riss, E. & Gouldbourt, U. 1973 Five year myocardial infarction incidence. II. Association of single variables to age and birth place. *J. chron. Dis.* **26**, 329–349.

Miller, O. V. & Gorman, R. R. 1979 Evidence for distinct PGI_2 and PGD_2 receptors in human platelets. *J. Pharmacl. exp. Ther.* **210**, 134–140.

Minkes, S., Stanford, M., Chi, M., Roth, G., Raz, A., Needleman, P. & Majerus, P. 1977 Cyclic adenosine 3′5′-monophosphate inhibits the availability of arachidonate to prostaglandin synthetase in human platelet suspensions. *J. clin. Invest.* **59**, 449–454.

Moncada, S., Gryglewski, R. J., Bunting, S. & Vane, J. R. 1976a An enzyme isolated from arteries transforms prostaglandin endoperoxides to an unstable substance that inhibits platelet aggregation. *Nature, Lond.* **263**, 663–665.

Moncada, S., Gryglewski, R. J., Bunting, S. & Vane, J. R. 1976b A lipid peroxide inhibits the enzyme in blood vessel microsomes that generates from prostaglandin endoperoxides the substance (prostaglandin X) which prevents platelet aggregation. *Prostaglandins* **12**, 715–733.

Moncada, S., Herman, A. G., Higgs, E. A. & Vane, J. R. 1977 Differential formation of prostacyclin (PGX or PGI_2) by layers of the arterial wall. An explanation for the anti-thrombotic properties of vascular endothelium. *Thromb. Res.* **11**, 323–324.

Moncada, S., Korbut, R., Bunting, S. & Vane, J. R. 1978 Prostacyclin is a circulating hormone. *Nature, Lond.* **273**, 767–768.

Moncada, S. & Vane, J. R. 1977 The discovery of prostacyclin – a fresh insight into arachidonic acid metabolism. In *Biochemical aspects of prostaglandins and thromboxanes* (ed. N. Kharasch & J. Fried), pp. 155–177. New York, San Francisco and London: Academic Press.

Moncada, S. & Vane, J. R. 1978 Unstable metabolites of arachidonic acid and their role in haemostasis and thrombosis. *Br. med. Bull.* **34**, 129–135.

Moncada, S. & Vane, J. R. 1979a Arachidonic acid metabolites and the interactions between platelets and blood vessel walls. *New Engl. J. Med.* **300**, 1142–1147.

Moncada, S. & Vane, J. R. 1979b The role of prostacyclin in vascular tissue. *Fedn Proc. Fedn Am. Socs. exp. Biol.* **38**, 62–66.

Moore, S., Pepper, D. S. & Cash, J. D. 1975 The isolation and characterization of a platelet-specific beta-globulin (β-thromboglobulin). *Biochim. biophys. Acta* **379**, 360–369.

Mullane, K. M., Dusting, G. J., Salmon, J. A., Moncada, S. & Vane, J. R. 1979 Biotransformation and cardiovascular effects of arachidonic acid in the dog. *Eur. J. Pharmac.* **54**, 217–228.

Mullane, K. M. & Moncada, S. 1980a Prostacyclin mediates the potentiated hypotensive effect of bradykinin following captopril treatment. *Eur. J. Pharmac.* **66**, 355–365.

Mullane, K. M. & Moncada, S. 1980b Prostacyclin release and the modulation of some vasoactive hormones. *Prostaglandins* **20**, 25–49.

Munday, B. R., Bewick, M., Moncada, S. & Vane, J. R. 1981 An experimental assessment of prostacyclin in the harvesting of kidneys for transplantation. *Transplantation.* (In the press.)

Munday, B. R., Bewick, M., Moncada, S. & Vane, J. R. 1980 Suppression of hyperacute renal allograft rejection in presensitized dogs with prostacyclin. *Prostaglandins* **19**, 595–603.

Mustard, J. F. & Packham, M. A. 1975 Platelets, thrombosis and drugs. *Drugs* **9**, 19–76.

Needleman, P. 1976 The synthesis and function of prostaglandins in the heart. *Fedn Proc. Fedn Am. Socs exp. Biol.* **35**, 2376–2381.

Needleman, P., Bronson, S. D., Wyche, A., Sivakoff, M. & Nicolaou, K. 1978 Cardiac and renal prostaglandin I_2. *J. clin. Invest.* **61**, 839–849.

Needleman, P., Marshall, G. R. & Sobel, B. E. 1975 Hormone interactions in the isolated rabbit heart: synthesis and coronary vasomotor effects of prostaglandins, angiotensin and bradykinin. *Circulation Res.* **37**, 802–808.

Needleman, P., Wyche, A. & Raz, A. 1979 Platelet and blood vessel arachidonate metabolism and interactions. *J. clin. Invest.* **63**, 345–349.

Neri Serneri, G. G., Masotti, G., Poggesi, L. & Galante, G. 1980 Release of prostacyclin into the bloodstream and its exhaustion in humans after local blood flow changes (ischaemia and venous stasis). *Thromb. Res.* **17**, 197–208.

Nijkamp, F. P., Moncada, S., White, H. L. & Vane, J. R. 1977 Diversion of prostaglandin endoperoxide metabolism by selective inhibition of thromboxane A_2 biosynthesis in lung, spleen or platelets. *Eur. J. Pharmac.* **44**, 179–187.

Nordoy, A., Svensson, B., Wiebe, D. & Hoak, J. C. 1978 Lipoproteins and the inhibitory effect of human endothelial cells on platelet function. *Circulation Res.* **43**, 527–534.

Nugteren, D. H. & Hazelhof, E. 1973 Isolation and properties of intermediates in prostaglandin biosynthesis. *Biochim. biophys. Acta* **326**, 448–461.

Oates, J. A., Falardeau, P., FitzGerald, G. A., Branch, R. A. & Brash, A. R. 1981 Quantification of urinary prostacyclin metabolites in man: estimates of the rate of secretion of prostacyclin into the general circulation. In *The clinical pharmacology of prostacyclin* (ed. P. J. Lewis & J. O'Grady). Raven Press. (In the press.)

Oelz, O., Seyberth, H. W., Knapp, H. R., Sweetman, B. J. & Oates, J. A. 1976 Effects of feeding ethyl-dihomo-γ-linolenate on prostaglandin biosynthesis and platelet aggregation in the rabbit. *Biochim. biophys. Acta* **431**, 268–277.

O'Grady, J. & Moncada, S. 1978 Aspirin: a paradoxical effect on bleeding time. *Lancet* ii, 780.

O'Grady, J., Warrington, S., Moti, M. J., Bunting, S., Flower, R. J., Fowle, A. S. E., Higgs, E. A. & Moncada, S. 1979 Effects of intravenous prostacyclin infusions in healthy volunteers – some preliminary observations. In *Prostacyclin* (ed. J. R. Vane & S. Bergström), pp. 409–417. New York: Raven Press.

Omini, C., Moncada, S. & Vane, J. R. 1977 The effects of prostacyclin (PGI_2) on tissues which detect prostaglandins (PG's). *Prostaglandins* **14**, 625–632.

Pace-Asciak, C. 1976 Isolation, structure and biosynthesis of 6-keto prostaglandin $F_{1\alpha}$ in the rat stomach. *J. Am. chem. Soc.* **98**, 2348–2349.

Pace-Asciak, C. R., Carrara, M. C., Rangaraj, G. & Nicolaou, K. G. 1978 Enhanced formation of PGI_2, a potent hypotensive substance, by aortic rings and homogenates of the spontaneously hypertensive rat. *Prostaglandins* **15**, 1005–1012.

Pomerantz, K., Sintetos, A. & Ramwell, P. 1978 The effect of prostacyclin on the human umbilical artery. *Prostaglandins* **15**, 1035–1044.

Rajah, S. M., Penny, S. & Kester, R. 1978 Aspirin and bleeding time. *Lancet* ii, 1104.

Remuzzi, G., Cavenaghi, A. E., Mecca, G., Donati, M. B. & De Gaetano, G. 1977 Prostacyclin (PGI_2) and bleeding time in uremic patients. *Thromb. Res.* **11**, 919–920.

Remuzzi, G., Misiani, R., Marchesi, D., Livio, M., Mecca, G., De Gaetano, G. & Donati, M. B. 1978 Haemolytic-uraemic syndrome: deficiency of plasma factor(s) regulating prostacyclin activity. *Lancet* ii, 871–872.

Robert, A., Hanchar, A. J., Lancaster, C. & Nezamis, J. E. 1979 Prostacyclin inhibits enteropooling and diarrhoea. In *Prostacyclin* (ed. J. R. Vane & S. Bergström), pp. 147–158. New York: Raven Press.

Rosenblum, W. I. & El-Sabban, F. 1978 Enhancement of platelet aggregation by tranylcypromine in mouse cerebral microvessels. *Circuln Res.* **43**, 238–241.

Roth, G. J. & Majerus, P. W. 1975 The mechanism of the effect of aspirin on human platelets. I. Acetylation of a particular fraction protein. *J. clin. Invest.* **56**, 624–632.

Roth, G. J. & Siok, C. J. 1978 Acetylation of the NH_2-terminal serine of prostaglandin synthetase by aspirin. *J. biol. Chem.* **253**, 3782–3784.

Saba, S. R. & Mason, R. G. 1974 Studies of an activity from endothelial cells that inhibits platelet aggregation, serotonin release and clot retraction. *Thromb. Res.* **5**, 747–757.

Saeed, S. A., McDonald-Gibson, W. J., Cuthbert, J., Copas, J. L., Schneider, C., Gardiner, P. J., Butt, N. M. & Collier, H. O. J. 1977 Endogenous inhibitor of prostaglandin synthetase. *Nature, Lond.* **270**, 32–33.

Salmon, J. A., Smith, D. R., Flower, R. J., Moncada, S. & Vane, J. R. 1978 Further studies on the enzymatic conversion of prostaglandin endoperoxide into prostacyclin by porcine aorta microsomes. *Biochim. biophys. Acta* **523**, 250–262.

Shimamoto, T., Kobayashi, M., Takahashi, T., Takashima, Y., Sakamoto, M. & Morooka, S. 1978 An observation of thromboxane A_2 in arterial blood after cholesterol feeding in rabbits. *Jap. Heart J.* **19**, 748–753.

Sim, A. K. & McCraw, A. P. 1977 The activity of γ-linolenate and dihomo-γ-linolenate methyl esters *in vitro* and *in vivo* on blood platelet function in nonhumans. *Thromb. Res.* **10**, 385–397.

Sinzinger, H., Feigl, W. & Silberbauer, K. 1979 Prostacyclin generation in atherosclerotic arteries. *Lancet* ii, 469.

Slater, T. F. 1972 *Free radical mechanisms in tissue injury.* London: Pion Ltd.

Steer, M. L., MacIntyre, D. E., Levine, L. & Salzman, E. W. 1980 Is prostacyclin a physiologically important circulating antiplatelet agent? *Nature, Lond.* **283**, 124–125.

Szczeklik, A., Gryglewski, R. J., Musial, J., Grodzinska, L., Serwonska, M. & Marcinkiewicz, E. 1978a Thromboxane generation and platelet aggregation in survivals of myocardial infarction. *Thromb. Diathes. haemorrh.* **40**, 66–74.

Szczeklik, A., Gryglewski, R. J., Nizankowski, R. & Musial, J. 1978b Pulmonary and antiplatelet effects of intravenous and inhaled prostacyclin in man. *Prostaglandins* **16**, 654–660.

Szczeklik, A., Gryglewski, R. J., Nizankowski, R., Skawinski, S., Gluszko, P. & Korbut, R. 1980 Prostacyclin therapy in peripheral artery disease. *Thromb. Res.* **19**, 191–199.

Szczeklik, A., Nizankowski, R., Skawinski, S., Szczeklik, J., Gluszko, P. & Gryglewski, R. J. 1979 Successful therapy of advanced arteriosclerosis obliterans with prostacyclin. *Lancet* i, 1111–1114.

Tansik, R. L., Namm, D. H. & White, H. L. 1978 Synthesis of prostaglandin 6-keto-$F_{1\alpha}$ by cultured aortic smooth muscle cells and stimulation of its formation in a coupled system with platelet lysates. *Prostaglandins* **15**, 399–408.

Tateson, J. E., Moncada, S. & Vane, J. R. 1977 Effects of prostacyclin (PGX) on cyclic AMP concentrations in human platetets. *Prostaglandins* **13**, 389–399.

Terashita, Z., Nishikawa, K., Terao, S., Nakagawa, M. & Hino, T. 1979 A specific prostaglandin I_2 synthetase inhibitor, 3-hydroperoxy-3-methyl-2-phenyl-3H Indole. *Biochem. biophys. Res. Commun.* **91**, 72–78.

Terragno, N. A., Terragno, D. A., Early, J. A., Roberts, M. A. & McGiff, J. C. 1978 Endogenous prostaglandin synthesis inhibitor in the renal cortex. Effects on production of prostacyclin by renal blood vessels. *Clin. Sci. molec. Med.* **55**, 199s–202s.

Terragno, N. A., Terragno, D. A. & McGiff, J. C. 1977 Contribution of prostaglandins to the renal circulation in conscious anaesthetized and laparatomized dogs. *Circuln Res.* **40**, 590–595.

Ubatuba, F. B., Moncada, S. & Vane, J. R. 1979 The effect of prostacyclin (PGI_2) on platelet behaviour, thrombosis formation *in vivo* and bleeding time. *Thromb. Diathes. haemorrh.* **41**, 425–434.

Vane, J. R. 1964 The use of isolated organs for detecting active substances in the circulating blood. *Br. J. Pharmac. Chemother.* **23**, 360–373.

Vane, J. R. & Ferreira, S. H. 1976 Interactions between bradykinin and prostaglandins. In *Chemistry and biology of the kallikrein-kinin system in health and disease (Fogarty International Center Proceedings*, no. 27) (ed. J. J. Pisano & K. F. Austen), pp. 255–266. Washington, D. C.: U.S. Government Printing Office.

Vane, J. R. & McGiff, J. C. 1975 Possible contributions of endogenous prostaglandins to the control of blood pressure. *Circuln Res.* **36–37**, suppl. 1, I-68–I-75.

Vargaftig, B. B. & Chignard, M. 1975 Substances that increase the cyclic AMP content prevent platelet aggregation and concurrent release of pharmacologically active substances evoked by arachidonic acid. *Agents Actions* **5**, 137–144.

Vermylen, J., Chamone, D. A. F. & Verstraete, M. 1979 Stimulation of prostacyclin release from vessel wall by BAYg6575, an antithrombotic compound. *Lancet* i, 518–520.

Verstraete, M. 1976 Are agents affecting platelet functions clinically useful? *Am. J. Med.* **81**, 897–914.

Villa, S., Livio, M. & De Gaetano, G. 1979 The inhibitor effect of aspirin on platelet and vascular prostaglandins in rats cannot be completely dissociated. *Br. J. Haemat.* **42**, 425–431.

Walker, I. D., Davidson, J. F., Faichney, A., Wheatley, D. & Davidson, K. 1980 Prostacyclin in cardiopulmonary bypass surgery. In *Abstracts, 6th Int. Congress on Thrombosis*, Monaco.

Warrington, S. & O'Grady, J. 1980 Cardiovascular effects of prostacyclin (PGI_2) in man. In *Advances in prostaglandin and thromboxane research* (ed. B. Samuelsson, P. W. Ramwell & R. Paoletti), vol. 7, pp. 619–624. New York: Raven Press.

Weiss, H. J. & Turitto, V. T. 1979 Prostacyclin (prostaglandin I_2, PGI_2) inhibits platelet adhesion and thrombus formation on subendothelium. *Blood* **53**, 244–250.

Weksler, B. B., Knapp, J. M. & Jaffe, E. A. 1977a Prostacyclin synthesized by cultured endothelial cells modulates polymorphonuclear leukocyte function. *Blood* **50**, 287.

Weksler, B. B., Ley, C. W. & Jaffe, E. W. 1978 Stimulation of endothelial cell prostacyclin production by thrombin, trypsin, and the ionophore A23187. *J. clin. Invest.* **62**, 923–930.

Weksler, B. B., Marcus, A. J. & Jaffe, E. A. 1977b Synthesis of prostaglandin I_2 (prostacyclin) by cultured human and bovine endothelial cells. *Proc. natn. Acad. Sci. U.S.A.* **74**, 3922–3926.

Whittle, B. J. R., Moncada, S. & Vane, J. R. 1978 Comparison of the effects of prostacyclin (PGI_2), prostaglandin E_1 and D_2 on platelet aggregation in different species. *Prostaglandins* **16**, 373–388.

Whitworth, J. A., D'Apice, A. J. F., Kincaid-Smith, P., Shulkes, A. A. & Skinner, S. L. 1978 Antihypertensive effect of plasma exchange. *Lancet* i, 1205.

Willis, A. L., Comai, K., Kuhn, D. C. & Paulsrud, J. 1974 Dihomo-γ-linolenate suppresses platelet aggregation when administered *in vitro* or *in vivo*. *Prostaglandins* **8**, 509–519.

Woodford, F. P., Bottcher, C. J. F., Oette, K. & Ahrens, E. H., Jr 1965 The artifactual nature of lipid peroxides detected in extracts of human aorta. *J. Atheroscler. Res.* **5**, 311–316.

Woods, H. F., Ash, G., Weston, M. J., Bunting, S., Moncada, S. & Vane, J. R. 1978 Prostacyclin can replace heparin in haemodialysis in dogs. *Lancet* ii, 1075–1077.

Wynalda, M. A. & Fitzpatrick, F. A. 1980 Albumins stabilize prostaglandin I_2. *Prostaglandins* **20**, 853–861.

S. MONCADA AND J. R. VANE

Discussion

ELSPETH B. SMITH (*Department of Chemical Pathology, University Medical Buildings, Foresterhill, Aberdeen, U.K.*). In the trial with low-dose aspirin [data not in published report] I was interested to see that there were two non-responders, both with the same initial. Were they members of the same family? Is there evidence of a familial factor in response to aspirin?

S. MONCADA. They were not members of the same family; there is no evidence of a familial factor in response to aspirin, although we have not looked at this in detail.

D. B. LONGMORE (*National Heart Hospital, London, U.K.*). In this very important paper, the possible role of prostacyclin in cross-species transplantation has been mentioned. In the mid-1960s at the National Heart Hospital, we attempted animal–man transplantation unsuccessfully. We used a pigs heart–lung as a supplementary organ system to boost the circulation in two patients whose cardiovascular system was inadequate to enable us to wean them off the heart–lung machine. There was total cessation of coronary flow within 4–6 minutes. We have recently tried pig–dog and dog–pig cross-species heart transplant experiments in our laboratories with prostacyclin. We have tried dose levels of PGI_2 varying between 8 and 15 ng kg^{-1} min^{-1}. We have achieved a lengthening of the time for vascular occlusion of up to 2 h. We wonder why, in spite of the PGI_2 infusion and the initially high flow rates through the transplanted organ, total occlusion of the vascular system should still occur relatively quickly. The addition of dipyridamole, a powerful coronary vasodilator in dogs, has not in our initial experiments made any difference to this acute intravascular clotting. PGI_2 is obviously helpful, but a survival time of an hour or two is of little value to the patient receiving a cross-species heart transplant. Has Dr Moncada any suggestions as to how we should try to extend the beneficial effect of PGI_2 in this difficult situation?

S. MONCADA. A lengthening of about 1 h in xenografts is already a great improvement since controls run for about 5–6 min. What we have to study now in detail is, first, whether prostacyclin is effective in other mechanisms apart from inhibiting platelet aggregation and second, whether by increasing prostacyclin doses we shall obtain a further prolongation in the time. This is, of course, difficult to do since the cardiovascular effects of prostacyclin prevent us from increasing the dose.

H. O. J. COLLIER (*Miles Laboratories Limited, U.K.*). May I call attention to a third factor that may affect the outcome of an interaction between prostacyclin and thromboxane A_2 at the platelet? Awareness of this factor derives from our observation that blood plasma or serum inhibits synthesis of the main prostaglandins from arachidonic acid *in vitro* (Saeed *et al.* 1977; Collier *et al.* 1980; Denning-Kendall *et al.* 1981). This ability of plasma can be expressed in its inhibition of arachidonate-induced aggregation of platelets. Thus, we have found that platelets suspended in plasma require about ten times more arachidonate to induce their aggregation than do washed platelets suspended in buffer (Collier & McDonald-Gibson 1980). This inhibitory effect on platelet aggregation can largely be attributed to plasma albumin, which is a potent inhibitor of prostaglandin synthesis (Collier & McDonald-Gibson 1980; Collier *et al.* 1981).

The authors have said that there is not enough prostacyclin in plasma to inhibit strongly

[112]

platelet aggregation in the circulating blood. If this is so, then the presence of free arachidonic acid in the blood, which might arise from its ingestion or from its liberation from store, would threaten to induce aggregation of circulating platelets, if another inhibitory mechanism did not operate. We have proposed that a hitherto unrecognized function of plasma albumin may be to make it harder for free arachidonic acid in the plasma to induce aggregation, since, in the presence of albumin, a greater amount of arachidonic acid, such as might be liberated at a damaged vessel wall, would be required to induce aggregation (Collier & McDonald-Gibson 1980).

References

Collier, H. O. J., Denning-Kendall, P. A., McDonald-Gibson, W. J. & Saeed, S. A. 1980 Plasma proteins that inhibit prostaglandin synthesis. In *Hemostasis, prostaglandins, and renal disease* (ed. G. Remuzzi, G. Mecca & G. de Gaetano), pp. 257–267. New York: Raven Press.

Collier, H. O. J., Denning-Kendall, P. A., McDonald-Gibson, W. J., Saeed, S. A., Brennecke, S. P. & Mitchell, M. D. 1981 Endogenous inhibitors of prostaglandin synthesis (EIPS) in blood plasma: possible identity and function. In *The role of chemical mediators in hemodynamic and metabolic failure in the critically-ill* (ed. R. McConn). New York: Raven Press. (In the press.)

Collier, H. O. J. & McDonald-Gibson, W. J. 1980 Plasma albumin inhibits arachidonate-induced aggregation of suspended platelets. *J. Physiol., Lond.* (In the press.)

Denning-Kendall, P. A., Saeed, S. A. & Collier, H. O. J. 1981 Comparison of the inhibition by human serum, albumin and haptoglobin of biosynthesis of various prostaglandins. *Biochem. Soc. Trans.* (In the press.)

Phil. Trans. R. Soc. Lond. B **294**, 331–338 (1981)

Printed in Great Britain

Role of the vascular endothelium

By J. C. Hoak, R. L. Czervionke, G. L. Fry,
D. L. Haycraft and A. A. Brotherton

*Cardiovascular Center and Specialized Center for Research in Atherosclerosis,
University of Iowa College of Medicine, Iowa City, Iowa 52242, U.S.A.*

The intact vascular endothelial surface is considered to be 'non-thrombogenic', and blood platelets usually fail to adhere to it. In this role, the endothelium serves to maintain the integrity of the vascular system by preventing the escape of blood and by preventing the build-up of solid thrombus within the vessel, which would compromise blood flow. A possible explanation for the non-thrombogenic effect of the endothelium is the presence of prostacyclin (PGI_2), the potent inhibitor of platelet aggregation and adherence, which is produced and released by the endothelium in response to various stimuli. Removal of PGI_2 from the endothelium by four different methods did not increase baseline platelet adherence, but did increase thrombin-induced platelet adherence from 4 to 60%. Addition of exogenous PGI_2, at low concentrations reversed the enhanced thrombin-induced platelet adherence under these conditions. Although it is unlikely that prostacyclin is the sole factor regulating platelet adherence to the endothelium, it appears to play a major role in the interaction of platelets with components of the blood vessel wall.

Introduction

A decade ago, it had been known for some time that the vascular endothelium functioned differently from other cells, but the remarkable capacity for the endothelial surface to maintain non-thrombogenic properties in the face of myriads of procoagulant substances and activated platelets, though appreciated, was poorly understood. During the previous two decades, many advances were recorded in our understanding of the ultrastructural features of endothelium, responses to vascular injury, exchange of fluid and nutrients across the endothelial layer and the migration of blood cells into the tissues (Majno 1965; Florey 1966). The past decade has witnessed a better understanding of endothelial cell biochemistry and physiology following the development of techniques that permitted these cells to be grown in tissue culture.

Normal functions of the endothelium

In general, three functions have been delineated for the vascular endothelium. It supplies small molecular nutrients to the subendothelial structures, acts as a barrier to large macromolecular substances, and presents a non-thrombogenic surface to circulating blood constituents. The endothelium forms a continuous monolayer, 0.5–1.2 μm in thickness. The long axis of the individual cells constituting this monolayer parallels the direction of blood flow. Each endothelial cell is sheet-like in character with an extremely high surface:volume ratio.

The luminal surface of the endothelium is covered by an ultrathin micropolysaccharide coat referred to as the glycocalyx. The cell's plasma membrane is a trilaminar structure similar to other biological membranes. Intercellular junctions are of three main varieties: (1) tight junctions are very localized areas of fusion of the two outer plasmalemmal leaflets of adjacent cells and are local permeability barriers to protein molecules; (2) gap junctions are areas of close cellular apposition that are not fused and are important in the intercellular transfer of ions; (3) the major portion of intercellular contact is an overlapping of peripheral cytoplasmic portions of neighbouring cells with an intercellular space of 15–20 nm.

Several different types of membrane-related structures are likely to be important in cellular transport. Vesicles known as caveolae intracellulares, measuring about 70 nm in diameter, are distributed along both luminal and basal plasma membranes. They are fused with the membrane to form flask-shaped structures; occasionally several may fuse to form a transcellular channel. Phosphatase activity has been demonstrated within these structures, but no relation with ADP-induced platelet aggregation has yet been reported. A second type of vesicle referred to as a 'pit' can be seen, which measures 80–120 nm in diameter. These pits function in the selective uptake of substances, particularly proteins, and include sites of enzyme activity and lipoprotein receptors.

NON-THROMBOGENIC FEATURES

The emphasis in this paper is on those properties of the vascular endothelium that enable it to maintain its normal non-thrombogenic surface. Possible factors and mechanisms that may be involved are listed in table 1.

TABLE 1. FACTORS IN ENDOTHELIAL NON-THROMBOGENICITY

electrostatic repulsion
surface ADPase
heparans–proteoglycans
plasminogen activator
thrombin binding
prostacyclin

Both the intact platelet and endothelial cell have negatively charged membranes at physiological pH and thus are mutually repelled by each other. It is believed that the surface of the endothelium is influenced by the presence of heparans and glycosoaminoglycans. Of particular interest has been the demonstration that the platelet contains an enzyme capable of liberating and degrading heparan sulphate associated with the surface of the endothelial cell (Buonassisi & Root 1975). Heparan sulphate is chemically related to heparin and at high concentrations shows anticoagulant activity. Thus, the platelet may be able, through an as yet unidentified stimulus, to modify directly an antithrombogenic property of the endothelial cell to enhance local haemostatic mechanisms.

An enzyme with ADPase activity has been found to be associated with the endothelial surface and would have an obvious role in preventing platelet aggregates from forming near intact endothelium (Heyns et al. 1974). The endothelium is known to produce an activator of plasminogen and carries the potential for activation of the fibrinolytic system to promote lysis of fibrin in clots or thrombi.

An interesting new role for the endothelium has been suggested by the recent work of Lollar & Owen (1980). These workers have demonstrated that the binding of thrombin to the endothelium is an important primary mechanism for the rapid removal of thrombin from the circulation and facilitates its subsequent association with anti-thrombin III (AT-III) to form a thrombin–AT-III complex.

Perhaps the most important non-thrombogenic property of the endothelium relates to its ability to produce and release prostacyclin. Moncada *et al.* (1976) have shown that arachidonate metabolic machinery exists in endothelial cells to convert arachidonic acid and cyclic endo-peroxides to prostacyclin, a most potent inhibitor of platelet aggregation and adhesion.

PLATELET ADHERENCE STUDIES

To delineate more clearly the role of prostacyclin, we have performed studies on a platelet adherence system with cultured vascular cell monolayers (table 2). Prostacyclin was measured in these studies by using a radioimmunoassay for 6-keto-$PGF_{1\alpha}$, the stable end product of prostacyclin (Czervionke *et al.* 1978, 1979).

TABLE 2. EFFECT OF BOVINE THROMBIN ON ADHERENCE OF PLATELETS
(PERCENTAGES)

(Monolayers were rocked with 1 ml incubation medium (i.m.), with or without 0.5 U bovine thrombin, and 0.5 ml ^{51}Cr-labelled platelets for 30 min at 37 °C. Adherence was determined by the method of Czervionke *et al.* (1978). Values given are means ± s.e. for at least six dishes.) These data are taken from Fry *et al.* (1980) *Blood* **55**, 271.

	control (i.m.)	bovine thrombin, 0.5 U
endothelium		
venous	1.5 ± 0.2	4.0 ± 0.5
haemangioendothelioma	2.6 ± 0.7	66.9 ± 1.9
arterial smooth muscle	2.4 ± 1.0	79.4 ± 0.3
arterial fibroblasts	1.3 ± 0.4	79.4 ± 0.9
empty dish	2.1 ± 0.1	77.7 ± 2.7

To test the effect of prostacyclin in the platelet adherence system we used four different approaches to eliminate it from the endothelium.

Aspirin (ASA) is known to acetylate the cyclo-oxygenase of the platelet and to inhibit thromboxane A_2 formation. Therefore, we chose to treat the endothelial monolayer with aspirin so that in a similar way the endothelial cyclooxygenase would be inhibited and prosta-cyclin production would cease. We tested this possibility by using our assay for 6-keto-$PGF_{1\alpha}$ and the thrombin-induced platelet adherence system.

The results are shown in figure 1. In the absence of thrombin, there was no increased platelet adherence despite inhibition of prostacyclin formation. In the presence of thrombin and in the absence of aspirin, 6-keto-$PGF_{1\alpha}$ increased and there was little platelet adherence. When the endothelium was treated with 0.01 mM aspirin, thrombin still caused significant release of 6-keto-$PGF_{1\alpha}$, and no increase in platelet adherence occurred. However, treatment of the endothelium with 1 mM aspirin prevented the formation of 6-keto-$PGF_{1\alpha}$ even in the presence of thrombin, and platelet adherence increased to 44%.

In additional studies we demonstrated that the effect of aspirin on the endothelium was temporary (figure 2). When the aspirin-treated endothelium was removed from contact with the aspirin and restored to culture conditions 2 h later, thrombin caused significant 6-keto-$PGF_{1\alpha}$ release, and platelet adherence returned to normal. When cycloheximide, an inhibitor of

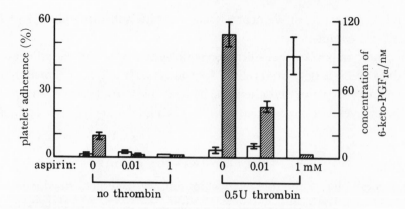

FIGURE 1. Platelet adherence (open columns) to untreated and aspirin (ASA)-treated endothelium compared with 6-keto-PGF$_{1a}$ release (shaded columns). ASA or buffer control was incubated with the monolayer for 30 min at 37 °C, with rocking. The preincubation solution was removed and the dish was washed twice. Thrombin or buffer control was added, followed immediately by ^{51}Cr-labelled platelets (for adherence) or unlabelled platelets (for PGI$_2$ determinations). The monolayer was rocked for 30 min at 37 °C. The percentage adherence was calculated by dividing counts per minute of cells attached to the monolayer, multiplied by 100, by total counts per minute added to the dish. 6-Keto-PGF$_{1a}$ released into the supernatant was determined by radioimmunoassay.

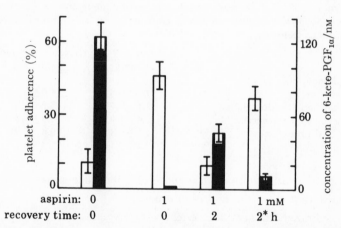

FIGURE 2. Duration of the aspirin effect on endothelium as reflected by 0.5 U thrombin-induced platelet adherence (open columns) and 6-keto-PGF$_{1a}$ release (solid columns). ASA or buffer control was incubated with the monolayer for 30 min at 37 °C, with rocking. The preincubation solution was removed and the monolayer was washed twice. The designated monolayers were layered with 2 ml cultured medium with and without 2.5 μg/ml cycloheximide, incubated in a 5% CO$_2$ atmosphere at 37 °C for 2 h (recovery period), and rewashed twice. All monolayers were then treated with thrombin and platelets. *, With cycloheximide. From Czervionke et al. (1979) J. clin. Invest. 63, 1089.

protein synthesis, was added to the endothelial culture during the recovery period, little 6-keto-PGF$_{1a}$ was released, and platelet adherence remained abnormal.

Prostacyclin was also removed from the platelet adherence system by using an incubation system containing a rabbit antibody against 6-keto-PGF$_{1a}$, which cross-reacts with prostacyclin. In the presence of the antibody, thrombin-induced platelet adherence to endothelium increased from 7.7% to 39.1%.

In the third set of experiments, the endothelium was subjected to repeated incubation with thrombin. As demonstrated by Czervionke et al. (1979), after the initial exposure to thrombin, the cultured endothelium was unable to respond to a second thrombin stimulus with a release of PGI_2. When platelet adherence studies were performed under these conditions in the absence of prostacyclin, platelet adherence was increased (see figure 3).

Using a culture of bovine pulmonary artery endothelium that did not produce prostacyclin, we performed additional platelet adherence studies (see table 3).

In the presence of thrombin, platelet adherence to the endothelial cells, which were unable to produce prostacyclin, was 78 %. Pretreatment of the endothelium with aspirin did not increase the platelet adherence.

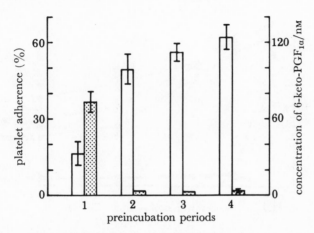

FIGURE 3. The 6-keto-$PGF_{1\alpha}$ release response with repeated exposure of the endothelial monolayer to thrombin. Five minutes after each addition of 0.5 U thrombin, the incubation mixture was completely removed. Fresh buffer containing thrombin was then added to the unwashed monolayer, which was reincubated, with rocking, for 5 min. This procedure was repeated 3 times. Platelet adherence (open columns) and 6-keto-$PGF_{1\alpha}$ concentrations (stippled columns) were determined. From Hoak *et al.* (1979) In *Florence International Meeting on Myocardial Infarction (Int. Cong. Ser.* no. 491), vol. 1, pp. 289–298. Excerpta Medica.

TABLE 3. RESPONSES OF BOVINE PULMONARY ARTERY ENDOTHELIUM,
NO PGI_2 PRODUCED

(Platelet adherence was performed as in figure 1, except that the source of endothelium was a bovine pulmonary artery that failed to produce prostacyclin.)

	platelet adherence (%)
control	3
thrombin (0.5 U)	78
thrombin + 100 mm PGI_2	16
ASA (1 mm) + thrombin	69
ASA + thrombin + PGI_2	14

In each of the four sets of experiments used to remove prostacyclin from the endothelium, baseline platelet adherence did not increase. However, when thrombin was added to the incubation system, in every instance platelet adherence increased significantly and this increase was prevented by the addition of exogenous prostacyclin to the incubation media. Thus, prostacyclin appeared to be an important component to maintain platelet adherence at a low value when thrombin was present in the incubation system with the endothelium.

In order to study the effect of exogenous prostacyclin on platelet adherence to different types of vascular cells, the monolayers were pretreated with 1 mm ASA to block endogenous production of prostacyclin by thrombin. In order to determine whether some cell types were more sensitive to prostacyclin, concentrations from 25 to 150 nM were used. Fibroblasts were chosen as a representative cell type from the subendothelium, since values for smooth muscle and fibroblasts were not significantly different. Mouse fibroblasts were used as a control for the haemangioendothelioma. Figure 4 shows that platelet adherence to the venous endothelium, and haemangioendothelioma, decreased markedly with as little as 25 nM prostacyclin. In contrast, the platelet adherence to fibroblasts in the presence of thrombin was extremely resistant to the effect of prostacyclin.

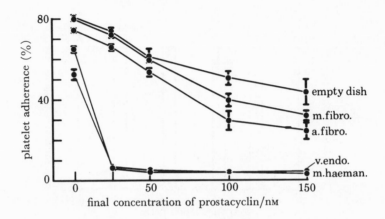

FIGURE 4. Inhibition by exogenous PGI_2 of 0.5 U thrombin-induced platelet adherence to 1 mM aspirin-treated cell layers. All monolayers were incubated for 30 min with 1 mM aspirin in incubation medium. After rinsing twice, platelet adherence was determined as described in the legend to figure 1. PGI_2 was added just before thrombin and platelets to achieve the concentrations shown. Abbreviations: a. fibro., arterial fibroblasts; v. endo., venous endothelium; m. haeman., mouse haemangioendothelioma; m. fibro., mouse L929 fibroblast. From Fry et al. (1980) Blood 55, 271.

TABLE 4. EFFECT OF DAPA ON ADHERENCE OF THROMBIN-INDUCED PLATELET

AGGREGATES

ASA (100 μM)	thrombin (0.067 U/ml)	DAPA (1.34 μM)	percentage adherence		
			endo.	fibro.	empty dish
.	×	.	38 ± 7	81 ± 4	86 ± 3
.	×	×	3 ± 4	71 ± 1	66 ± 1
×	×	.	68 ± 10	82 ± 2	85 ± 1
×	×	×	11 ± 6	67 ± 7	66 ± 3

In studies designed to test whether the effects of the thrombin were entirely on the platelets in the adherence system, we have obtained additional results suggesting that prostacyclin is not completely responsible for the non-thrombogenic character of the endothelium. DAPA (dansyl-arginine-N-(3-ethyl-1,5-pentanediyl) amide, an inhibitor of the active site of thrombin (Nesheim et al. 1979) was added to platelet aggregates that had formed when thrombin was added to ^{51}Cr-labelled platelets in an aggregometer. After the DAPA was mixed with the platelet aggregates, they were transferred to vascular cell monolayers to determine their adherence (see table 4).

DAPA prevented thrombin-induced platelet adherence to the endothelium, but failed to influence platelet adherence to fibroblasts or to the surface of the empty dish control. Even when ASA-treated endothelium was used, the presence of DAPA prevented significant adherence to the endothelium.

Our studies to date suggest a significant role for prostacyclin in the maintenance of a normally functioning endothelium. We have been concerned with control mechanisms for prostacyclin production and release.

Prostacyclin formation and release

Preincubation of cultured endothelial cells with 1 mM TMB-8 (Malagodi & Chiou 1974), an antagonist of intracellular calcium ions, or with 4 mM 3-isobutyl-1-methylxanthine (IBMX), an inhibitor of cyclic nucleotide phosphodiesterase activity, blocked prostacyclin release

TABLE 5. EFFECT OF PGI_2 AND 3-ISOBUTYL-1-METHYLXANTHINE (IBMX) ON THE AMOUNT OF CYCLIC AMP (PICOMOLES) IN ENDOTHELIAL CELL MONOLAYERS

treatment	number of experiments	amount of cAMP in 4.5×10^5 cells	
		control	IBMX (4 mM)
control	7	2.16 ± 0.26	5.55 ± 0.57
PGI_2 (400 nM)	7	2.86 ± 0.46	11.81 ± 1.93

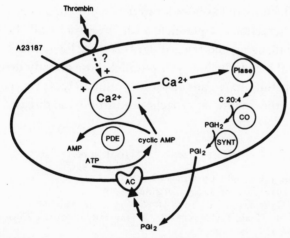

FIGURE 5. Hypothetical mechanisms involved in prostacyclin production and release. Abbreviations: AC, adenylate cyclase; CO, cyclo-oxygenase; PDE, phosphodiesterase; PGI_2, prostacyclin; Plase, phospholipase; SYNT, prostacyclin synthetase.

induced by thrombin or the calcium ionophore A23187, decreased arachidonic acid-induced release by about 50 %, but had no effect on PGH_2-induced release (Brotherton & Hoak 1980). Radioimmunoassay of cyclic AMP in the endothelium showed that the basal level (2.16 ± 0.26 pmol of cyclic AMP per 4.5×10^5 cells) was increased by an average of 2.6-fold with 4 mM IBMX. As table 5 shows, prostacyclin (0.4 μM) had no significant effect on cyclic AMP levels in the absence of IBMX, but caused a twofold increase with 4 mM IBMX.

These findings suggest that an increase in the intracellular concentration of cyclic AMP antagonizes the effect of agents that require calcium ions for the induction of prostacyclin release. In addition, high cyclic AMP phosphodiesterase activity in the endothelium may protect against a negative feedback mechanism involving activation of adenylate cyclase by released prostacyclin. Figure 5 is a diagram of hypothetical reactions involved in prostacyclin control mechanisms.

CONCLUSION

The endothelium has a number of important functions. In this presentation, its normal role in platelet – vessel wall interactions has been emphasized. Prostacyclin appears to play a key role in preventing the aggregation of platelets and their adherence to the vascular wall cells when a thrombogenic stimulus such as thrombin is present.

The failure of high concentrations of prostacyclin to completely block thrombin-induced platelet adherence to smooth muscle cells and fibroblasts suggests that these cells either lack a component normally found in endothelium or produce a substance that promotes adherence. Possible differences include collagen production (type and amount) by smooth muscle and fibroblasts or, for endothelium, interactions at the surface that enhance the effect of prostacyclin. Monolayers derived from normal endothelium or from a malignant type of endothelium (haemangioendothelioma) exhibit some property in addition to prostacyclin that prevents thrombin-induced platelet adherence. Therefore, despite its ability to decrease adherence to all of the cell types tested, it is unlikely that prostacyclin is the sole factor regulating platelet adherence.

We are in an era in which there has been a rapid accumulation of new information about the endothelium and the interactions of platelets with the vessel wall. One can expect that the future will be equally challenging and rewarding. It is quite likely that discoveries of congenital and acquired defects of the endothelium will parallel those already described for platelet and coagulation factors. Hopefully, these advances will ultimately be reflected in the development of better preventive and therapeutic approaches to thrombotic disease.

REFERENCES (Hoak et al.)

Brotherton, A. F. A. & Hoak, J. C. 1980 *Circulation* 62 (2), 165.
Buonassisi, V. & Root, M. 1975 *Biochim. biophys. Acta* 385, 1–10.
Czervionke, R. L., Hoak, J. C., & Fry, G. L. 1978 *J. clin. Invest.* 62, 847–856.
Czervionke, R. L., Smith, J. B., Hoak, J. C. Fry, G. L. & Haycraft, D. 1979 *Thromb. Res.* 14, 781–786.
Florey, H. W. 1966 *Br. med. J.* 2, 487–490.
Heyns, A. D. P., VanDenBerg, D. J., Potgieter, G. M. & Retief, F. 1974 *Thromb. Diath. haemorrh.* 32, 417–431.
Lollar, P. & Owen, W. G. 1980 *J. clin. Invest.* 66, 1222–1230.
Majno, G. 1965 In *Handbook of physiology*, §2 (*Circulation*), vol. 3 (ed. W. F. Hamilton & P. Dow), pp. 2293–2375. Washington, D.C.: American Physiological Society.
Malagodi, M. H. & Chiou, C. Y. 1974 *Eur. J. Pharmac.* 27, 25–33.
Moncada, S., Gryglewski, R., Bunting, S. & Vane, J. R. 1976 *Nature, Lond.* 263, 663–665.
Nesheim, M. E., Prendergast, & Mann, K. G. 1979 *Biochemistry, Wash.* 18, 996–1003.

Phil. Trans. R. Soc. Lond. B **294**, 339–342 (1981)
Printed in Great Britain

Platelet and vascular prostaglandins in uraemia, thrombotic microangiopathy and pre-eclampsia

By G. de Gaetano†, M. Livio†, M. B. Donati† and G. Remuzzi‡

† *Laboratory of Cardiovascular Clinical Pharmacology, Istituto di Ricerche Farmacologiche*
'Mario Negri', via Eritrea 62, 20157 Milan, Italy
‡ *Division of Nephrology and Dialysis, Ospedali Riuniti, Bergamo, Italy*

The metabolism of arachidonic acid in platelets and vascular cells is often altered in clinical conditions associated with haemorrhagic or thromboembolic complications.

We have focused on the one hand on uraemia as a condition frequently complicated by bleeding episodes and, on the other, on thrombotic microangiopathy (thrombotic thrombocytopenic purpura, t.t.p.; haemolytic–uraemic syndrome, h.u.s.) and pre-eclampsia as conditions characterized by uncontrolled intravascular platelet activation.

The observation that prostaglandin synthesis may be regulated by factors present in normal human plasma (Saeed *et al.* 1977; MacIntyre *et al.* 1978) prompted us to investigate whether such plasmatic control was altered in the clinical situations mentioned.

Venous specimens removed from uraemic patients during the institution of an artero-venous shunt for haemodialysis generated significantly more prostacyclin (prostaglandin I_2, PGI_2) than control vessels (Remuzzi *et al.* 1977). Similar findings were subsequently reported in aortic tissue from nephrectomized rats and in arterial tissue from uraemic patients (Leithner *et al.* 1978). Uraemic plasma showed a greater capacity for stimulating PGI_2 synthesis by vascular rings or endothelial cultured cells (Remuzzi *et al.* 1978; Defreyn *et al.* 1980).

This suggests that altered prostacyclin generation in vessel walls from uraemic patients is mediated by plasma. In contrast, both malondialdehyde (MDA) and thromboxane B_2 generated in response to relatively high concentrations of arachidonic acid or thrombin were significantly lower in platelets from uraemic patients than from controls. Uraemic plasma inhibited MDA generation in normal platelets, and normal plasma partly corrected the defect in uraemic platelets (Remuzzi *et al.* 1980*a*).

This suggests that an imbalance in the plasmatic regulation of prostaglandin metabolism in platelets and vessel wall from uraemic patients may contribute to their tendency to bleed.

Thrombotic microangiopathy is characterized by thrombocytopenia, haemolytic anaemia, neurological abnormalities and/or renal failure. Microthrombi occluding arterioles and capillaries of different organs are found on pathological examination. This reflects the occurrence of widespread intravascular platelet aggregation, a crucial event in the pathogenetic sequence of thrombotic microangiopathy.

In three patients with t.t.p. or h.u.s. that we studied (Remuzzi *et al.* 1978; Donati *et al.* 1980), no prostacyclin activity was released from vascular specimens obtained during the acute phase of the disease, which suggested that prostacyclin might be the physiological inhibitor of platelet aggregation, postulated as defective in a patient with t.t.p. described by Byrnes & Khurana (1977). Plasma taken from all three patients on admission had very low capacity, if any, for stimulating vascular prostacyclin synthesis. Treatment with plasma exchange or infusion led to a rapid clinical improvement, and each patient's plasma recovered its capacity to stimulate prostacyclin generation. A deficiency of the plasma factor(s) stimulating vascular PGI_2 activity was therefore suggested as having some role in the pathogenetic sequence of thrombotic micro-angiopathy (Remuzzi *et al.* 1978). This 'missing factor' hypothesis has gained further support from more recent observations that plasma levels of 6-keto-$PGF_{1\alpha}$ (the chemically inactive derivative of PGI_2) were very low or undetectable in patients with t.t.p. or h.u.s. (Hensby *et al.* 1979; Machin *et al.* 1980; Webster *et al.* 1980). In a patient described recently (Remuzzi *et al.* 1980*c*), the deficiency of the plasma factor persisted for at least a year after clinical remission from h.u.s. without recurrence. A similar deficiency was detected in two of this patient's four offspring, who had never suffered from microangiopathic episodes.

This suggests that, at least in some cases of h.u.s. the plasma defect might be genetically determined. Deficient PGI_2-stimulating activity in plasma would not normally result in any clinical sign of disturbed platelet function as long as no aetiological agent such as an endotoxin triggers the pathogenetic sequence of thrombotic microangiopathy (Donati *et al.* 1980).

Preliminary data in two patients studied during the acute phase of h.u.s. indicate that an increased tendency of activated platelets to generate thromboxane A_2 might be an additional factor favouring disseminated intravascular platelet aggregation in this syndrome. Whether plasma modulates the exaggerated metabolism of arachidonic acid in platelets from patients with h.u.s. has not yet been clarified.

Pre-eclampsia is a major cause of morbidity and death for the pregnant woman and her foetus. Signs of consumptive coagulopathy frequently accompany hypertension, oedema and proteinuria, the triad characteristic of this syndrome. Pathological examination may show placental and glomerular vessels occluded by microthrombi, and utero-placental ischaemia appears to play a central role in the pathogenesis.

We have recently reported that PGI_2 production is significantly depressed in umbilical and placental vessels from patients with severe pre-eclampsia in comparison with a normal pregnancy (Remuzzi *et al.* 1980*b*). Reduced PGI_2 production has now been confirmed in umbilical artery (Downing *et al.* 1980), in amniotic fluid (Bodzenta *et al.* 1980) and in plasma (Bussolino *et al.* 1980). Thus maternal hypertension, platelet consumption and reduced placental perfusion could be triggered or maintained by a defect of the mechanism(s) leading in normal pregnancy to increased levels of PGI_2. Indeed, in normal human pregnancy, both foetal and maternal vessels produce larger amounts of PGI_2 than vessels from non-pregnant women (Remuzzi *et al.* 1979; Lewis *et al.* 1980). This implies that an increase in vasodilatory PGI_2 may account for the low peripheral resistance and the high renin activity of normal pregnancy.

This pathogenetic interpretation is reinforced by earlier observations that pregnant rats fed with a vitamin E-deficient fat diet developed eclamptic crises (Stamler 1959). Indeed, vitamin E deficiency has recently been reported to impair PGI_2 production in rats (Okuma *et al.* 1980). Moreover, administration of indomethacin to sheep is followed by a marked increase in the resistance of uterine and placental vascular beds (Rankin *et al.* 1979).

Plasmatic regulation of vascular PGI_2 generation in pregnancy has recently been studied (Remuzzi *et al.* 1981). No significant difference was found between non-pregnant and pregnant women during early pregnancy, but a significant reduction of prostacyclin-stimulating activity was observed in plasma during late normal pregnancy. In patients with severe pre-eclampsia this plasmatic activity was within the range of control non-pregnant women, but significantly higher than comparable women with normal pregnancy.

These results are surprising and apparently difficult to reconcile with the good correlation between high plasmatic activity and high vascular PGI_2 in uraemic patients and low plasmatic activity and low vascular PGI_2 in patients with thrombotic microangiopathy. Possibly more than one mechanism operates in the control of vascular prostacyclin production in normal pregnancy. Perhaps the striking similarity between the behaviour of 'plasma factor' and the response of blood pressure to angiotensin II in normal and complicated pregnancies (Ferris 1978) offers a key to a better understanding of the role of prostacyclin and its regulation in pregnancy. It seems pertinent to mention here that in women with recurrent spontaneous abortion a plasmatic activity (linked to the IgG fraction) inhibiting the release of PGI_2 from aortic rings has recently been found (Carreras et al. 1980).

CONCLUSIONS

The nature of the plasma component(s) modulating platelet and vascular prostaglandin synthesis in uraemia, thrombotic microangiopathy and pregnancy is unknown. Whether such factor(s) are identical to the endogenous modulator(s) described in normal plasma has still to be clarified.

A crucial step in this phenomenon might lie in the balance between free radical formation and removal in plasma (for detailed discussion, see Donati et al. (1980)). An imbalance in the synthesis of metabolites of endogenous arachidonic acid in some clinical conditions such as those discussed in this paper is not necessarily corrected either by the removal of the products generated in excess (achievable for instance by using aspirin or more selective prostaglandin synthesis inhibitors) or by replacement of the defective compound (for instance by infusion of prostacyclin or one of its stable analogues). Indeed, beneficial effects of intravenous infusion of prostacyclin in t.t.p. or h.u.s. have been reported in some patients (Webster et al. 1980) but not in others (Hensby et al. 1979; Budd et al. 1980). On the other hand, patients with pre-eclampsia reportedly benefit from aspirin treatment at doses presumably inhibiting prostacyclin generation (Crandon & Isherwood 1979).

Thus, although any new therapeutic attempt to improve the natural course of these diseases must be encouraged, it would be premature to draw any pharmacological implications from pathogenetic hypotheses still awaiting full confirmation.

Work mentioned in this paper was performed with the support of the Associazione Bergamasca per lo studio delle malattie renali, and of Italian National Research Council ('Farmacologia Clinica e Malattie Rare' and Gruppo Nazionale di Ricerca 'Tecniche sostitutive di funzioni d'organo').

REFERENCES (de Gaetano et al.)

Bodzenta, A., Thomson, J. M. & Poller, L. 1980 Prostacyclin activity in amniotic fluid in pre-eclampsia. *Lancet* ii, 650.

Budd, G. T., Bukowski, R. M., Lucas, F. V., Cato, A. E. & Cocchetto, D. M. 1980 Prostacyclin therapy of thrombotic thrombocytopenic purpura. *Lancet* ii, 915.

Bussolino, F., Benedetto, C., Massobrio, M. & Camussi, G. 1980 Maternal vascular prostacyclin activity in pre-eclampsia. *Lancet* ii, 702.

Byrnes, J. J. & Khurana, M. 1977 Treatment of thrombotic thrombocytopenic purpura with plasma. *New Engl. J. Med.* **297**, 1386–1389.

Carreras, L. D., Defreyn, G., Machin, S. J. & Vermylen, J. 1980 Inhibition of prostacyclin release from rat aorta by IgG from a patient with lupus anticoagulant and recurrent thrombosis. In *Abstracts, Sixth International Congress on Thrombosis*, Monte Carlo, October, no. 187.

Crandon, A. J. & Isherwood, D. M. 1979 Effect of aspirin on incidence of pre-eclampsia. *Lancet* i, 1356.

Defreyn, G., Vergara Dauden, M., Machin, S. J. & Vermylen, J. 1980 A plasma factor in uraemia which stimulates prostacyclin release from cultured endothelial cells. *Thromb. Res.* **19**, 695–700.

Donati, M. B., Misiani, R., Marchesi, D., Livio, M., Mecca, G., Remuzzi, G. & de Gaetano, G. 1980 Hemolytic-uremic syndrome, prostaglandins, and plasma factors. In *Hemostasis, prostaglandins and renal disease* (ed. G. Remuzzi, G. Mecca & G. de Gaetano), pp. 283–290. New York: Raven Press.

Downing I., Shepherd, G. L. & Lewis, P. J. 1980 Reduced prostacyclin production in pre-eclampsia. *Lancet* ii, 1374.

Ferris, T. F. 1978 Postpartum renal insufficiency. *Kidney Int.* **14**, 383–392.

Hensby, C. N., Lewis, P. J., Hilgard, P., Mufti, G. J., Hows, J. & Webster, J. 1979 Prostacyclin deficiency in thrombotic thrombocytopenic purpura. *Lancet* ii, 748.

Leithner, C., Winter, M., Silberbauer, K., Wagner, O., Pinggera, W. & Sinzinger, H. 1978 Enhanced prostacyclin availability of blood vessels in uraemic humans and rats. In *Dialysis, transplantation, nephrology* (ed. B. H. B. Robinson & J. B. Hawkins), pp. 418–422. Tunbridge Wells, Kent: Pitman Medical.

Lewis, P. J., Boylan, P., Friedman, L. A., Hensby, C. N. & Downing, I. 1980 Prostacyclin in pregnancy. *Br. med. J.* **280**, 1581–1582.

Machin, S. J., Defreyn, G., Chamone, D. A. F. & Vermylen, J. 1980 Plasma 6-keto-PGF$_{1\alpha}$ levels after plasma exchange in thrombotic thrombocytopenic purpura. *Lancet* i, 661.

MacIntyre, D. E., Pearson, J. D. & Gordon, J. L. 1978 Localisation and stimulation of prostacyclin production in vascular cells. *Nature, Lond.* **271**, 549–551.

Okuma, M., Takayama, H. & Uchino, H. 1980 Generation of prostacyclin-like substance and lipid peroxidation in vitamin E-deficient rats. *Prostaglandins* **19**, 527–536.

Rankin, J. H. G., Berssenbrugge, A., Anderson, D. & Phernetton, T. 1979 Ovine placental vascular responses to indomethacin. *Am. J. Physiol.* **236**, H61–H64.

Remuzzi, G., Cavenaghi, A. E., Mecca, G., Donati, M. B. & de Gaetano, G. 1977 Prostacyclin-like activity and bleeding in renal failure. *Lancet* ii, 1195–1197.

Remuzzi, G., Marchesi, D., Livio, M., Schieppati, A., Mecca, G., Donati, M. B. & de Gaetano, G. 1980a Prostaglandins, plasma factors and hemostasis in uremia. In *Hemostatis, prostaglandins and renal disease* (ed. G. Remuzzi, G. Mecca & G. de Gaetano), pp. 273–281. New York: Raven Press.

Remuzzi, G., Marchesi, D., Zoja, C., Muratore, D., Mecca, G., Misiani, R., Rossi, E., Barbato, M., Capetta, P., Donati, M. B. & de Gaetano, G. 1980b Reduced umbilical and placental vascular prostacyclin in severe pre-eclampsia. *Prostaglandins* **20**, 105–110.

Remuzzi, G., Mecca, G., Livio, M., de Gaetano, G., Donati, M. B., Pearson, J. D. & Gordon, J. L. 1980c Prostacyclin generation by cultured endothelial cells in haemolytic uraemic syndrome. *Lancet* i, 656–657.

Remuzzi, G., Misiani, R., Marchesi, D., Livio, M., Mecca, G., de Gaetano, G. & Donati, M. B. 1978 Haemolytic–uraemic syndrome: deficiency of plasma factor(s) regulating prostacyclin activity? *Lancet* ii, 871–872.

Remuzzi, G., Misiani, R., Muratore, D., Marchesi, D., Livio, M., Schieppati, A., Mecca, G., de Gaetano, G. & Donati, M. B. 1979 Prostacyclin and human foetal circulation. *Prostaglandins* **18**, 341–348.

Remuzzi, G., Zoja, C., Marchesi, D., Schieppati, A., Mecca, G., Misiani, R., Donati, M. B. & de Gaetano, G. 1981 Plasmatic regulation of vascular prostacyclin in pregnancy. *Br. med. J.* **282**, 512–514.

Saeed, S. A., McDonald-Gibson, W. J., Cuthbert, J., Copas, J. L., Schneider, C., Gardiner, P. J., Butt, N. M. & Collier, H. O. J. 1977 Endogenous inhibitor of prostaglandin synthetase. *Nature, Lond.* **270**, 32–36.

Stamler, F. W. 1959 Fatal eclamptic disease of pregnant rats fed anti-vitamin E stress diet. *Am. J. Path.* **35**, 1207–1231.

Webster, J., Rees, A. J., Lewis, P. J. & Hensby, C. N. 1980 Prostacyclin deficiency in haemolytic–uraemic syndrome. *Br. med. J.* **281**, 271.

Phil. Trans. R. Soc. Lond. B **294**, 343–353 (1981)
Printed in Great Britain

Interactions between stimulated platelets and endothelial cells
in vitro

By A. J. Marcus, M. J. Broekman, B. B. Weksler, E. A. Jaffe,
L. B. Safier, H. L. Ullman and K. Tack-Goldman
*Veterans Administration Hospital, New York, New York 10010, U.S.A., and
Cornell University Medical College, New York, New York, 10021, U.S.A.*

Prostaglandins and hydroxy acids are synthesized mainly from the essential poly-unsaturated fatty acid arachidonate, and these substances have been identified in almost all mammalian tissues. Prostaglandins, thromboxane A_2 (TXA_2) and pro-stacyclin (PGI_2) are autocoids that appear to function in the regulation of vascular tone, cell secretion and contractile processes. So far, hydroxy acids have been found to function as chemotactic agents and in the formation of slow-reacting substances. Other actions of hydroxy acids will certainly be defined in future research. The endoperoxides PGG_2 and PGH_2 represent common precursors of all prostaglandin end-products. In studying the prostaglandin metabolism of a specific tissue, the total profile of endo-peroxide transformation should be determined. In platelets the endoperoxides are transformed mainly into TXA_2, a potent vasoconstrictor and inducer of platelet aggre-gation. Endothelial cells convert endoperoxides to PGI_2, a vasodilator and inhibitor of platelet aggregation. In addition, endothelial cells can utilize endoperoxides from stimulated plates to form PGI_2. The concept that platelets and endothelial cells can share common precursors for the production of modulating substances may be applicable to other cell types.

Introduction

From the standpoint of both basic and clinical research, there is currently a great deal of interest in prostacyclin (PGI_2) and thromboxane A_2 (TXA_2), the principal products of the cyclo-oxygenase pathways in endothelial cells and platelets, respectively (tables 1 and 2). PGI_2 induces strong vasodilatation and inhibits platelet aggregation by stimulating adenylate cyclase, which in turn elevates cyclic AMP and blocks platelet calcium mobilization. TXA_2 is a vasoconstrictor, inducing platelet aggregation via inhibition of adenylate cyclase and promotion of platelet calcium mobilization. Both PGI_2 and TXA_2 are derived enzymically from a common precursor, the prostaglandin endoperoxide PGH_2. The concept of reciprocal regulation of platelet cyclic AMP levels by PGI_2 and TXA_2 has interesting implications. As originally proposed by Bunting *et al.* (1976), a biochemical interaction between platelets and vessel walls may take place in which endoperoxides released in the immediate vicinity of stimu-lated platelets might be used by vessels to form PGI_2. This in turn would elevate platelet cyclic AMP. In this way a balance between the pro-aggregatory effect of TXA_2 and the anti-aggregatory activity of PGI_2 might be achieved (Marcus 1979).

In this paper we summarize recent research in our laboratory on interactions between stimulated platelets and cultured human endothelial cells. In addition, some aspects of arachi-donic acid metabolism in platelets are discussed.

[127]

TABLE 1. ARACHIDONATE METABOLITES FROM THROMBIN-STIMULATED
ENDOTHELIAL CELLS

product	count/min	percentage
6-keto-PGF$_{1\alpha}$	116008	65.5
PGF$_{2\alpha}$	30484	17.2
PGE$_2$	6060	3.4
PGD$_2$	2119	1.2
hydroxy acids	6559	3.7
free 20:4	3220	1.8

TABLE 2. ARACHIDONATE METABOLITES FROM THROMBIN-STIMULATED
PLATELETS

product	count/min	percentage
PGF$_{2\alpha}$	469	2.2
TXB$_2$	9268	43.1
PGE$_2$	467	2.2
PGD$_2$	607	2.8
hydroxy acids	9855	45.8
free 20:4	229	1.1

ARACHIDONIC ACID METABOLISM IN HUMAN PLATELETS

Arachidonic acid (20:4) is a polyunsaturated fatty acid, which mammals synthesize from linoleic acid (18:2), which cannot be synthesized by mammals and so must be obtained from the diet. Prolonged feeding of diets lacking in 18:2 and 18:3 to experimental animals results in a well characterized disorder known as essential fatty acid deficiency (for review see Marcus 1978).

Mechanical or biochemical stimulation of platelets initiates a series of biochemical events culminating in the transformation of arachidonic acid to TXA$_2$ and hydroxy fatty acids. Arachidonate composes about 30 % of the fatty acids in platelet phospholipids (Marcus et al. 1969). Although arachidonic acid is present in all platelet subcellular compartments, i.e. membranes, granules and cytosol (Marcus et al. 1969; Broekman et al. 1976), the precise source of arachidonate for thromboxane synthesis is still not known. Arachidonic acid cannot be processed to TXA$_2$ or hydroxy fatty acids unless it is first rendered available in an unesterified form. Currently, two mechanisms for hydrolysis of platelet phospholipids to yield free 20:4 have received general acceptance. One involves the activity of a phospholipase C on platelet phosphatidylinositol, followed by hydrolysis of the resulting diglyceride by diglyceride lipase to yield unesterified arachidonic acid, which then becomes available to the cyclo-oxygenase and lipoxygenase enzymes (Bell & Majerus 1980; Broekman et al. 1980). The other mechanism involves a phospholipase A$_2$, which acts on arachidonate in the 2-position of one or more platelet phospholipids (Bills et al. 1977; Broekman et al. 1980). It is of interest that after platelet stimulation, far more 20:4 is available than is actually used by the cyclo-oxygenase and lipoxygenase enzymes. The insertion of molecular oxygen and subsequent rearrangement of arachidonate are catalysed by platelet cyclo-oxygenase. Arachidonic acid is the most important substrate for the cyclo-oxygenase, and Lands (1979) has proposed that hydroperoxide(s) is required for activation of cyclo-oxygenase. Some of the free arachidonate is bound to other proteins in the platelet cytoplasm, additional amounts are released into the surrounding medium, and some of the 20:4 becomes reacylated. These alternative pathways for the free arachidonate have not yet been investigated in human platelets.

Free arachidonate is also oxygenated by platelet lipoxygenase. The lipoxygenase is a cytoplasmic enzyme that catalyses formation of 12-hydroxy acids in the platelet. The rate of lipoxygenase catalysis is slower than that of cyclo-oxygenase. Thus, 12-hydroxy acids such as HETE appear in the milieu of stimulated platelets later than TXA_2 (Hamberg *et al.* 1974). HETE is a chemotactic molecule, and its late appearance may correlate with the delayed entry of leucocytes in haemostatic plugs and arterial thrombi.

Endoperoxide formation generates an interesting by-product, 12-L-hydroxy-5,8,10-heptadecatrienoic acid (HHT). This compound contains 17 carbon atoms, the other three being accounted for by malondialdehyde. As might have been anticipated, HHT and malondialdehyde do not form when platelets are pretreated with aspirin or indomethacin. Chemotactic activity is the only biological function to have been determined for HHT. Malondialdehyde was identified as thiobarbituric acid-positive material generated during thrombin-induced platelet aggregation (Hamberg *et al.* 1974), and is a highly reactive molecule that induces cross-linking of proteins and disturbances in enzyme function both *in vivo* and *in vitro*. Why this potentially harmful material is produced during platelet stimulation is not known.

PHOSPHOLIPID METABOLISM IN STIMULATED HUMAN PLATELETS

Studies of endogenous phospholipid metabolism in stimulated platelets have recently been reported from our laboratory (Broekman *et al.* 1980). After platelets had been stimulated with thrombin or collagen, a phosphorus assay of the major and minor platelet phospholipids separated by means of two-dimensional thin-layer chromatography, was carried out. Endogenous platelet phosphatidylinositol (PI) rapidly decreased following thrombin addition. It was expected that the PI decrease would be accompanied by an increase in phosphatidic acid (PA). However, this correlation was not quantitative. One explanation for the discrepancy was that a transient intermediate in platelet PI metabolism, such as diglyceride formed by a PI-specific phospholipase C (Rittenhouse-Simmons 1979) was no longer available for PA formation as catalysed by diglyceride kinase. The transient diglyceride could have been hydrolysed by a diglyceride lipase, as recently described by Bell *et al.* (1979). The latter hydrolytic step would have yielded free arachidonate for subsequent transformation to products of cyclo-oxygenase and lipoxygenase activity. In addition, Broekman *et al.* (1980) noted accumulation of both choline and ethanolamine lysophosphoglycerides in stimulated platelets. Thus, after the addition of thrombin, lysophosphatidylethanolamine accumulated rapidly, reaching plateau levels within 15–20 s after stimulation. Analysis of the fatty acids and aldehydes of the lysophosphatidylethanolamine suggested the presence of platelet phospholipase A_2 activity with an apparent preference for diacylethanolamine phosphoglycerides. Broekman *et al.* also demonstrated that collagen stimulation of platelets was accompanied by changes in PI, PA and lysophospholipids, which occurred concomitantly with the aggregation response and consumption of oxygen indicative of prostaglandin endoperoxide formation. At present it is not unequivocally certain that arachidonate is released from platelet phospholipids by the pathway proposed by Bell *et al.* (1979), i.e. the action of a diglyceride lipase upon the product of phospholipase C hydrolysis of PI. The presence of a diglyceride lipase, combined with the well characterized loss in PI content due to phospholipase C (Rittenhouse-Simmons 1979) is suggestive, but more work remains to be done in this area. Our data on lysophosphoglycerides (Broekman *et al.* 1980) indicate that the Bell pathway is accompanied by classical phospholipase A_2 activity. On the other hand, our data showing incomplete recovery, as PA, of the loss in PI support the hypothesis of a diversion of an intermediate in the PI cycle, such as the action of diglyceride lipase on diglyceride produced by phospholipase C. However, other mechanisms are also possible, such as phospholipase(s) A_2 acting on PI and/or PA. These mechanisms are currently under study. Since the amounts of intermediate diglyceride are far less than the amounts of PI and PA, the diglyceride lipase would have to be far more active than possible phospholipase(s) A_2 acting on PI and/or PA. As yet no data have been presented supporting a turnover number that is sufficiently high. This should be viewed in the light of studies by Lapetina & Cuatrecasas (1979), who showed that PA may be the first lipid product formed after platelet stimulation. Further evidence supporting an important role for PA has been presented (Billah *et al.* 1979; Lapetina *et al.* 1980) and centres on the activity of diglyceride kinase. Obviously, competition between diglyceride kinase and diglyceride lipase could be crucial to the fate of diglyceride. Membrane perturbation with deoxycholate inhibits diglyceride kinase, leading to accumulation of diglyceride (Billah *et al.* 1979). Presumably diglyceride lipase activity was also blocked. Large concentrations of indomethacin (140 µM) inhibit diglyceride lipase more specifically, without inhibiting the kinase (Rittenhouse-Simmons 1980). To what extent these somewhat divergent sets of data are due to methodological and/or species differences is unknown. Our studies (Broekman *et al.* 1980) support phospholipase A_2 activity on PE and PC. In the absence of conclusive data we would suggest that both the Bell hypothesis and a role for PA are possible in human platelets. Whether PA may additionally function as a 'natural ionophore', as proposed by Gerrard *et al.* (1979), is an interesting question. Clearly more experimental data, both in intact platelets and in lysates, are necessary to establish a more definitive rank order for these interesting hypotheses.

ENZYMIC CONVERSION OF ARACHIDONIC ACID AND ENDOPEROXIDE PGH_2 TO PROSTACYCLIN BY CULTURED HUMAN ENDOTHELIAL CELLS

Prostacyclin (PGI_2), the major prostaglandin produced by vascular tissues, is a strong vasodilator and the most powerful inhibitor of platelet aggregation yet described (for review see Marcus 1979). Formation of PGI_2 from the endoperoxide PGH_2 has been demonstrated in fresh arterial and venous tissues in several laboratories (for review see Moncada & Vane 1979).

In 1977, Weksler *et al.* demonstrated that cultured endothelial cells from human umbilical veins and bovine aorta generated an inhibitor of platelet aggregation. Microsomal fractions from these endothelial cells were then shown to synthesize PGI_2 after incubation with [³H]-arachidonic acid (Weksler *et al.* 1977). Marcus *et al.* (1978) then carried out experiments in which exogenous radiolabelled PGH_2 or arachidonic acid was added to intact, unstimulated endothelial cell monolayers. Products of this reaction were studied in detail. The salient features of these studies are summarized here.

Incubation of endothelial cell monolayers with [1-¹⁴C]*arachidonate*

When endothelial cell monolayers were incubated with radioactive arachidonate for 20 min, the major product in the supernatant was 6-keto-$PGF_{1\alpha}$, the chemically stable end-product of PGI_2 breakdown. Small quantities of $PGF_{2\alpha}$ and PGE_2 were also noted. The supernatant fluid from these unstimulated monolayers also contained a large quantity of unconverted arachidonic acid. In contrast to the supernatants of the incubated cells, only traces of prostaglandins were detectable in extracts of the cells *per se*. Radioactivity associated with the cells was identified only in the phospholipid fraction and in the area on the thin-layer plates corresponding to unconverted arachidonic acid.

TABLE 3. QUANTITATIVE RADIO-T.L.C. ANALYSES OF SUPERNATANT PRODUCTS FORMED AFTER INCUBATION OF ENDOTHELIAL CELL MONOLAYERS WITH $[1-^{14}C]PGH_2$ AND $[1-^{14}C]20:4$

(After separation on t.l.c. plates, areas co-chromatographing with appropriate standards and representing radioactive peaks were scraped from the plates and counted. Numbers in the table represent the quantity of counts (± s.d.) in each peak as a percentage of the total counts recovered from the plate. The sum of the percentages does not equal 100 because there were scattered areas of insignificant radioactivity on the plate that did not correspond to known lipids.)

	cells			no cells	
product	20:4	20:4 + aspirin	PGH_2	20:4	PGH_2
6-keto-$PGF_{1\alpha}$	9.0 ± 3.0	0.7	14.6 ± 0.5	0.3	1.1†
$PGF_{2\alpha}$	3.4 ± 1.9	0.5	6.5 ± 2.0	0.2	2.0
PGE_2	4.8 ± 1.1	1.1	35.2 ± 2.3	0.3	46.3
PGD_2	—	—	18.2 ± 1.9	—	21.4
HHT	—	—	12.4 ± 5.0	—	12.9
Unconverted 20:4	65.6 ± 12.4	87.7	—	93.5	—

† Counts in the 6-keto-$PGF_{1\alpha}$ area of this plate did not represent a peak.

Incubation of endothelial cell monolayers with $[1-^{14}C]PGH_2$

In these experiments, endogenous prostaglandin synthesis was blocked by pretreatment of the cells with 100 μM acetylsalicylic acid. The radiolabelled PGH_2 was biosynthesized in our laboratory by the method of Gorman *et al.* (1977). Radiolabelled PGH_2 (2 μM) was added to the aspirin-treated endothelial cells for 5 min. Approximately 15% of the recoverable counts in the cell supernatants was accounted for by 6-keto-$PGF_{1\alpha}$, $PGF_{2\alpha}$, PGE_2, PGD_2 and HHT were also identified. Results obtained with the PGH_2 incubations were in contrast to those observed with arachidonate in that only 0.4% of the radioactivity recovered from the supernatants, plus the cells, were associated with the cells themselves.

Non-enzymic transformation of PGH_2 was studied by incubating radiolabelled PGH_2 in flasks that did not contain endothelial cells. No 6-keto-$PGF_{1\alpha}$ was identified in this system, but spontaneous formation of $PGF_{2\alpha}$, PGE_2, PGD_2 and HHT was observed. Results of the above experiments are summarized in table 3.

We proposed two hypotheses to explain the observed production of PGI_2 by resting endothelial cell monolayers (Marcus *et al.* 1978): (*a*) radiolabelled PGH_2 entered the cell, was converted to prostacyclin and other products, and was then released into the surrounding medium; (*b*) the radiolabelled PGH_2 was enzymatically and non-enzymatically transformed to PGI_2 and other prostaglandins at the cell surface. In any case, it was then of interest to extend these studies with the use of a natural source of PGH_2: the stimulated platelet. These studies have recently been completed and will be summarized in the next section. (Marcus *et al.* 1980).

USE OF PLATELET ENDOPEROXIDES FOR PGI_2 PRODUCTION
BY ENDOTHELIAL CELLS

The experiments were carried out under conditions wherein stimuli were added to mixtures of platelets and endothelial cells. It was also necessary that the endothelial cells were unable to transform endogenous or exogenous arachidonic acid to prostaglandins or hydroxy acids. In control experiments, endothelial cells that had not been treated with aspirin were stimulated with thrombin in the presence of tritiated arachidonic acid (AA). Under these conditions, 66 % of the supernatant AA metabolites was 6-keto-$PGF_{1\alpha}$. Also present were $PGF_{2\alpha}$ (17 %), PGE_2 (3 %), PGD_2 (1 %), hydroxy acids (4 %), and unconverted arachidonic acid (2 %). When the endothelial cells were treated with aspirin (1 mM, 30 min) and then stimulated with thrombin in the presence of tritiated arachidonic acid, no radiolabelled 6-keto-$PGF_{1\alpha}$ was found as measured by radiochromatography and radioimmunoassay. These control experiments were carried out before, during and at the end of each experiment to ascertain that recovery from aspirin treatment did not occur.

An additional experiment to monitor endothelial cell recovery from aspirin treatment was performed as follows: radiolabelled platelets were pretreated with aspirin and then stimulated with thrombin in the presence of aspirin-inhibited endothelial cell suspensions. Thrombin stimulation resulted in the release of free arachidonate from the platelets, but this arachidonate was not used by the aspirin-treated endothelial cells, as shown by our failure to detect 6-keto-$PGF_{1\alpha}$.

PGI_2 synthesis from platelet endoperoxides

These experiments were carried out with the use of radiolabelled platelet suspensions $(2 \times 10^5/\mu l)$ combined with 3000–6000/μl aspirin-treated endothelial cells, also in suspension. The mixtures were stimulated with ionophore A23187, thrombin or collagen in platelet aggregometry cuvettes. In this way, platelet aggregation responses and the formation of PGI_2 and TXA_2 were studied in the same sample.

Two additional controls were carried out, demonstrating that in the absence of an endoperoxide source, aspirin-treated endothelial cells did not form PGI_2. First, when endothelial cells were removed from the system, no 6-keto-$PGF_{1\alpha}$ was detected. Secondly, when unstimulated radiolabelled platelets were incubated with aspirin-treated endothelial cells, no PGI_2 production resulted.

When platelets and aspirin-treated endothelial cell suspensions were stimulated with ionophore, platelet aggregation was inhibited, and the radioactivity in thin-layer chromatograms of lipids derived from these incubation mixtures indicated formation of 6-keto-$PGF_{1\alpha}$. In addition, ionophore-treated platelets produced almost twice as much thromboxane B_2 (TXB_2) in the absence of endothelial cells than they did in their presence. The radiolabelling experiments were corroborated by the demonstration of significant quantities of 6-keto-$PGF_{1\alpha}$ by radioimmunoassay. Thus, a mixture of aspirin-treated endothelial cells (2×10^6) and platelets (10^8) produced 1.7 ng of 6-keto-$PGF_{1\alpha}$ after stimulation with ionophore. Despite the detection of 21 ng of TXB_2 in this mixture, no platelet aggregation occurred in the presence of endothelial cells.

In comparison with control samples, platelet aggregation in response to thrombin was always markedly reduced in the presence of aspirin-treated endothelial cell suspensions, and, concomitantly, PGI_2 synthesis was demonstrable in these systems. Radioimmunoassay results indicated that 0.5 ng of 6-keto-$PGF_{1\alpha}$ and 7.6 ng of TXB_2 had formed after thrombin addition (table 4). As in the ionophore experiments, thrombin-stimulated platelets produced more TXB_2 (1.4-fold) in the absence of aspirin treated endothelial cells than in their presence.

In the presence of aspirin-treated endothelial cells, inhibition of the platelet aggregation response to collagen was comparable with that observed with thrombin. The quantities of 6-keto-$PGF_{1\alpha}$ and TXB_2 detected after collagen exposure were smaller than those observed with thrombin or ionophore. Thus, the quantitative profile of endothelial cell PGI_2 production in the presence of platelets was: ionophore > thrombin > collagen. The pattern of TXB_2 production by the platelets in these combined suspensions followed the same order.

TABLE 4. RADIOIMMUNOASSAY OF 6-KETO-$PGF_{1\alpha}$ AND TXB_2 PRODUCED BY SUSPENSIONS OF PLATELETS AND ASPIRIN-TREATED ENDOTHELIAL CELLS

product	ionophore	thrombin	collagen
6-keto-$PGF_{1\alpha}$/ng	1.7	0.5	0.1
TXB_2/ng	21.3	7.6	2.5

TABLE 5. PLATELET CONTRIBUTION TO PGI_2 FORMATION BY ENDOTHELIAL CELLS

components	6-keto-$PGF_{1\alpha}$/ng
endothelial cells + thrombin	7.7
endothelial cells + platelets + thrombin	19.2
aspirin-treated endothelial cells + platelets + thrombin	8.4

Contribution of platelet endoperoxides to PGI_2 formation by endothelial cells

Addition of thrombin to 3×10^6 endothelial cells in the absence of aspirin resulted in production of 8 ng of 6-keto-$PGF_{1\alpha}$. When 10^8 platelets were mixed with endothelial cells not treated with aspirin and stimulated with thrombin, 19.2 ng of 6-keto-$PGF_{1\alpha}$ was measured by radioimmunoassay. Thus the quantity of PGI_2 approximately doubled. Endothelial cells from the identical cultures were then treated with aspirin and added to platelets, the only source of endoperoxide. When this mixture was stimulated with thrombin, 8.4 ng of 6-keto-$PGF_{1\alpha}$ were detected, and this quantity was derived solely from platelet endoperoxides. This amount (8.4 ng) was similar to that produced by endothelial cells that had not been treated with aspirin. It was therefore concluded that in this system approximately half of the PGI_2 produced by platelet – endothelial cell mixtures originated from endoperoxides synthesized by platelets. These results are summarized in table 5.

Role of platelet concentration in the production of prostacyclin by aspirin-treated endothelial cells

A group of experiments were carried out wherein 1.45×10^6 endothelial cells (2900/μl) were combined with either 10^8 or 15.5×10^8 platelets (i.e. 2 or 31×10^5/μl), and each mixture was stimulated with ionophore, thrombin or collagen. The mixtures in which platelet concentrations were increased produced greater amounts of both 6-keto-$PGF_{1\alpha}$ and TXB_2. However, the increase in platelets resulted in the production of much more TXB_2 than 6-keto-$PGF_{1\alpha}$. The ratio of TXB_2 to 6-keto-$PGF_{1\alpha}$ was increased fourfold to sevenfold. The effects of increasing platelet concentrations in the setting of constant quantities of endothelial cells on the aggregation response were also evaluated. When 2×10^5 platelets/μl were combined with 3850 aspirin-treated endothelial cells/μl and the mixture was stimulated with thrombin (5 U/ml), platelet aggregation did not occur. On the other hand, when platelet concentrations were increased to 5×10^5/μl, the inhibitory effect of the aspirin-treated endothelial cells on platelet aggregation was lost and the responses were normal.

Comparison of studies involving platelets and endothelial cell monolayers with endothelial cell suspensions

When radiolabelled platelets were added to aspirin-treated endothelial cell monolayers and then stimulated with ionophore, less PGI_2 production occurred than when the experiment was carried out with platelets and endothelial cell suspensions (respectively, radioactive counts of 491 and 782/min). Comparable results were obtained when thrombin was the stimulus. When platelets and aspirin-treated endothelial cell monolayers were studied in the presence of thromboxane synthetase inhibitors such as imidazole or U54701, an increase in PGI_2 production occurred, as reported by other laboratories (Moncada et al. 1977; Needleman et al. 1979; Baenziger et al. 1979). Presumably these results were obtained as a consequence of an accumulation of platelet endoperoxides, thus facilitating PGI_2 synthesis by the aspirin-treated endothelial cells. These observations with thromboxane synthetase inhibitors suggested that endothelial cell synthesis of PGI_2 from platelet endoperoxides could indeed occur under appropriate experimental conditions.

The effects of imidazole and U54701 were readily apparent when platelets and aspirin-treated endothelial cell suspensions were used in place of the endothelial cell monolayers. Radioactive counts in the 6-keto-$PGF_{1\alpha}$ area of the thin-layer chromatograms increased from 782 to 12030/min in the presence of imidazole, and to 10847/min with U54701.

Possible significance of interactions between platelets and endothelial cells in vitro

There may be two mechanisms for PGI_2 synthesis by vascular tissues, and in particular human endothelial cells. The first involves synthesis of PGI_2 from endogenous precursors under conditions of perturbation of vascular surfaces. The second occurs from endoperoxides, which the endothelial cells can process when stimulated platelets are in close proximity. Specific conditions under which one or both of these mechanisms may be operative in vivo or even in vitro remain to be established.

In the studies reported, two independent methods for detection of 6-keto-$PGF_{1\alpha}$ were employed: radiolabelling and radioimmunoassay. The radiometric studies allowed us to trace the metabolism of platelet-derived endoperoxides by aspirin-treated endothelial cells. The radioimmunoassay experiments provided quantitative information on the total amount of 6-keto-$PGF_{1\alpha}$ generated by the endothelial cells. Furthermore, the radioimmunoassays allowed us to compare the quantity of 6-keto-$PGF_{1\alpha}$ synthesized endogenously by endothelial cells alone with that derived from platelet endoperoxides.

The use of [^{3}H]arachidonate of high specific activity in the radiolabelling experiments allowed us to study platelets in the concentration range of 2×10^5/μl and markedly increased the sensitivity of the thin-layer chromatographic detection system. The use of endothelial cell suspensions in preference to monolayers facilitated platelet – endothelial cell proximity by concentrating the components in a small volume and allowing adequate mixing. Under these conditions we were able to study aggregation responses and analyse the products generated in the same test sample.

It was also of interest that stimulated platelets synthesized less TXB_2 when mixed with aspirin-treated endothelial cells than when present in the incubation system alone. One explanation is that some of the available platelet endoperoxides were diverted to PGI_2 synthesis when aspirin-treated endothelial cells were present with the platelets. In addition, it is plausible that the PGI_2 formed by the endothelial cells led immediately to inhibition of platelet aggregation and therefore to a decrease in additional thromboxane production.

SUMMARY

1. We have demonstrated that aspirin-treated endothelial cells that were unable to synthesize prostacyclin from endogenous sources were capable of utilizing platelet endoperoxides for PGI_2 synthesis.

2. PGI_2 formation was demonstrable by radio-thin-layer chromatographic analysis and radioimmunoassay.

3. Inhibition of platelet aggregation took place in mixtures of aspirin-treated endothelial cells and platelet suspensions in which PGI_2 formation could be demonstrated.

4. Increasing the ratio of platelets to endothelial cells decreased the ratio of 6-keto-$PGF_{1\alpha}$ to thromboxane, and platelet aggregation occurred.

5. PGI_2 synthesis was more apparent in suspensions of platelets and aspirin-treated endothelial cells than it was when endothelial cell monolayers were studied.

6. PGI_2 synthesis was not attributable to recovery of endothelial cells from aspirin treatment.

7. Endothelial cells are capable of utilizing platelet endoperoxides for as much as one-half of their PGI_2 production.

This work was supported by grants from the Veterans Administration, the National Institutes of Health (HL 18828 05 SCOR), the New York Heart Association and the A. R. Krakower Foundation.

REFERENCES (Marcus *et al.*)

Bell, R. L., Kennerly, D. A., Stanford, N. & Majerus, P. W. 1979 Diglyceride lipase: a pathway for arachidonate release from human platelets. *Proc. natn. Acad. Sci. U.S.A.* **76**, 3238–3241.

Bell, R. L. & Majerus, P. W. 1980 Thrombin-induced hydrolysis of phosphatidylinositol in human platelets. *J. biol. Chem.* **255**, 1790–1792.

Billah, M. M., Lapetina, E. G. & Cuatrecasas, P. 1979 Phosphatidyl-inositol-specific phospholipase-C of platelets: association with 1,2-diacylglycerol-kinase and inhibition by cyclic AMP. *Biochem. biophys. Res. Commun.* **90**, 92–98.

Bills, T. K., Smith, J. B. & Silver, M. J. 1977 Selective release of arachidonic acid from the phospholipids of human platelets in response to thrombin. *J. clin. Invest.* **60**, 1–6.

Broekman, M. J., Handin, R. I., Derksen, A. & Cohen, P. 1976 Distribution of phospholipids, fatty acids, and platelet factor 3 activity among subcellular fractions of human platelets. *Blood* **47**, 963–971.

Broekman, M. J., Ward, J. W. & Marcus, A. J. 1980 Phospholipid metabolism in stimulated human platelets. Changes in phosphatidylinositol, phosphatidic acid, and lysophospholipids. *J. clin. Invest.* **66**, 275–283.

Bunting, S., Gryglewski, R., Moncada, S. & Vane, J. R. 1976 Arterial walls generate from prostaglandin endoperoxides a substance (prostaglandin X) which relaxes strips of mesenteric and coeliac arteries and inhibits platelet aggregation. *Prostaglandins* **12**, 897–913.

Gerrard, J. M., Kindom, S. E., Peterson, D. A., Peller, J., Krantz, K. E. & White, J. G. 1980 Lysophosphatidic acids. Influence on platelet aggregation and intracellular calcium flux. *Am. J. Path.* **96**, 423–438.

Gorman, R. R., Sun, F. F., Miller, O. V. & Johnson, R. A. 1977 Prostaglandin-H_1 and prostaglandin-H_2 – convenient biochemical synthesis and isolation – further biological and spectroscopic characterization. *Prostaglandins* **13**, 1043–1053.

Hamberg, M., Svensson, J. & Samuelsson, B. 1974 Prostaglandin endoperoxides. A new concept concerning the mode of action and release of prostaglandins. *Proc. natn. Acad. Sci. U.S.A.* **71**, 3824–3828.

Lands, W. E. M. 1979 The biosynthesis and metabolism of prostaglandins. *A. Rev. Physiol.* **41**, 633–652.

Lapetina, E. G., Billah, M. M. & Cuatrecasas, P. 1980 Stimulation of the phosphatidylinositol-specific phospholipase-C and the release of arachidonic acid in activated platelets. In *The regulation of coagulation* (*Developments in biochemistry*, vol. 8) (ed. K. G. Mann & F. B. Taylor), pp. 491–497. New York: Elsevier.

Lapetina, E. G. & Cuatrecasas, P. 1979 Stimulation of phosphatidic acid production in platelets precedes the formation of arachidonate and parallels the release of serotonin. *Biochim. biophys. Acta* **573**, 394–402.

Marcus, A. J. 1978 The role of lipids in platelet function: with particular reference to the arachidonic acid pathway. *J. Lipid Res.* **19**, 793–826.

Marcus, A. J. 1979 The role of prostaglandins in platelet function. *Prog. Hemat.* **11**, 147–171.

Marcus, A. J., Ullman, H. L. & Safier, L. B. 1969 Lipid composition of subcellular particles of human blood platelets. *J. Lipid Res.* **10**, 108–114.

Marcus, A. J., Weksler, B. B. & Jaffe, E. A. 1978 Enzymatic conversion of prostaglandin endoperoxide H_2 and arachidonic acid to prostacyclin by cultured human endothelial cells. *J. biol. Chem.* **253**, 7138–7141.

Marcus, A. J., Weksler, B. B., Jaffe, E. A. & Broekman, M. J. 1980 Synthesis of prostacyclin from platelet-derived endoperoxides by cultured human endothelial cells. *J. clin. Invest.* **66**, 979–986.

Moncada, S. & Vane, J. R. 1979 Arachidonic acid metabolites and the interactions between platelets and blood-vessel walls. *New Engl. J. Med.* **300**, 1142–1147.

Rittenhouse-Simmons, S. 1979 Production of diglyceride from phosphatidylinositol in activated human platelets. *J. clin. Invest.* **63**, 580–587.

Weksler, B. B., Marcus, A. J. & Jaffe, E. A. 1977 Synthesis of prostaglandin I_2 (prostacyclin) by cultured human and bovine endothelial cells. *Proc. natn. Acad. Sci. U.S.A.* **74**, 3922–3926.

Discussion

I. F. SKIDMORE (*Glaxo Group Research, Ware, U.K.*).

1. In his graph of PI breakdown and PA accumulation Dr Marcus implied that the difference between the two might account for the arachidonic acid released. Is it possible to calculate how much arachidonic acid is released? Does the difference between PI breakdown and PA accumulation account for it, and if not, what other mechanisms are involved?

2. Some workers have claimed that lyso PC accumulates in activated platelets but Dr Marcus's data indicates that lyso PE is the major lysophosphatide found. How is this difference explained? Can it be attributed to differences in the time of sampling after activation?

3. Would Dr Marcus consider specific transacylation from PC (or PE) to PI as described by Irvine & Dawson (*Biochem. biophys. Res. Commun.* **91**, 1399–1405) as a reasonable alternative for the generation of lysophosphatides to a mechanism involving phospholipase A_2?

A. J. MARCUS.

1. These are very interesting, indeed intriguing, questions. We inferred from our measurements of phosphate content that the difference between the loss in PI and the gain in PA might possibly contribute to the quantities of arachidonate hydrolysed from platelet phospholipids. Our calculations indicate that it probably can account for a maximum of two-thirds of the arachidonate liberated if we postulate that the quantities of diglyceride and other intermediates are negligible. Thus, other mechanisms, such as the phospholipase A_2 activity that we demonstrated on PE and PC, must also be contributing to the liberation of arachidonate. It is further possible to postulate pathways whereby PI is the sole source of the liberated arachidonate, with the loss of 20:4 from other phospholipids being channelled directly towards synthesis of PA and/or PI.

2. Technical differences, including sampling time and composition of the medium in which the platelets were suspended, are most likely responsible for this apparent discrepancy. Time-course studies, which are of course difficult to carry out, are critical in some of these determinations.

3. This may indeed be a reasonable alternative but, it should be emphasized that Irvine & Dawson's work was carried out on rat liver microsomes. Nevertheless, this is a very interesting and, of course, energy-efficient process, which is currently under investigation in our laboratory.

G. HORNSTRA (*Department of Biochemistry, Rijksuniversiteit Limburg, The Netherlands*). Some time ago we published a study (Hornstra *et al.* 1979) in which we demonstrated that:

(*a*) the PGI_2 production of vascular tissue is not significantly different on incubation in either platelet-poor plasma (p.p.p.) or platelet-rich plasma (p.r.p.);

(*b*) indomethacin-treated tissue does not produce prostacyclin upon short-term incubation in p.p.p. or p.r.p., whereas it does so on incubation with PGH_2;

(*c*) vascular tissue pretreated with indomethacin is unable to produce prostacyclin even if it is incubated in a suspension of collagen-activated endoperoxide-producing blood platelets;

(*d*) PGI_2 formation of vascular tissue is not different upon incubation in collagen-activated p.r.p. of normal or arachidonic acid-deficient rats producing very different amounts of endoperoxides.

We also demonstrated that the restoration of prostacyclin production occurring upon long-term incubation of indomethacin-treated vessel walls as observed by Bunting *et al.* (1976) is due to the removal of indomethacin from the cyclo-oxygenase enzyme system, which is consequently reactivated.

Recently we have shown that the presence of blood platelets does not significantly accelerate the course of this restoration.

It might be true that our negative results are due to the fact that the ratio between the number of platelets and endothelial cells was too high to allow platelet-derived endoperoxides to reach the vascular tissue. However, it should be realized that such a high ratio will also exist at the site of mural thrombus formation. Nevertheless, Dr Marcus has very convincingly shown that under favourable conditions endoperoxides can indeed escape platelets and serve as a substrate for vascular prostacyclin formation. The question that remains to be answered is: does this also happen under conditions less artificial than used so far?

Reference

Hornstra, G., Haddeman, E. & Don, J. A. 1979 Blood platelets do not provide endoperoxides for vascular prostacyclin production. *Nature, Lond.* **279**, 66–68.

Phil. Trans. R. Soc. Lond. B **294**, 355–371 (1981)
Printed in Great Britain

Platelet – vessel wall interaction: role of blood clotting

By G. Hornstra

Department of Biochemistry,
State University of Limburg, P.O. Box 616,
600 200 MD Maastricht, The Netherlands

Vascular damage initiates not only the adhesion and aggregation of blood platelets but also coagulation, which is of mixed (intrinsic and extrinsic) origin. Evidence is presented that thrombin, generated as a result of the injury, is a prerequisite for platelet aggregation.

Platelets, after activation, in their turn promote coagulation. Prostaglandin I_2 (PGI_2 or prostacyclin) inhibits coagulation induced by damaged vascular tissue. This effect of PGI_2 is mediated by the inhibition of platelets in their participation in the generation of factor X_a and thrombin. Dietary cod liver oil, by changing plasma coagulability, decreases the procoagulation activity of vessel walls, and arterial thrombosis. Another fish oil with similar effects on plasma coagulability and some other haemostatic parameters does not modify vessel wall-induced clotting, nor does it significantly lower arterial thrombosis tendency; this indicates the physiological relevance of vessel wall-induced clotting in arterial thrombus formation. Some evidence is also given for the importance of vessel wall-induced clotting in primary haemostasis.

1. Introduction

The major event triggering haemostasis and thrombosis is disruption of vascular endothelium. Exposure of the blood to subendothelium results in the simultaneous occurrence of two closely interrelated processes: platelet activation and blood clotting. Platelet activation may lead to the formation of a fragile platelet thrombus by a process reviewed by Mustard & Packham (1970), Weiss (1975), and many others. In brief, circulating platelets adhere to subendothelial tissue – collagen, microfibrils, basement membrane – which may become exposed to the blood after vessel trauma, rupture of an atherosclerotic plaque, etc. Adhered platelets release some of their constituents, such as adenine nucleotides, serotonin, Ca^{2+} and adrenalin. Adenosine diphosphate (ADP), released by this reaction, causes passing platelets to aggregate and stick to the adhered ones, thus forming a mural platelet thrombus which, being unstable, is easily embolized. The platelet-release reaction is also induced by platelet aggregation; so the formation of mural and circulating platelet thrombi is a self-propagating process.

Since vascular tissue has thromboplastic activity (Nemerson & Pitlick 1972), vessel wall damage is likely to trigger extrinsic clotting. Moreover, subendothelial collagen, while interacting with one of the contact factors (factor XII) (Niewiarowski *et al.* 1965; Wilner *et al.* 1968) or with platelets (Walsh 1972*a*), triggers the intrinsic coagulation system, which is also initiated by platelets *per se* when activated by small amounts of ADP (Walsh 1972*b*). Coagulation is accelerated by platelet factor 3 (PF_3), a phospholipoprotein entity that is normally inactive (Fantl & Ward 1958) but which becomes available upon platelet activation (Sixma & Nijessen 1970; Joist *et al.* 1974).

The contribution of coagulation to arterial thrombus formation has long been thought to be of secondary importance, being confined to reinforcement by fibrin of the fragile white platelet thrombus. However, as will be demonstrated below, there is evidence that coagulation is of primary importance here, because thrombin formation appeared to be necessary for the platelet response to vessel wall damage *in vitro*.

2. Measurement of vessel wall-induced clotting

Rats are bled under ether anaesthesia by puncturing the abdominal aorta. The blood is collected in citrate; platelet-rich plasma (p.r.p.) and platelet-poor plasma (p.p.p.) are prepared by differential centrifugation. The aortas are rapidly removed, cleaned of adhering

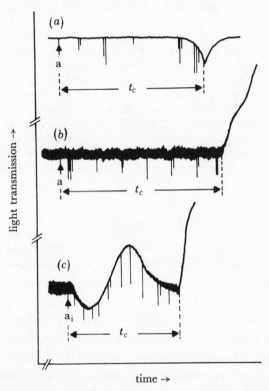

FIGURE 1. Clotting-induced changes in light transmission in platelet-poor plasma (*a*) and platelet-rich plasma preceded (*c*) or not (*b*) by platelet shape change and aggregation. Abbreviations: a, aorta; a_i, aorta pretreated with indomethacin; t_c, clotting time.

tissue, opened longitudinally and kept in an ice-cold Krebs–Henseleit (K.H.) buffer. P.r.p. or p.p.p. (50 μl) and 450 μl Ca^{2+}-containing saline ($CaCl_2$, 0.65 μmol/l, in NaCl, 0.154 mol/l) are placed into the cuvette of an aggregometer. The temperature is maintained at 37.5 °C and the stirring speed is 600–700 rev/min. After 3 min, a small piece of tissue, 3 mm in diameter, is punched out of the aorta and transferred into the cuvette, where light transmission is recorded continuously. Fibrin formation is indicated by a decrease in light transmission, which is very clearly observed in p.p.p. (figure 1*a*). This decrease is followed by a rapid increase when the fibrin fibres become twisted around the stirring bar. When the vascular tissue passes the light beam, the tracing shows spikes. In p.r.p., fibrin formation is not always clearly visible, owing to the high turbidity of the solution. However, the subsequent increase in transmission is more pronounced than in p.p.p., because platelets are trapped in the fibrin strands twisting around the stirring bar (figure 1 b). The time lapse (in seconds) between tissue addition and the moment of clotting is called the clotting time, t_c, which, for statistical reasons, is indicated by the clotting index $S = 1000/t_c$. The higher S, the higher is the clotting tendency of the plasma. So far, vessel wall-induced clotting has been observed with material from rabbits, rats, dogs and man. Most of the experiments to be described here have been performed with material from rats.

The tissue is punched out of a blood vessel; therefore our model may be more related to haemostasis than to thrombosis since in the latter process vascular damage is more superficial. However, the basic processes in haemostasis and thrombosis may be similar; therefore our findings may be relevant for both haemostasis and thrombosis.

3. Tentative characterization of the clotting process initiated by damaged vascular tissue

The process of blood clotting can be activated via two different routes (figure 2). (For a review see Suttie & Jackson (1977).) In the intrinsic pathway, which can be measured by the a.p.t.t. test (activated partial thromboplastin time), only blood-borne clotting factors are involved. Extrinsic clotting is initiated by a tissue thromboplastin and, moreover needs clotting factor VII. It can be measured by the p.t. test (prothrombin time).

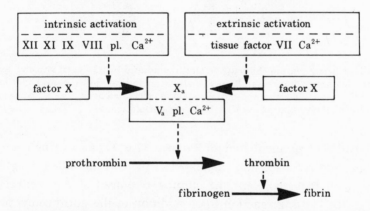

Figure 2. Simplified diagram of coagulation pathways; pl., platelets or phospholipids.

So far, only preliminary investigations have been carried out on the vessel wall-induced clotting process. When compared with rat-brain thromboplastin, damaged tissue of rat aorta induced similar clotting indices in human VII-deficient plasma, which were about 60% lower than in a standard plasma (figure 3). When human vascular tissue was used (obtained from surgical patients), the clotting response in human VII-deficient plasma was about 40% lower than that obtained with a standard plasma. Both results indicate that the vessel wall activates the extrinsic clotting mechanism. This is in line with the fairly well documented tissue-factor activity of the vessel wall (for review see Nemerson & Pitlick 1972).

This finding was confirmed in preliminary experiments with a rabbit-raised fibrinogen-free and complement-free antiserum against human brain thromboplastin (prepared and provided by Dr K. van Ginkel, Amsterdam), which was shown to be ineffective in the a.p.t.t. test.

Pieces of vascular tissue from rat or man were incubated in 50 μl antithromboplastin or control serum, diluted with 450 μl Tris buffer (10 mmol/l) in saline (pH 7.3), containing Ca^{2+} at 4 mmol/l, in a stirred cuvette at 700 rev/min and 37 °C. After incubation for 3 and 15 min, 50 μl portions of the incubate were transferred into an aggregometer cuvette, containing 450 μl Tris–saline buffer with Ca^{2+} (4 mmol/l) and 50 μl standard rat or human platelet-

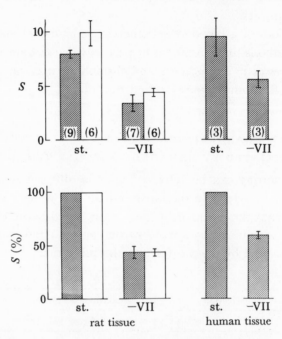

FIGURE 3. Effect of VII-deficient plasma (human) on clotting induced by damaged vascular tissue (shaded bars) and rat brain thromboplastin (open bars). Upper row, clotting indicated by the mean clotting index $S \pm$ s.e.m. (standard error of the mean); lower row, clotting responses calculated as $\% \pm$ s.e.m. compared with standard plasma (100 %). St., standard plasma; − VII, VII-deficient plasma.

free plasma, which had been preincubated for 3 min at 37.5 °C at a stirring rate of 700 rev/min. The clotting response was recorded and calculated as the clotting index, S (§2).

In figure 4, the open bars represent the clotting responses of the control incubate. The shaded bars refer to the clotting reaction upon addition of the antithromboplastin incubate. The difference between these responses as a percentage of the control S is indicated by the black bars and it can be seen that the clotting potency of rat and human tissue is greatly diminished (but not blocked) upon preincubation with antithromboplastin antibodies. The fact that neither the VII-deficient plasma nor the thromboplastin antibodies are able to prevent vessel wall-induced clotting completely suggests that in this clotting process an intrinsic component is also involved. This is supported by studies of VIII-, IX-, XI and XII-deficient plasmas (human), which showed a lower clotting response with rat aortic tissue than a human standard plasma. The combined character of vessel wall-induced clotting (intrinsic and extrinsic) is also underlined by the significant correlation existing between vessel wall-induced clotting and p.t. as well as a.p.t.t., as was observed in a study of dietary fish-oil induced changes in vessel wall-induced clotting (see §9). However, more experiments are needed for a further analysis of this clotting process.

4. VESSEL WALL-INDUCED PLATELET REACTIONS:
ROLE OF THROMBOXANE A_2 AND ADP

The clotting of p.r.p., brought about by a piece of vascular tissue producing little or no pro-stacyclin, is preceded by platelet shape change and aggregation (figure 1c). The time course of these platelet reactions very much resembles that of collagen-induced aggregation, which is known to be mediated by ADP (Hovig & Holmsen 1963) and by thromboxane A_2, (TXA_2) (Hamberg et al. 1975) which are derived from activated blood platelets and which can be inhibited by aspirin (O'Brien 1968; Weiss et al. 1968; Zucker & Peterson 1970).

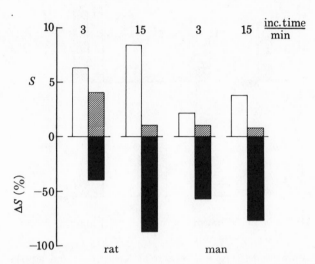

FIGURE 4. Effect of an antithromboplastin antiserum on the clotting index (S) of rat and human tissue. Open bars, tissue incubated with control serum; shaded bars, tissue incubated with antiserum; solid bars, difference in clotting response occurring upon tissue incubating in control and antiserum respectively (ΔS).

To investigate the role of platelet ADP and TXA_2 in the aggregation of p.r.p. after exposure to damaged vascular tissue, p.r.p. was preincubated with aspirin (0.55 mmol/l in saline) or with saline for 1 h at room temperature. Subsequently, aggregation was measured in 50 µl p.r.p. diluted with 440 µl Ca^{2+}-containing saline (Payton Dual Channel aggregometer), on addition of one piece of indomethacin-treated vascular tissue (with 10 µl saline), 10 µl ADP (0.25 µmol/l, final concentration), 10 µl of a suspension of collagen in saline (5.6 µg protein/ml, final concentration) or 10 µl thrombin (0.09 N.I.H. units/ml, final concentration).

The results of this study are shown in figure 5a, from which it is evident that the aggregation induced by injured vascular tissue and by thrombin is not significantly affected by aspirin treatment of the p.r.p. The collagen- and ADP-induced aggregation was significantly impaired, thus showing the effectiveness of the aspirin dose used to block platelet TXA_2 production. These results strongly suggest that vessel wall-induced aggregation is not primarily mediated by TXA_2 and/or ADP.

However, it has been shown repeatedly that the aspirin effect can be overcome by simply increasing the trigger strength, thereby inducing the release of ADP independently of platelet thromboxane production (Zucker & Peterson 1970; Fukami et al. 1976). Therefore, the aspirin experiment was repeated with p.r.p. obtained from Fawn Hooded (FH) rats. This strain of rats has a hereditary defect of the platelet release reaction: their dense granules, which in normal animals contain ATP, ADP, Ca^{2+}, serotonin, pyrophosphate and antiplasmin (Holmsen 1978), seem to be empty. This defect is thought to be the cause of the bleeding tendency observed in these animals, because the collagen-induced aggregation is greatly impaired (Raymond & Dodds 1975; Tschopp & Zucker 1972). However, collagen-induced platelet TXA_2 production is normal in FH rats, judging from the production of a TXA_2 metabolite, malondialdehyde (MDA), upon supramaximal triggering with collagen (FH, 1.33 ± 0.048; Wistar strain, 1.30 ± 0.069 nmol MDA/10^9 platelets; $n = 9$).

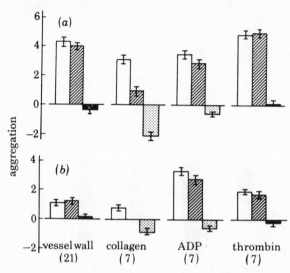

FIGURE 5. Aggregation (arbitrary units, $\pm$ s.e.m.) of normal (open bars) and aspirin-treated (hatched bars) p.r.p. induced by different stimuli. (a) Wistar rats; (b) Fawn Hooded rats. Solid black bars, difference between normal and aspirin-treated p.r.p. not significant ($p_2 > 0.05$); stippled bars, difference significant ($p_2 < 0.01$); numbers in parentheses, n.

As shown in figure 5b, the results obtained with FH p.r.p. are identical to those obtained with Wistar rats. Preincubation of p.r.p. with an aspirin dose large enough to block the collagen-induced aggregation completely and inhibit the ADP-induced aggregation significantly did not modify vessel-wall and thrombin-induced aggregation.

The role of released ADP was further investigated by measuring the aggregation of p.r.p. induced by a piece of indomethacin-treated rat aorta in the presence and absence of the ADP dephosphorylating enzyme apyrase (Ardlie et al. 1971) and the ADP transphosphorylating system creatine phosphate and creatine phosphokinase (Izrael et al. 1974). These ADP scavengers appeared to inhibit platelet aggregation only in doses about double those needed to block a comparable degree of aggregation induced by added ADP.

These results demonstrate that neither TXA_2 nor ADP plays a primary role in the aggregation of platelets induced by damaged vascular tissue.

5. VESSEL WALL-INDUCED PLATELET REACTIONS: ROLE OF THROMBIN

As shown in figure 5a, b, the aggregation induced by damaged vascular tissue closely resembles that of thrombin as far as the effect of aspirin is concerned. Since the p.r.p.–vessel-wall interaction triggers a clotting response, the preceding platelet reactions may be mediated by thrombin formed during this clotting response. We tested this hypothesis by measuring vessel wall-induced aggregation and clotting of p.r.p. in the presence of increasing amounts of hirudin (from Pentapharm, Basle, Switzerland), which is a specific thrombin-inactivating polypeptide and does not modify platelet aggregation induced by ADP. It appeared that this substance very effectively blocked platelet aggregation when added to p.r.p. in doses only slightly effective in lowering the clotting response (figure 6).

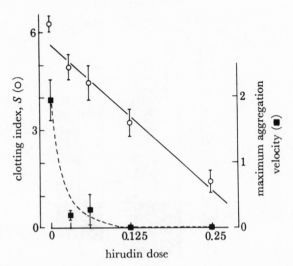

FIGURE 6. Effect of hirudin (final concentrations in antithrombin units per millilitre) on clotting (○) and platelet aggregation (■) induced by damaged vascular tissue; mean values ±s.e.m.; $n = 5$.

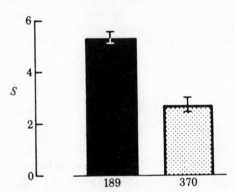

FIGURE 7. Effect of blood platelets on vessel wall-induced clotting ($S\pm$s.e.m.). Figures below bars are clotting times (seconds) calculated from mean S values; $n = 28$. Solid bar, clotting occurring in p.r.p.; stippled bar, clotting occurring in p.p.p.

It is therefore concluded that platelet aggregation after exposure to damaged vascular tissue is mediated by thrombin, generated during vessel wall-induced clotting. Since ADP scavengers had also some inhibitory effect on vessel wall-induced platelet reactions, a supporting role of ADP, released from erythrocytes, adherent platelets and/or from non-adherent platelets activated by the generated thrombin, is probable (Packham *et al.* 1973).

[145]

6. Role of blood platelets in vessel wall-induced clotting

When vessel wall-induced clotting in p.r.p. and p.p.p. was compared, it appeared that the clotting response in p.r.p. is significantly greater than that in p.p.p. (figure 7; $p_2 < 0.01$, Student's t-test). Although the pieces of vascular tissue used provide a thrombogenic surface, especially along their edges, platelets not in direct contact with the vessel wall are not activated, as can be concluded from the absence of platelet shape change and aggregation (figure 1b).

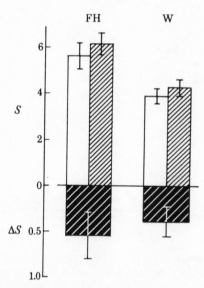

Figure 8. Effect of ADP-induced platelet aggregation on vessel wall-induced clotting ($S \pm$ s.e.m.) of p.r.p. Experiments carried out with material from Fawn Hooded rats (FH) and Wistar rats (W); $n = 12$. Open bars, clotting of p.r.p. without ADP added; upper hatched bars, clotting of p.r.p. when aggregation is induced by adding ADP; lower hatched bars, difference in clotting ($\Delta S \pm$ s.e.m.) resulting from ADP-induced aggregation.

This would indicate that, for their clot-promoting effect, platelets need not become activated. However, it is likely that the adhered and thereby activated platelets are responsible for the clot-promoting effect observed. When, immediately upon tissue addition, aggregation is triggered by adding ADP 0.35 µmol/l, final concentration), coagulation is significantly enhanced ($p_2 < 0.05$) (figure 8). Since ADP in itself has never been shown to affect blood clotting, this strongly suggests that activated platelets have a stronger clot-promoting effect than non-activated ones. As is also evident from figure 8, vessel wall-induced clotting in FH rats (see §4) is significantly ($p_2 < 0.01$, Student's two-samples test) higher than in normal Wistar rats. This has been confirmed in later experiments and requires further investigation.

7. Effect of vascular prostacyclin on vessel wall-induced clotting

Vascular tissue produces prostacyclin (PGI_2), which is a very active inhibitor of platelet activation (Moncada *et al.* 1976) and may therefore be expected to inhibit the participation of blood platelets in vessel wall-induced clotting. When vascular prostacyclin formation is blocked by pretreatment of the tissue with indomethacin, aspirin or tranylcypromine, the clotting response is enhanced; moreover, it is preceded by a generalized activation of the platelets in the cuvette as indicated by their shape change and aggregation. Indeed, this finding suggests that vascular prostacyclin, by diminishing platelet activation, inhibits vessel wall-induced clotting. However, an alternative explanation may be that the compounds used to prevent prostacyclin generation affect vessel wall induced clotting in a direct, prostacyclin-independent way. We therefore measured vessel wall-induced clotting with material taken from arachidonic acid (AA) deficient animals. Vascular tissue of these animals produces only very small amounts of prostacyclin (Hornstra *et al.* 1978). Consequently, if PGI_2 does indeed play a regulating role, vessel wall-induced clotting might be expected to be enhanced in AA

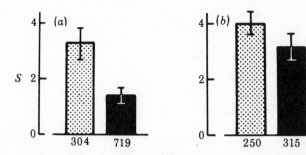

FIGURE 9. Vessel wall-induced clotting ($S \pm$ s.e.m.) observed with material obtained from AA-deficient (stippled bars) and control (solid black bars) animals. (*a*) Untreated tissue incubated in autologous p.r.p. ($n = 10$); (*b*) indomethacin-treated tissue, incubated in autologous p.r.p. ($n = 12$). Figures below bars are clotting times (seconds) calculated from mean S values.

deficiency. This indeed appeared to be so: clotting induced by AA-deficient tissue is significantly higher than with control material (figure 9*a*). Only in the AA-deficient group, clotting was preceded by platelet shape change and aggregation.

When the tissue was pretreated with indomethacin, thereby preventing any role of vascular prostacyclin, the difference between both groups was greatly reduced (figure 9*b*). These and other findings (Hornstra & Hemker 1979) demonstrate that vascular prostacyclin inhibits vessel wall-induced clotting.

8. MECHANISM BY WHICH PGI_2 INHIBITS VESSEL WALL-INDUCED CLOTTING

S. Bunting & S. Moncada (personal communication) and Ts'ao *et al.* (1979) demonstrate that clotting tests performed in the absence of platelets are not modified by PGI_2. Moreover, vessel wall-induced clotting in p.p.p. is not affected by pretreatment of the tissue with indomethacin. Only in the presence of platelets has prostacyclin been demonstrated to inhibit clotting. Therefore, any effect of prostacyclin on vessel wall-induced clotting is probably mediated by its effect on blood platelets.

Platelets contribute to blood coagulation in various ways (figure 10): when activated with collagen or ADP they initiate the intrinsic pathway of coagulation (Walsh 1974). Moreover, they contribute to the intrinsic activation of factor X and the conversion of prothrombin into thrombin. (For a review see Zwaal (1978)). This latter activity is known as platelet factor 3 (PF_3) and has been shown to reflect procoagulant phospholipids (mainly phosphatidyl serine) becoming available at the platelet surface. For the expression of PF_3 activity, intact platelets must become activated and it appeared that of all physiologically relevant platelet activators only a combination of collagen and thrombin is able to make these activities available (Zwaal *et al.* 1980). Recently the same was shown to hold for the role of platelets in the activation of factor X

(G. van Dieijen, personal communication). Since this combined trigger is likely to be present at the site of a vascular injury (collagen from the subendothelium and thrombin as a result of vessel wall-induced clotting), it is conceivable that the effect of blood platelets on vessel wall-induced clotting is at least partly due to their stimulation of X_a-generation, prothrombin conversion, or both. Consequently, PGI_2 may inhibit vessel wall induced clotting by inhibiting these platelet functions. This is currently under investigation with the use of the following

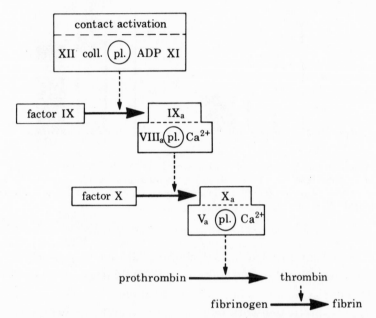

FIGURE 10. Simplified diagram to indicate the participation of platelets (pl.) in the various stages of coagulation.

assay system. A mixture of the appropriate amounts of Ca^{2+} and of the various purified clotting factors is incubated with washed platelets preactivated with collagen and thrombin in the presence of different amounts of PGI_2. After a given incubation time the reaction is interrupted and the amount of X_a or thrombin formed is measured spectrophotometrically, by using X_a or thrombin-specific chromogenic substrates and standard curves obtained with purified X_a and thrombin (Rosing et al. 1980; van Dieijen et al. 1981).

When no platelets are present, or when the platelets are not properly activated, X_a generation is hardly measurable. However, the presence of activated platelets greatly accelerates X_a formation, and preliminary results (figure 11) clearly indicate that this process is inhibited by PGI_2 in a dose-dependent way. No inhibition is observed when the procoagulant phospholipids are added as lipid vesicles or when lysed platelets are used as a source of these phospholipids. This demonstrates that prostacyclin does not interfere with X_a formation as such, but specifically inhibits the process by which collagen and thrombin stimulate platelets to expose procoagulant phospholipids.

Essentially similar, although quantitatively different, results were obtained for the participation of platelets in the generation of thrombin. As shown in figure 11, a rather high dose of PGI_2 is required to inhibit those platelet-procoagulant activities; moreover the inhibition is only partial. This partial inhibition is also observed, although to a lesser extent, when the aggregation of blood platelets and their ATP release is measured in response to a mixture of collagen and thrombin. Although each trigger can on its own be effectively blocked by PGI_2, their combined action cannot be inhibited completely. It is tempting to speculate that the rest-activity is due to platelets that have adhered to the collagen, despite the high PGI_2 concentration. From our preliminary data it seems that platelet thrombotic functions (aggregation

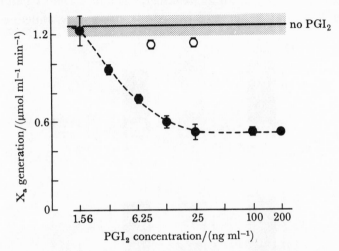

FIGURE 11. Effect of prostacyclin (PGI_2) on the participation of washed platelets (2.7×10^7/ml), activated with a mixture of collagen and thrombin, in the generation of factor X_a. Means of 2–6 determinations $\pm$ s.e.m. Open circles refer to measurements performed with platelet lysates, diluted to obtain about the same X_a generation as the platelet preparation under investigation (value without PGI_2: 1.12 ± 0.02 µmol X_a ml^{-1} min^{-1}).

and release) are about 10 times more sensitive to inhibition by prostacyclin than the platelet procoagulant activities under investigation. Further experiments are in progress to explore these phenomena.

9. EFFECT OF DIETARY FISH OIL ON VESSEL WALL-INDUCED CLOTTING

From the experiments with AA-deficient animals (see §7) it appeared that vascular prostacyclin inhibits vessel wall-induced clotting. As with AA deficiency, feeding fish oil also results in a diminished production of vascular prostacyclin (Hornstra & Hemker 1979; Ten Hoor et al. 1980). Moreover, feeding fish oils to rats does not result in the formation of prostaglandin I_3 (Hornstra et al. 1981). Because of this low production of PGI, vessel wall-induced clotting may be expected to be enhanced by fish oil feeding. However, as has been demonstrated before for FH rats (Hornstra & Hemker 1979), feeding cod liver oil results in a significant inhibition of this vascular clotting response, which appeared to be due to some plasma condition. This cod liver oil effect has been confirmed with Wistar rats; it is not produced by fish oils in general since feeding another fish oil did not result in a lower vessel wall-induced clotting response (figure 12). Because cod liver oil and the other fish oil lowered platelet and vascular prostaglandin production to about the same extent (Hornstra 1981), vascular prostacyclin is unlikely to be involved. Moreover, the cod liver oil effect is likely to act through the plasma, excluding any other vascular factor. We therefore measured plasma coagulability in animals fed with fish oil and compared it with that of plasma obtained from animals fed either a commercial stock diet or a diet enriched with sunflower seed oil. To investigate the intrinsic pathway of coagulation, a.p.t.ts were measured in platelet-free plasma (p.f.p.) prepared by high-speed contrifugation (16000 g for 20 min) of p.p.p. The test was performed in p.f.p., diluted to 20% with a Tris buffer (10 mmol/l in saline) at pH 7.35. The activation mixture consisted of inositin, 50 mg/ml (0.2 ml); kaolin, 100 mg; and Tris–saline buffer (19.8 ml). Clotting was measured in an aggregometer (Payton Dual Channel) at 37.5 °C in siliconized glass tubes. Transmitted light was recorded continuously while the reaction mixture

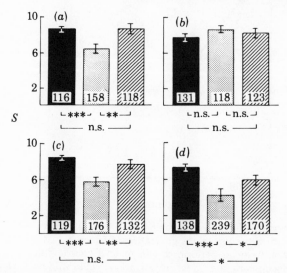

FIGURE 12. Vessel wall-induced clotting ($S\pm$s.e.m., $n = 10$) measured with vascular tissue, p.r.p. and p.p.p. of rats fed on diets containing 50 % of its digestible energy as sunflower seed oil (black bars), cod liver oil (shaded bars), and another fish oil (hatched bars). Figures in bars represent clotting times (seconds) calculated from mean S values. (a) Vascular tissue in autologous p.r.p.; (b) vascular tissue in p.r.p. of stock animals; (c) vascular tissue of stock animals in different p.r.ps; (d) vascular tissue of stock animals in various p.f.ps. Significance levels: n.s., $p_2 > 0.10$; *, $0.05 < p_2 < 0.10$; **, $0.001 < p_2 < 0.01$; ***, $p_2 < 0.001$.

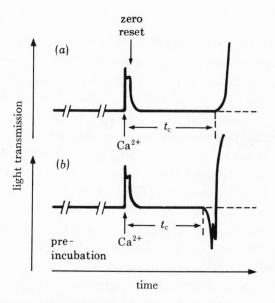

FIGURE 13. Diagram of aggregometer tracings obtained when measuring a.p.t.t. (a) and p.t. (b) in platelet-free plasma dilutions; t_c, clotting times.

[150]

was stirred with a siliconized metal bar at 500 rev/min; 0.1 ml Tris–saline buffer, 0.1 ml plasma dilution and 0.1 ml activation mixture were incubated for 2 min, after which 0.1 ml $CaCl_2$ (0.033 mol/l) was added. Clotting times were calculated from the recorder tracings as indicated in figure 13. Because of skew distribution, these clotting times (t_c, seconds) were converted to the clotting index, $S = 1000/t_c$ (see §2).

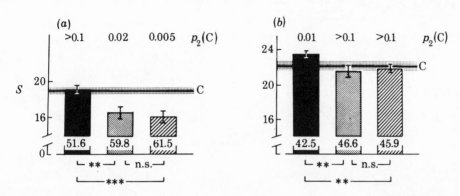

FIGURE 14. Intrinsic (a.p.t.t., (a)) and extrinsic (p.t., (b)) clotting ($S \pm$ s.e.m., $n = 10$) measured in platelet free plasma dilutions of rats fed on diets containing 50% of their digestible energy as sunflower seed oil (black bars), cod liver oil (shaded bars), and another fish oil (hatched bars). Figures in bars indicate clotting times (seconds) calculated from mean S values. C, Results obtained with plasma of control animals fed a commercial stock diet (heavy line, mean; shaded area, s.e.m.); p_2(C), significance level compared with control group; n.s., $p_2 > 0.10$; **, $0.001 < p_2 < 0.01$; ***, $p_2 < 0.0001$.

Extrinsic clotting was measured with the one-stage p.t. test by using rat-brain thromboplastin prepared according to a procedure described by Owren & Aas (1951). The preparation was diluted with Michaelis buffer to give a clotting time of about 14 s ($S = 71.4$) with undiluted standard rat p.f.p. P.t. measurements were performed on p.f.p., diluted to 20% by volume with the Tris–saline buffer. Plasma dilution (0.15 ml) and 0.15 ml of the rat-brain thromboplastin preparation were incubated for 1 min at 37.5 °C at a stirring rate of 500 rev/min in a siliconized glass cuvette of the Payton Dual Channel aggregometer. Coagulation was triggered by adding 0.15 ml $CaCl_2$ (0.033 mol/l). Clotting times were calculated from the aggregometer tracings as shown in figure 13 and converted to S values as discussed for a.p.t.ts.

As illustrated in figure 14a, intrinsic clotting is reduced in both fish oil groups compared with the control group, whereas extrinsic clotting is not significantly altered by fish oil feeding (figure 14b). Compared with sunflower seed oil, both intrinsic clotting and extrinsic clotting are reduced in both fish oil groups.

In fact, a significant correlation was observed between vessel wall-induced clotting and plasma extrinsic and intrinsic coagulability (figure 15). This supports the view that vessel wall-induced clotting is of mixed intrinsic and extrinsic origin (see §3). However, these results do not explain the difference between the two fish oils in their effect on vessel wall-induced clotting. This difference therefore needs further investigation.

10. PHYSIOLOGICAL RELEVANCE OF VESSEL WALL-INDUCED CLOTTING

As stated in §2, vessel wall-induced clotting may be important in haemostasis and thrombosis. As far as primary haemostasis is concerned, supporting evidence was obtained from experiments with the AA-deficient animals and those fed on cod liver oil. As shown in table 1, both groups of animals show a striking similarity in platelet and vascular prostaglandins and platelet aggregation. However, the bleeding time in the animals fed with cod liver oil is prolonged, whereas in AA-deficient rats it is normal. It might very well be that the enhanced vessel wall-induced clotting observed in AA-deficient animals has effectively counteracted the reduced platelet aggregation after collagen activation, leading to a normal bleeding time,

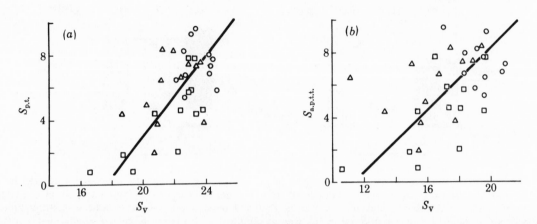

Figure 15. Relation between vessel wall-induced clotting (S_v) and extrinsic (p.t., (a)) and intrinsic (a.p.t.t., (b)) clotting measured in platelet-free plasma of animals fed on diets containing 50 % of its digestible energy as sunflower seed oil (O), cod liver oil (□) or another fish oil (△). (a) $y = -21.67 + 1.23x$, $n = 35$, $r = 0.64$, $p < 0.001$; (b) $y = -10.73 + 0.95x$, $n = 35$, $r = 0.50$, $0.001 < p < 0.01$.

TABLE 1. COMPARISON BETWEEN COD LIVER OIL FEEDING AND ARACHIDONIC ACID (AA) DEFICIENCY IN THEIR EFFECT ON VARIOUS HAEMOSTATIC PARAMETERS IN RATS

(+, enhanced compared with control animals; −, diminished compared with control animals; O, not significantly different from control animals.)

parameter	cod liver oil	AA deficiency
platelet and vascular prostaglandins	−	−
aggregation induced by:		
ADP	O	O
collagen	−	−
thrombin	+	+
bleeding time	+	O
vessel wall-induced clotting	−	+

whereas the reduced vessel wall-induced clotting observed in the cod liver oil group may have potentiated the effect of the diminished collagen-induced aggregation, resulting in a prolongation of the bleeding time. In this respect it is also relevant to recall that the lengthening of the bleeding time by aspirin is greatly increased in hypocoagulation (haemophilia, oral anticoagulation, etc.)

Vessel wall-induced clotting is also likely to be important in arterial thrombosis. A first indication was obtained from a study with rats in which different thrombosis tendencies were induced by feeding various dietary fats. After 3 months, arterial thrombosis tendency was measured in 50 % of the animals, whereas the other animals were used for the measurement of vessel wall-induced clotting. It then appeared that both parameters were strikingly correlated: the higher the vessel wall induced clotting, the higher the tendency towards arterial thrombosis (Hornstra & Hemker 1979).

A second indication of the importance of vessel wall-induced clotting in thrombogenesis is obtained from our fish oil studies. We repeatedly observed that cod liver oil feeding results in a significant lowering of the tendency towards arterial thrombosis, whereas feeding the other fish oil has little effect. This discrepancy between the two fish oils cannot be ascribed to any difference in platelet and vascular prostaglandins, platelet aggregability or plasma coagulability, which are about equal in both groups, as are the bleeding times (Hornstra 1981). Only vessel wall-induced clotting appeared different: it is reduced by feeding with cod liver oil, whereas it is not affected by feeding with the other fish oil (figure 12). It is tempting to speculate that this difference is responsible for the different effects on arterial thrombosis tendency produced by feeding the various fish oils.

As has been pointed out by Loeliger (1976), the preventive effect of oral anticoagulation on myocardial (re)infarction improves with level of anticoagulation. Recently, a well designed study was undertaken to investigate the effect of anticoagulant withdrawal from postmyocardial infarction patients aged 60 years and over. A significantly higher reinfarction rate was observed in the group in which anticoagulant therapy was discontinued. Bleeding complications were only slightly enhanced in the group in which treatment was continued, resulting in a lower overall mortality in this group (de Vries *et al.* 1980). Since vessel wall-induced clotting is closely correlated with plasma coagulability (see §9), these findings in man also support the importance of vessel wall-induced clotting in arterial thrombus formation. Therefore, further investigations into the phenomenon of vessel wall-induced clotting seem worthwhile.

Thanks are due to Mr C. Gardien and Mr J. S. W. Kleinekoort (Unilever Research, Vlaardingen, the Netherlands) for preparing the illustrations (C.G.) and for supervising the rat feeding experiments (J.S.W.K.). Dr G. van Dieijen and Dr E. Bevers cooperated in the measurements of the PGI_2 effects on X_a and thrombin generation (§8). Miss A. D. Muller made the rat brain thromboplastin preparation (§3).

REFERENCES (Hornstra)

Ardlie, N. G., Perry, D. W., Packham, M. A. & Mustard, J. F. 1971 Influence of apyrase on stability of suspensions of washed rabbit platelets. *Proc. Soc. exp. Biol. Med.* **136**, 1021–1023.

van Dieijen, G., Tans, G., Rosing, J. & Hemker, H. C. 1981 The role of phospholipid and factor VIII$_a$ in the activation of bovine factor X. *J. biol. Chem.* (in the press.)

Fantl, P. & Ward, H. A. 1958 The thromboplastic component of intact blood is present in masked form. *Aust. J. exp. Biol. med. Sci.* **36**, 499–504.

Fukami, H. M., Holmsen, H. & Bauer, J. 1976 Thrombin-induced oxygen consumption, malondialdehyde formation and serotonin-secretion in human platelets. *Biochim. biophys. Acta* **428**, 253–256.

Hamberg, M., Svensson, J. & Samuelsson, B. 1975 Thromboxanes, a new group of biologically active compounds, derived from prostaglandin endoperoxides. *Proc. natn. Acad. Sci. U.S.A.* **72**, 2994–2998.

Holmsen, H. 1978 Platelet secretion. Current concepts and methodological aspects. In *Platelet function testing* (D.H.E.W. Publication no. (N.I.H.) 78-1087), pp. 112–132. U.S. Department of Health, Education and Welfare.

ten Hoor, F., de Deckere, E. A. M., Haddeman, E., Hornstra, G. & Quadt, J. F. A. 1980 Dietary manipulation of prostaglandin and thromboxane synthesis in heart, aorta and blood platelets of the rat. *Adv. Prost. Thrombox. Res.* **8**, 1771–1781.

Hornstra, G. 1981 (In preparation.)

Hornstra, G. & Hemker, H. C. 1979 Clot-promoting effect of platelet–vessel wall interaction: influence of dietary fats in relation to arterial thrombus formation in rats. *Haemostasis* **8**, 211–226.

Hornstra, G., Christ-Hazelhof, E., Haddeman, E., Nugteren, D. H. & ten Hoor, F. 1981 Fish oil feeding lowers thromboxane and prostacyclin production by rat platelets and aorta and does not result in the formation of prostaglandin I₃. *Prostaglandins*. (In the press.)

Hornstra, G., Haddeman, E. & Don, J. A. 1978 Some investigations into the role of prostacyclin in thromboregulation. *Thromb. Res.* **12**, 367–374.

Hovig, T. & Holmsen, H. 1963 Release of a platelet-aggregating substance (adenosine diphosphate) from rabbit blood platelets induced by saline 'extracts' of tendon. *Thromb. Diathes. haemorrh.* **9**, 264–278.

Izrael, V., Zawilska, K., Jaisson, F., Levy-Toledano, S. & Caen, J. 1974 Effect of vast removal of plasmatic ADP by the creatine phosphate and creatine phosphokinase system on human platelet function *in vitro*. In *Platelets: production, function, transfusion and storage*, pp. 187–196. New York: Grune & Stratton.

Joist, J. H., Dolezel, G., Lloyd, J. V., Kinlough-Rathbone, R. L. & Mustard, J. F. 1974 Platelet factor-3 availability and the platelet release reaction. *J. Lab. clin. Med.* **84**, 474–482.

Loeliger, E. A., Hensen, A., Kroes, F., van Dijk, L. M., Fekkes, N. de Jonge, H. & Hemker, H. C. 1967 A double-blind trial of long-term anticoagulant treatment after myocardial infarction. *Acta med. scand.* **182**, 549–566.

Moncada, S., Gryglewski, R. J., Bunting, S. & Vane, J. R. 1976 An enzyme isolated from arteries transforms prostaglandin endoperoxides to an unstable substance that inhibits platelet aggregation. *Nature, Lond.* **263**, 663–665.

Mustard, J. F. & Packham, M. A. 1970 Factors influencing platelet function: adhesion, release and aggregation. *Pharmac. Rev.* **22**, 97–187.

Nemerson, Y. & Pitlick, F. A. 1972 The tissue factor pathway of blood coagulation. In *Progress in haemostasis and thrombosis* (ed. T. H. Spaet), vol. 1, pp. 1–37. New York and London: Grune & Stratton.

Niewiarowski, S., Bankowski, E. & Rogowicka, I. 1965 Studies on the absorption and activation of the Hageman factor (factor XII) by collagen and elastin. *Thromb. Diathes. haemorrh.* **14**, 387–400.

O'Brien, J. R. 1968 Effects of salicylates on human platelets. *Lancet* i, 779–783.

Owren, P. A. & Aas, K. 1951 The control of dicumarol therapy and the quantitative determination of prothrombin and proconvertin. *Scand. J. clin. Invest.* **3**, 201–208.

Packham, M. A., Guccione, M. A., Chang, P. L. & Mustard, J. F. 1973 Platelet aggregation and release: effects of low concentrations of thrombin or collagen. *Am. J. Physiol.* **225**, 38–47.

Raymond, S. L. & Dodds, W. J. 1975 Characterization of the Fawn-Hooded rat as a model for hemostatic studies. *Thromb. Diathes. haemorrh.* **33**, 361–369.

Rosing, J., Tans, G., Govers-Riemslag, J. W. P., Zwaal, R. F. A. & Hemker, H. C. 1980 The role of phospholipids and factor Vₐ in the prothrombinase complex. *J. biol. Chem.* **255**, 274–283.

Sixma, J. J. & Nijessen, J. G. 1958 Characteristics of platelet factor 3 release during ADP-induced aggregation. Comparison with 5-hydroxytryptamine release. *Thromb. Diathes. haemorrh.* **24**, 206–213.

Suttie, J. W. & Jackson, C. M. 1977 Prothrombin structure, activation and biosynthesis. *Physiol. Rev.* **57**, 1–70.

Ts'ao, C.-H., Holly, C. M., Serieno, M. A. & Galluzzo, T. S. 1979 Generation of a PGI₂-like activity by deendothelialized rat aorta. *Thromb. Haemostas.* **42**, 873–884.

Tschopp, T. B. & Zucker, M. B. 1972 Hereditary defect in platelet function in rats. *Blood* **40**, 217–226.

de Vries, W. A., Tyssen, J. P. G., Loeliger, E. A. & Roos, J. 1980 A double-blind trial to assess long term oral anticoagulant therapy in elderly patients after myocardial infarction. *Lancet* ii, 909–994.

Walsh, P. N. 1972a The effect of collagen and kaolin on the intrinsic coagulant activity of platelets. Evidence for an alternative pathway in intrinsic coagulation not requiring Factor XII. *Br. J. Haemat.* **22**, 393–405.

Walsh, P. N. 1972b The role of platelets in the contact phase of blood coagulation. *Br. J. Haemat.* **22**, 237–254.

Walsh, P. N. 1974 Platelet coagulant activities and haemostasis: a hypothesis. *Blood* **43**, 597–605.

Weiss, H. J., Aledort, L. M. & Kochwa, S. 1968 The effects of salicylates on the hemostatic properties of platelets in man. *J. clin. Invest.* **47**, 2169–2180.

Weiss, H. J. 1975 Platelet physiology and abnormalities of platelet function. *New Engl. J. Med.* **293**, 531–541; 580–588.

Wilner, G. D., Nossel, H. L. & Le Roy, E. C. 1968 Activation of Hageman factor by collagen. *J. clin. Invest* **47**, 2608–2615.

Zucker, M. B. & Peterson, J. 1970 Effect of acetylsalicylic acid, other nonsteroidal anti-inflammatory agents and dipyridamole on human blood platelets. *J. Lab. clin. Med.* **76**, 66–75.

Zwaal, R. F. A. 1978 Membrane and lipid involvement in blood coagulation. *Biochim. biophys. Acta* **515**, 165–207

Zwaal, R. F. A., Rosing, J., Tans, G., Bevers, E. M. & Hemker, H. C. 1980 Topological and kinetic aspects of phospholipids in blood coagulation. In *The regulation of coagulation* (ed. K. G. Mann & F. B. Taylor, Jr), pp. 95–115. Elsevier/North Holland.

Discussion

C. R. W. GRAY (*Thoracic Unit, Westminster Hospital, London, U.K.*). Dr Hornstra's results do not support the conclusion that endoperoxides pass from platelets to endothelium to increase its production of prostacyclin. The experiment by Begent & Born (1970) demonstrated rapid embolization of platelet thrombi after the iontophoretic application of ADP to small venules was stopped. This could indicate that ADP stimulates the production of endothelial prostacyclin.

Reference

Begent, N. & Born, G. V. R. 1970 Growth rate *in vivo* of platelet thrombi, produced by iontophoresis of ADP, as a function of mean blood flow velocity. *Nature, Lond.* **227**, 926–930.

G. HORNSTRA. In a series of experiments performed under a variety of conditions, we were unable to demonstrate that activated platelets produce endoperoxides for vascular prostacyclin formation (Hornstra *et al.* 1979). As demonstrated in §§7 and 8, prostacyclin inhibits vessel wall-induced clotting by diminishing platelet activation. If ADP did stimulate vascular PGI_2 production, it would also be expected to reduce vessel wall-induced clotting. However, ADP stimulates the vessel wall-induced clotting response (figure 8). This observation does not exclude the suggested interaction between ADP and the vessel wall since the clot-promoting effect of ADP-treated platelets (Walsh 1972*b*) may be more pronounced than the coagulation-inhibiting effect resulting from a possibly stimulated prostacyclin formation. Nevertheless, our findings do not in themselves support the concept that ADP enhances vascular PGI_2 production.

Reference

Hornstra, G., Haddeman, E. & Don, J. A. 1979 Blood platelets do not provide endoperoxides for vascular prostacyclin production. *Nature, Lond.* **279**, 66–68.

Phil. Trans. R. Soc. Lond. B **294**, 373–381 (1981)
Printed in Great Britain

Platelet – vessel wall interaction: influence of diet

By J. Dyerberg

*Department of Clinical Chemistry, Aalborg Hospital, Section North,
DK-9000 Aalborg, Denmark*

The interaction of platelets with the vessel wall is influenced by the diet. Of major importance is the dietary polyunsaturated fatty acids (PUFA). Epidemiological evidence from Greenland Eskimos with low incidences of acute myocardial infarction has drawn attention to the role of the $n-3$ PUFA family.

Experiments *in vitro* have demonstrated an anti-aggregatory effect of eicosapentaenoic acid (EPA). However, EPA does not inhibit vascular prostacyclin production. Antiaggregatory substances generated from EPA have not yet been demonstrated *in vivo*.

Studies *in vivo* in both animals and humans have demonstrated an antithrombotic effect of EPA. In a study where volunteers were given 6 g EPA per day for 3 weeks, moderate decreases in collagen-induced and ADP-induced platelet aggregation, lower thromboxane B_2 (TXB_2) synthesis and prolongation of bleeding time were found.

These observations indicate that dietary factors modulate the interaction of platelets and the vessel wall. Dietary advice aiming at lowering the incidence of ischaemic diseases must include this aspect. This necessitates a re-evaluation of advice hitherto given to the population in general.

Introduction

Attempts have been made for two or three decades to influence the alarmingly high incidence of mortality from ischaemic heart disease (i.h.d.) in western societies by dietary advice. The so-called lipid hypothesis, based on epidemiological evidence of a causal role of high blood cholesterol and, in later years, low levels of high-density lipoproteins in the pathogenesis of ischaemic heart disease has, however, proved unprofitable in spite of the effort made at its implementation. One of the main points in lipid lowering régimes has been the recommendation of a high intake of polyunsaturated fatty acids, which has been synonymous with a high intake of linoleic acid, the principal member of the $n-6$ family. The inconsistency of the scientific data supporting this recommendation has led the Food and Nutrition Board (1980) under The National Academy of Science in U.S.A. in its report *Toward healthful diets* to state that 'the benefit of altering the diet (towards a higher P:S ratio) has not been established'. In his comment on this report, Olson (1980) states, 'the Lipid Hypothesis is not proved and has failed as a strategy for reduction of IHD. New excitement has been generated about the "Platelet Hypothesis". Feeding aspirin and marine oils may provide a new strategy for prevention of coronary disease.'

Great differences in the incidence of ischaemic heart disease exist, however, between different societies, and many observations point to environmental causes for this difference. Thus, the study of different populations and their way of life may still prove useful in identifying the factors leading to ischaemic heart disease.

Some observations indicate that this difference in morbidity pattern may be associated with differences in platelet – vessel wall interaction, and that differences in this balance may be attributed to differences in dietary habits.

I shall illustrate this by referring to studies on Greenland Eskimos and to the experimental evidence that we have, elucidating the mechanisms involved in the Eskimo pattern of morbidity. Finally I shall discuss the results of an experiment designed to see if the platelet – vessel wall interaction can be changed by dietary alterations.

THE GREENLAND ESKIMOS: STUDIES ON THE MECHANISM OF THEIR LOW INCIDENCE OF I.H.D.

It has been known (but not documented) for decades that myocardial infarction in Greenland Eskimos is very rare. Recently this common knowledge has gained support from medical statistics as reported in *The state of health in Greenland*, an annual report from the chief medical officer in Greenland (1978), from which it can be calculated that the overall mortality from ischaemic heart diseases in the years 1973–6 averaged 3.5%. This is not due to short life expectancy, for the average life span of Greenlanders is now about 60 years as reported by the Ministry of Greenland (1979). We have had the opportunity of investigating this problem during four expeditions to northwestern Greenland in the years 1970–8. First we examined the plasma lipid and lipoprotein concentrations (Bang & Dyerberg 1972; Dyerberg *et al.* 1977) and table 1 shows the average differences in plasma lipid and lipoprotein concentrations between 130 Greenlanders and 470 Danish controls, matched for age and sex.

The Eskimos had lower cholesterol and triglyceride concentrations owing to lower LDL and VLDL levels and also higher HDL concentrations. Such differences are documented by several epidemiological studies as associated with a lower risk of developing i.h.d. The differences were, however, not large enough to explain satisfactorily the difference in mortality due to i.h.d., which is about 50% in Denmark.

In investigating the fatty acid pattern of the plasma lipids (Dyerberg *et al.* 1975), we found that the distribution of polyunsaturated fatty acids was dominated by those belonging to the linolenic class or the $n-3$ class in contrast to the $n-6$ class, which is the prevailing type in Danes. This is illustrated in table 2 in which the fatty acid distribution in the plasma phospholipids is given.

During two expeditions to the same area in Greenland in 1972 and 1976 we examined the diet of Greenlanders (Bang *et al.* 1980). The total consumption of fat was no greater than in Danes, whereas the protein content due to the higher meat consumption was higher and the carbohydrate content correspondingly lower. Of the fat in the diet (table 3), the $n-3$ class was the prevailing type of polyunsaturated fat, in contrast with the $n-6$ class in Danes.

This dominance was due to a high content of eicosapentaenoic acid (EPA), docosapentaenoic acid and docosahexaenoic acid (table 4), and we calculated that approximately 5–6 g of EPA was eaten per day.

At the time of our work it was found by Samuelsson's group in Sweden (Hamberg *et al.* 1975) and Vane's group in Beckenham (Moncada *et al.* 1976) that unstable metabolites of arachidonic acid were generated by platelets and the vessel wall respectively and that these metabolites had opposite effects on platelet – vessel wall interactions. It was further postulated that a balanced effect between these substances regulated haemostasis (Moncada & Vane 1978). By combining these findings with our observations of a shift from arachidonic acid into

TABLE 1. AVERAGE DIFFERENCES IN PLASMA LIPID AND LIPOPROTEIN CONCENTRATIONS BETWEEN CAUCASIAN DANES AND GREENLAND ESKIMOS

cholesterol	1.15 mmol/l
triglycerides	0.66 mmol/l
LDL	0.76 g/l
VLDL	0.86 g/l
HDL	−0.66 g/l

TABLE 2. FATTY ACID COMPOSITION OF PLASMA PHOSPHOLIPIDS IN GREENLAND ESKIMOS (G.E., $N = 16$) AND DANISH CONTROLS (D., $N = 20$)

(Values are means as a percentage of total.)

	G.E.	D.		G.E.	D.
8:0–15:0	4.2	0.3	20:4	3.8	7.4
16:0	32.2	30.0	20:5	7.4	1.8
16:1	4.3	0.8	22:0–22:5	2.2	2.2
16:2–17:1	—	0.7	22:6	3.6	2.2
18:0	17.0	14.6	24:0–24:1	2.5	4.2
18:1	14.9	12.4	saturated	54.5	47.3
18:2	5.4	22.3	monoenes	24.4	15.3
18:3	0.1	0.2	polyenes	21.1	34.2
18:4–20:3	3.3	0.7	20:5/20:4	1.95	0.24

TABLE 3. DIETARY FAT TYPES IN ESKIMO AND DANISH FOOD

	Eskimos	Danish
saturated (percentage of total fatty acids)	22.8	52.7
monounsaturated (percentage of total fatty acids)	57.3	34.6
polyunsaturated (percentage of total fatty acids)	19.2	12.7
P:S ratio	0.84	0.24
linoleic class $(n-6)/(g/day/3000\ kcal)$	5.4	10.0
linolenic class $(n-3)/(g/day/3000\ kcal)$	13.7	2.8
monoenes, except 16:1 and 18:1/(g/day/3000 kcal)	29.6	2.1

TABLE 4. FATTY ACID COMPOSITION OF FOOD LIPIDS IN GREENLAND ESKIMOS, 1976 (G.E., $N = 178$) AND IN DANISH FOOD, 1972 (D.)

(Values are means as a percentage of total.)

	G.E.	D.		G.E.	D.
12:0	4.8	13.4	20:1	14.7	0.4
16:0	13.6	25.5	20:4	0.4	—
16:1	9.8	3.8	20:5	4.6	0.5
16:2–17:1	0.4	—	22:1	8.0	1.2
18:0	4.0	9.5	22:5–22:6	8.5	0.3
18:1	24.6	29.2	saturated	22.8	52.7
18:2	5.0	10.0	monoenes	57.3	34.6
18:3	0.6	2.0	polyenes	19.2	12.7
20:0	0.1	4.3	20:5/18:2	0.92	0.05

eicosapentaenoic acid, the precursor of the prostaglandin-3 family in Eskimos, we hypothesized that such a shift may alter haemostasis and thrombosis tendency towards an antithrombotic direction and thereby give an additional explanation to the low morbidity of acute myocardial infarction in Eskimos. An indication of such a shift was found in nosographic reports from Greenland, in which throughout the centuries we find descriptions of an enhanced bleeding tendency in Eskimos ascribed by many to the heavy intake of blubber (Bang & Dyerberg

TABLE 5. FATTY ACID COMPOSITION OF PLATELET LIPIDS IN GREENLAND ESKIMOS,
1978 (G.E., $N = 24$) AND DANISH CONTROLS (D., $N = 20$)

(Values are means as a percentage of total.)

	G.E.	D.		G.E.	D.
12:0–14:0	0.2	0.1	22:0–24:1	8.8	5.9
16:0–16:1	23.8	20.4	22:5	3.4	1.0
18:0	12.0	17.2	22:6	6.1	1.5
18:1	18.2	17.2	(unidentified	1.0	3.6)
18:2	4.0	8.2	saturated	35.6	41.3
20:0–20:1	5.6	2.3	monoenes	32.8	21.8
20:4	8.9	22.1	polyenes	30.3	33.0
20:5	8.3	0.5	20:5/20:4	0.93	0.02

1980). We hypothesized that this was due to the influence of EPA on the balance between pro- and antiaggregatory conditions in the platelet and vessel wall, and we demonstrated that EPA inhibits platelet aggregation (Dyerberg & Bang 1978). Furthermore, we suggested that EPA in the vessel wall could be converted into an antiaggregatory substance (Dyerberg *et al.* 1978). Consequently the haemostasis in Greenlanders was examined (Dyerberg & Bang 1979). We found that the bleeding time in Eskimos averaged 8.05 min, which was significantly longer than in Danes (4.76 min). This difference was due to a decreased platelet aggregability, as measured by ADP and collagen induced aggregation. It was paralleled by a difference in fatty acid composition of the platelet lipids (table 5), the Eskimos being dominated by the $n-3$ class, especially $20:5$, $n-3$ (EPA) to which we in our hypothesis ascribed the platelet hypoaggregability.

We concluded from our studies that the low incidence of ischaemic heart disease in Eskimos was associated with platelet hypoaggregability and high content of EPA in structural and transport lipids, coming from a dietary intake of 5–6 g of this substance per day. Furthermore, the Eskimos showed no sign whatsoever of deficiency of essential fatty acids. I mention this because Gudbjarnason & Oskarsdottir (1975) found that rats fed with a marine oil diet showed a higher mortality after isoproterenol injection than control animals. The diet was, however, also rich in vitamin D, which is known to increase the sensitivity of these animals to isoproterenol. It was also rich in long-chain monoenoic acids, which in rats (in contrast to several other species) produce cardiac muscle degeneration. In investigating human hearts the same authors actually found a higher content of arachidonic acid in persons dying a sudden cardiac death than in controls (Gudbjarnason & Hallgrimsson 1975).

Another epidemiological observation should be mentioned in this context. During the World War II a distinct decline in mortality from i.h.d. was observed in Oslo, Norway (Strøm & Jensen 1951) followed by a marked rise after the war. In this period the consumption of food containing fish increased very substantially owing to a shortage of dairy products. We have calculated (Bang & Dyerberg 1981) that this resulted in an average daily EPA intake comparable with that of the Eskimos. No conclusion can, of course, be drawn from such figures.

The mechanism of action of EPA on platelet – vessel wall interaction

The mechanism by which EPA may influence platelet – vessel wall interaction is only partly clarified. EPA inhibits platelet aggregation (Dyerberg & Bang 1978; Silver *et al.* 1973). This inhibition may be due to a competitive inhibition of the conversion of arachidonic acid into thromboxane A_2 (TXA_2) (Lands *et al.* 1973; Culp *et al.* 1979). This mechanism, however, is not the only one. Gryglewski *et al.* (1979) have found that EPA very effectively blocks TXA_2 receptors in the platelet membrane, and we and others have demonstrated that it blocks

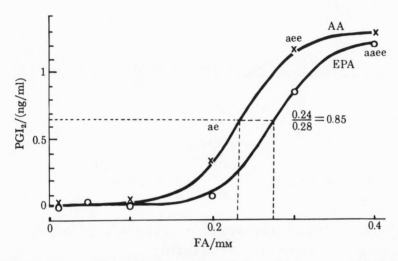

FIGURE 1. Production of PGI-like material in human umbilical vascular tissue measured by bioassay. The production of PGI-like material in mixed incubates is indicated by the letters a and e; ae means 0.1 mM AA + 0.1 mM EPA, aee means 0.1 mM AA + 0.2 mM EPA in the incubation mixture, and so on. AA and EPA are 20:4, $n-6$ and 20:5, $n-3$, respectively (Dyerberg & Jørgensen 1980).

prostaglandin-independent thrombin receptors too (Jakubowski & Ardlie 1979). The conversion of EPA into prostaglandins of the 3-series seem to be low and thromboxane A_3 (TXA_3) has low proaggregatory properties (Needleman *et al.* 1979; Whitaker *et al.* 1979). It is not known whether EPA is converted by human vascular tissue into PGI_3 or PGD_3, which are both powerful antiaggregatory substances. We have data suggesting such a conversion, and from the same set of experiments there is a clear indication that EPA does not inhibit the conversion of arachidonic acid into PGI_2 (Dyerberg & Jørgenson 1980). These data are given in figure 1. Powdered washed human vascular tissue was incubated with either arachidonic acid (AA) or EPA, or the two in combination. The prostacyclin produced was then measured by bioassay. We could not demonstrate any inhibition by EPA of the production of antiaggregatory material from AA. This situation contrasts with that of the platelets where the conversion of AA is markedly depressed.

The present knowledge of the influence of EPA on haemostatic functions is summarized in table 6.

EPA inhibits TXA_2 formation in platelets, whereas it does not inhibit PGI_2 synthesis in human vascular tissue *in vitro*. EPA blocks prostaglandin-dependent and prostaglandin-independent platelet membrane receptors. If any metabolic conversion of EPA takes place, TXA_3 is a very weak proaggregatory substance whereas PGD_3 and PGI_3 are powerfully antiaggregatory. Thus, the effect of incorporating EPA into structural lipids would appear as a shift in the haemostatic balance in an antithrombotic direction, which was exactly what we found in Eskimos. We thus felt encouraged to look further into the question of whether a supplement of EPA to the food would influence thrombogenesis.

TABLE 6. EFFECTS OF EPA ON HAEMOSTASIS

1. *blocks prostaglandin synthesis (competition)*

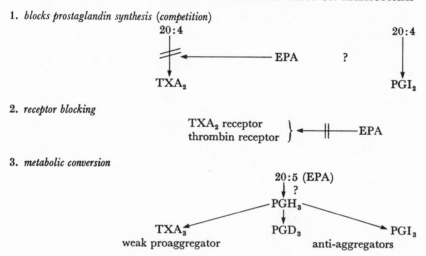

2. *receptor blocking*

3. *metabolic conversion*

FEEDING EXPERIMENTS INTENDED TO ALTER PLATELET – VESSEL WALL INTERACTION

Di-homo-γ-linolenic acid $(20:3, n-6)$ has been suggested as a dietary antiaggregatory substance (Kernoff *et al.* 1977; Willis *et al.* 1974). Reports on its effect have, however, been inconclusive (Oelz *et al.* 1976; O'Brien 1980).

Prostaglandin synthesis from $20:3, n-6$ results in eicosanoids of the 1-family. TXA_1 is without proaggregatory properties and no PGI compound can be synthesized owing to the lack of a double bond in the 5-position. Another aspect that should, however, be kept in mind is that $20:3, n-6$ is readily metabolized to AA $(20:4, n-6)$ in man.

The Western diet contains very little AA, whereas it is rich in linoleic acid $(18:2, n-6)$, which is converted into AA with di-homo-γ-linolenic acid as an intermediate. The almost indetectable amount of $20:3, n-6$ in human body lipids indicates the facility of this conversion.

Feeding experiments with the $n-3$ family are very scarce and in this context I must again refer to the lifelong experiment that the Greenland Eskimos represent. Another fact to be remembered is that in short-term experiments, thrombotic tendency is often measured very indirectly by haemostatic variables. In an interesting experiment by Black *et al.* (1979) a group of cats were given 8 % of their dietary calories as fish oil for 3 weeks, after which cerebral infarction was induced by ligation of the left middle cerebral artery. Both the neurological deficit and the volume of brain infarction in the group of cats given fish oil was significantly less than that of the control group.

Seiss *et al.* (1980) gave 5–800 g of mackerel daily to seven volunteers for a week. A shift in $20:5/20:4$ ratio in platelet lipids was paralleled by a decrease in platelet aggregability and TXB_2 formation. Sanders *et al.* (1980) have reported on the effect on bleeding time of giving

TABLE 7. COMPOSITION OF EPA ETHYL ESTER CONCENTRATE

(Values are percentage of total.)

18:1	4.2	22:1	5.1
18:2	0.7	22:5	0.2
18:3	0.7	22:6	5.4
20:1	9.3	saturated	0
20:2	2.3	monoenes	18.6
20:4	4.0	polyenes	80.1
20:5	66.6	20:5/20:4	16.7

TABLE 8. CHANGES IN PLASMA LIPIDS AND LIPOPROTEINS DURING 3 WEEKS OF INTAKE OF 10 ml PER DAY OF A 60% EPA ETHYL ESTER CONCENTRATE, $N = 20$

	before $\overline{X}$	s.e.m.	during $\overline{X}$	s.e.m.	significance of difference
total lipids/(g/l)	5.64	0.18	5.12	0.17	$p < 0.01$
cholesterol/(mmol/l)	4.87	0.17	4.67	0.16	$p < 0.05$
triglycerides/(mmol/l)	1.02	0.10	0.69	0.06	$p < 0.01$
LDL/(g/l)	3.85	0.17	3.73	0.17	n.s.
VLDL/(g/l)	1.10	0.14	0.78	0.08	$p < 0.01$
HDL/(g/l)	2.95	0.12	2.71	0.11	n.s.

TABLE 9. PLATELET TOTAL FATTY ACID DISTRIBUTION DURING 3 WEEKS OF DAILY INTAKE OF 10 ml OF A 60% EPA ETHYL ESTER CONCENTRATE, COMPARED WITH BASELINE VALUES, $N = 20$

	before	during	significance of difference
12:0–14:0	0.11	0.08	n.s.
16:0–16:1	19.8	19.5	n.s.
18:0	16.9	15.6	$p < 0.01$
18:1	17.7	16.4	$p < 0.01$
18:2	10.4	8.1	$p < 0.01$
18:3	0.01	0.31	$p < 0.01$
20:0–20:2	1.7	2.4	$p < 0.01$
20:4	21.1	16.3	$p < 0.01$
20:5	0.01	4.5	$p < 0.01$
22:0–24:1	6.5	9.2	$p < 0.01$
22:5	1.4	4.3	$p < 0.01$
22:6	1.5	1.4	n.s.
saturated	42.5	42.0	n.s.
monoenes	20.4	20.9	n.s.
polyenes	34.3	34.4	n.s.
20:5/20:4	0	0.28	$p < 0.01$

TABLE 10. CHANGES IN HAEMOSTATIC VARIABLES DURING 3 WEEKS OF DAILY INTAKE OF 10 ml OF A 60% EPA ETHYL ESTER CONCENTRATE, COMPARED WITH BASELINE VALUES, $N = 20$

platelet aggregation:

ΔO.D.$_{max}$ ADP, rel.	−13.1%	$p < 0.05$
ΔO.D.$_{max}$ collagen, rel.	−11.1%	$p < 0.01$
Δt O.D.$_{50\%}$ collagen, rel.	+13.0%	$p < 0.01$
change in TXB$_2$, collagen	−15.5 ng/ml	$p < 0.05$
change in bleeding time, Ivy, rel.	+11.1%	$p < 0.05$

volunteers 5 g of cod-liver oil four times daily for 6 weeks. A significant increase in bleeding time of 1.8 min was observed.

In collaboration with the Wellcome Research Laboratories, we have recently performed a study on 20 volunteers, giving them a daily dose for 3 weeks of 10 ml of an EPA-ethyl ester concentrate made from cod-liver oil. This concentrate was properly tested for toxicity on monkeys and rats given a tenfold dose per kilogram body mass. The composition of the oil is shown in table 7.

The volunteers were examined once a week for 2 weeks before the study, during the study, and for 2 weeks after the cessation of oil supplement. During this period they were asked to refrain from any intake of alcohol or medicine as this may affect platelet function.

Modest but significant decreases in plasma cholesterol, triglyceride and VLDL concentrations were found (table 8).

The oil intake led to an increase in EPA content of plasma lipids and of the fatty acids of the platelet lipids, increasing from almost undetectable amounts to an average of 4.5% (table 9). This increase was seen during the first week of treatment and did not increase further during the feeding period.

Haemostasis was measured by platelet aggregation, bleeding time determinations (by the technique of Ivy) and by TXB_2 formation in platelet-rich plasma during collagen-induced aggregation. The results are given in table 10.

A significant fall in ADP- and collagen-induced aggregation was found, measured both as the $O.D._{max}$ obtained and as the time elapsed for reaching 50% of maximal aggregation response. TXB_2 formation was also decreased. The bleeding time was prolonged by a factor comparable with the alteration in platelet aggregability. This could be interpreted as indicating unaltered vessel wall function. The modest alterations do not, however, warrant far-reaching conclusions.

Does diet influence platelet – vessel wall interaction? The data summarized in this survey and the experimental results presented indicate that it does. As it is generally accepted that the haemostatic process influences thrombogenesis and atherogenesis, this means that dietary advice given to the public aiming at lowering the incidence of ischaemic heart disease must include this aspect. It does not indicate the sort of advice that should be given, but it opens up new possibilities in an area rich in disappointments.

This study was supported by grants from Statens Lægevidenskabelige Forskningsfond and The Danish Heart Association.

REFERENCES (Dyerberg)

Bang, H. O. & Dyerberg, J. 1972 *Acta. med. scand.* **192**, 85–94.
Bang, H. O. & Dyerberg, J. 1980 *Dan. med. Bull.* **27**, 202–205.
Bang, H. O. & Dyerberg, J. 1981 *Acta med. scand.* (In the press.)
Bang, H. O., Dyerberg, J. & Sinclair, H. M. 1980 *Am. J. clin. Nutr.* **33**, 2657–2611.
Black, K. L., Culp, B., Madison, D., Randall, O. S. & Lands, W. E. M. 1979 *Prostaglandins Med.* **3**, 269–278.
Culp, B. R., Titus, B. G. & Lands, W. E. M. 1979 *Prostaglandins Med.* **3**, 257–268.
Dyerberg, J. & Bang, H. O. 1978 *Lancet* i, 152.
Dyerberg, J. & Bang, H. O. 1979 *Lancet* ii, 433–435.
Dyerberg, J. & Jørgensen, K. A. 1980 *Artery* 8, 12–17.
Dyerberg, J., Bang, H. O. & Hjørne, N. 1975 *Am. J. clin. Nutr.* **28**, 958–966.
Dyerberg, J., Bang, H. O. & Hjørne, N. 1977 *Dan. med. Bull.* **24**, 52–55.
Dyerberg, J., Bang, H. O., Stoffersen, E., Moncada, S. & Vane, J. R. 1978 *Lancet* ii, 117–119.

Food and Nutrition Board 1980 *Toward healthful diets*. Washington, D.C.: National Academy of Sciences.

Gryglewski, R. J., Salmon, J. A., Ubatuba, F. B., Weatherly, B. C., Moncada, S. & Vane, J. R. 1979 *Prostaglandins* 18, 453–478.

Gudbjarnason, S. & Hallgrimsson, J. 1975 *Acta med. scand. suppl. no.* 578, pp. 17–26.

Gudbjarnason, S. & Oskarsdottir, G. 1975 In *Recent advances in studies on cardiac structure and metabolism*, vol. 6 (ed. A. Fleckenstein & G. Rona), pp. 193–203. Baltimore: University Park Press.

Hamberg, M., Svensson, J. & Samuelsson, B. 1975 *Proc. natn. Acad. Sci. U.S.A.* 72, 2994–2998.

Jakubowski, J. A. & Ardlie, N. G. 1979 *Thromb. Res.* 16, 205–217.

Kernoff, P. B., Willis, A. L., Stone, K. J., Davies, J. A. & McNicol, G. P. 1977 *Br. med. J.* ii, 1441–1444.

Lands, W. E. M., Le Tellier, P. E., Rome, L. H. & Vanderhock, J. Y. 1973 *Adv. Biosci.* 9, 15–28.

Ministry of Greenland 1978 *The state of health in Greenland (Annual report from the Chief Medical Officer in Greenland for the years 1973–76)*. Copenhagen.

Ministry of Greenland 1979 *Greenland 1978*. Copenhagen.

Moncada, S., Gryglewski, J. R., Bunting, S. & Vane, J. R. 1976 *Nature, Lond.* 263, 663–665.

Moncada, S. & Vane, J. R. 1978 *Br. med. Bull.* 34, 129–138.

Needleman, P., Raz, A., Minkes, M. S., Ferrendelli, J. A. & Sprecher, H. 1979 *Proc. natn. Acad. Sci. U.S.A.* 76, 944–948.

O'Brien, J. R. 1980 *Lancet* i, 981–982.

Oelz, O., Seyberth, H. W., Knapp, H. R., Sweetman, B. J. & Oates, J. A. 1976 *Biochim. biophys. Acta* 431, 268–277.

Olson, R. E. 1980 *Nutrition Today* 15, 12–19.

Sanders, T. A. B., Naismith, D. J., Haines, A. P. & Vickers, M. 1980 *Lancet* i, 1189.

Seiss, W., Roth, P., Scherer, B., Kurzmann, I., Böhlig, B. & Weber, P. C. 1980 *Lancet* i, 441–444.

Silver, M. J., Smith, J. B., Ingerman, C. & Kocsis, J. J. 1973 *Prostaglandins* 4, 863–875.

Strøm, A. & Jensen, R. A. 1951 *Lancet* i, 126–129.

Whitaker, M. O., Wyche, A., Fitzpatrick, F., Sprecher, H. & Needleman, P. 1979 *Proc. natn. Acad. Sci. U.S.A.* 76, 5919–5923.

Willis, A. L., Comai, K., Kuhn, D. C. & Paulsrud, J. 1974 *Prostaglandins* 8, 509–519.

Discussion

J. McMichael, F.R.S. (2 *North Square, London, U.K.*). Comparisons between countries can be very insecure. Africans die from their infestations and few reach the coronary age. When medical care is substandard, the accuracy of diagnosis is poor. Of the coronary deaths in this country, 85% are over the age of 65 years, and less than 10% below 60 years. Low wartime recording of coronary deaths in Norway could be ascribed to an absence of doctors.

J. Dyerberg. I would agree. However, Eskimos do live to the coronary age.

Phil. Trans. R. Soc. Lond. B **294**, 383–388 (1981)
Printed in Great Britain

Prostacyclin and vascular disease

By R. J. Gryglewski, A. Szczeklik, H. Żygulska-Mach
and E. Kostka-Trąbka

*Ophthalmological Clinic, Institute of Internal Medicine, Department of Pharmacology, N. Copernicus
Academy of Medicine in Kraków, 31–531 Kraków, Grzegórzecka 16, Poland*

We hypothesize that prostacyclin (PGI_2) is an anti-atherosclerotic hormone and that atherosclerosis develops when endothelial PGI_2 synthetase is inhibited by lipid peroxides. Serum lipid peroxides occur in low-density lipoproteins (LDL). LDL lipid peroxides are elevated in common types of hyperlipoproteinaemias, PGI_2 generation is impaired in atherosclerosis, and infusion of synthetic PGI_2 into patients alleviates symptoms resulting from arteriosclerosis obliterans, central retinal vein occlusion or spontaneous angina.

Introduction

Prostacyclin (PGI_2) is a potent stimulator of platelet adenylate cyclase (Gorman *et al.* 1977; Tateson *et al.* 1977). Therefore, it inhibits platelet aggregation (Gryglewski *et al.* 1976, Moncada *et al.* 1976a) and disaggregates platelet clumps (Gryglewski *et al.* 1978a). PGI_2 is also a vasodilator, especially in the pulmonary circulation (Kadowitz *et al.* 1980) and stimulates the release of a plasminogen activator from the lungs (Hechtman *et al.* 1980). PGI_2 is generated by arterial walls (Bunting *et al.* 1976; Gryglewski *et al.* 1976; Moncada *et al.* 1976a, b), lungs (Gryglewski 1978b, c, 1979a, b; Moncada *et al.* 1978), kidneys (Whorton *et al.* 1977; Remuzzi *et al.* 1978; Silberbauer *et al.* 1979), uterus (Vesin *et al.* 1979; Williams *et al.* 1978) and the other organs (Pace-Asciak & Rangaraj 1977). The lungs continuously secrete PGI_2 into arterial circulation (Gryglewski *et al.* 1978b, c; Moncada *et al.* 1978) and this secretion is stimulated by hyperventilation (Gryglewski *et al.* 1978b) or activation of chemoreceptors (Gryglewski *et al.* 1978b), or activation of chemoreceptors (Gryglewski *et al.* 1980a) as well as by angiotensin II (Gryglewski 1979a; Gryglewski *et al.* 1979, 1980b), bradykinin (Mullane & Moncada 1980) and acetylcholine (Gryglewski *et al.* 1980a).

Lipid peroxides, including 15-hydroperoxyeicosatetraenoic acid (15-HPETE, 15-HPAA), inhibit PGI_2 synthetase in porcine aortic microsomes (Gryglewski *et al.* 1976; Moncada *et al.* 1976b; Salmon *et al.* 1978). 15-HPETE inactivates the enzyme also in rabbit arterial slices (Bunting *et al.* 1976) and in cultured human endothelial cells (Marcus *et al.* 1978), possibly as the result of peroxidative reduction of lipid hydroperoxides and the release of $[O_x]$ (Kuehl *et al.* 1980). We believe that PGI_2 is a natural anti-atherosclerotic hormone (Gryglewski 1979a), and its removal from the body may initiate atherosclerotic process (Gryglewski 1980).

Indeed, the generation of PGI_2 by aorta, mesenteric arteries, heart (Dembińska-Kieć *et al.* 1977; Gryglewski *et al.* 1978d), lungs and kidneys (Dembińska-Kieć *et al.* 1979) in experimental atherosclerosis in rabbits, and this can be detected within a week of feeding the rabbits an atherogenic diet (Masotti *et al.* 1979). In atherosclerosis, arachidonic acid metabolism may be diverted from PGI_2 to other prostaglandins (Dembińska-Kieć *et al.* 1979) or to thromboxane A_2 (Szczeklik & Gryglewski 1978; Szczeklik *et al.* 1978a; Żmuda *et al.* 1977).

Although there exists no direct evidence that human atherosclerosis is causally associated with an increased lipid peroxidation, lipid peroxides have been found in human atherosclerotic arteries (Glavind *et al.* 1952; Hartroft & Prta 1965). Human atheromatic plaques generate very little PGI_2 (Angelo *et al.* 1978). Atherogenic low-density lipoproteins (LDL) were reported to inhibit the generation of an anti-aggregatory principle by cultured human endothelial cells (Nordøy *et al.* 1978) and to damage them (Henriksen *et al.* 1979), while anti-atherogenic high-density lipoproteins (HDL) prevented the deleterious action of LDL (Henriksen *et al.* 1979; Nordøy *et al.* 1978). We have recently found (Szczeklik & Gryglewski 1980) that lipid peroxides occur mainly in LDL while HDL are free from them.

The above indirect evidence for involvement of lipid peroxidation and PGI_2 deficiency in pathogenesis of atherosclerosis stimulated clinical trials with PGI_2 in arteriosclerosis obliterans. In 1978 we infused PGI_2 into healthy volunteers (Gryglewski *et al.* 1978 *e*, Szczeklik *et al.* 1978 *b*) and found that pharmacologically active doses of PGI_2 are within the range 1–20 ng kg^{-1} min^{-1}, intravenously. Moderate lowering of diastolic blood pressure, prolongation of bleeding time, reddening of the face and palms as well as inhibition of platelet aggregation and dissipation of circulating platelet aggregates were the most prominent pharmacological actions of PGI_2. A year later PGI_2 was administered to the first five patients suffering from arteriosclerosis obliterans (Szczeklik *et al.* 1979), and the number of the treated patients has now considerably increased (Szczeklik *et al.* 1980 *a*). Patients with central retinal vein occlusion were also treated with PGI_2 (Żygulska-Mach *et al.* 1981).

PATIENTS AND METHODS

Fifty patients (44 men and 6 women) were treated with PGI_2. Arteriosclerosis obliterans was diagnosed in 36 patients (46–76 years old) and thrombangiitis obliterans in 12 (33–44 years old). Two women (24 and 26 years old) suffered from Takayasu disease of the lower extremities. In all but 3 patients the diagnosis was confirmed by angiographic examination.

Ischaemia at rest was recorded in 44 patients as evidenced by rest pain, ischaemic ulceration or necrosis. Only in 6 patients was physical exercise (walking) necessary to induce pain. Of the 50 patients, 7 had undergone vascular reconstructive surgery, 8 perivascular sympathectomy, 5 amputation of toe or foot and 5 amputation of leg beneath knee. In the past, therapy with vasodilators (Complamin, Tolazoline, Bamethan) was tried without success.

Sodium salt of PGI_2 (Upjohn Co., Kalamazoo, U.S.A. and Wellcome Research Laboratories, Beckenham, U.K.) was dissolved in 0.1 M glycine buffer at pH 10·5 and infused into the femoral artery (33 patients) or subclavian vein (17 patients) at a dose of 2–10 ng kg^{-1} min^{-1} for 72 h. The infusion rates of PGI_2 were maintained at as high a level as the patients could tolerate. In 20 patients the PGI_2 therapy was repeated 2–4 times every 1–20 weeks. The total observation period for 50 patients studied was 3–17 months. No pharmacological treatment other than PGI_2 was prescribed.

Three patients (1 man and 2 women, 63–72 years old) with a sudden unilateral loss of vision resulting from the occlusion of the central retinal vein were infused with PGI_2 into a subclavian vein, at the doses indicated above. PGI_2 was administered 24 h, 48 h or 7 days after the first symptom of the disease had been reported by the patient.

RESULTS

Infusions of PGI_2 made the affected leg become dry and hot. Erythema usually appeared. Platelet aggregability was suppressed for up to 3 h after the termination of the infusion of PGI_2. Side effects of the PGI_2 therapy were, in diminishing order of frequency: pain in the infused leg, headache, jaw articular pain, nausea, lowering of diastolic arterial pressure, cardiac ventricular arrhythmias. Moderate hyperglycemia was recorded in several patients, especially in those with otherwise balanced diabetes. Because of rest pain, 23 patients had to rely on narcotic or non-narcotic pain-killers administered several times daily. In 15 of those 23 patients, the pain was abolished for a period of 4 weeks to 16 months, the day after termination of the infusion of PGI_2. In half of the 32 patients with ischaemic ulcers, partial or complete healing was observed, while in 7 patients with deep penetrating necrosis, no improvement occurred. In 5 out of 6 patients with intermittent claudication, PGI_2 caused a sustained increase in walking distance (4 km/h) by at least 50 %.

Patients with central retinal vein occlusion suffered from generalized atherosclerosis or hypertension. Their visual acuity in the affected eye was 1/50–2/50, while ophthalmoscopic examination revealed venous dilation and tortuosity, oedema of various regions of the retina, and punctate and small round haemorrhages scattered in the fundus. A dramatic improvement was observed in two patients to whom PGI_2 had been administered 24 and 48 h after the sudden diminution of vision.

Two months later their visual acuity was 0.2 and 0.5 and the regression of retinal oedema, haemorrhages and other lesions was nearly complete.

No improvement was observed in the patient who had received the treatment on the seventh day of the disease. Five months later his visual acuity was still 1/50, with oedema of the optic disc and retina, and haemorrhages and dilatation of the retinal vein.

DISCUSSION

The effectiveness of the PGI_2 therapy in arteriosclerosis obliterans seemed to depend on the localization of the obliterating lesions in arteries, the existence of collateral circulation and the advancement of the disease (Szczeklik *et al.* 1980*a*). Our group of patients was not homogeneous; nevertheless, 88 % of them suffered from the symptoms of ischaemia at rest, including focal necrosis, ischaemic ulcers and pain. In those patients, anticoagulant or vasodilator drugs are of little value (Coffman 1979), as we have confirmed in our patients. In 40 % of this group of patients, single or repeated courses of the PGI_2 therapy resulted in a long-term clinical improvement. We therefore assume, from the benefit derived, that in those patients PGI_2 substituted the lacking anti-atherosclerotic endogenous hormone. The results of our clinical trials fully support the initiation of controlled clinical studies on the effectiveness of PGI_2 in arteriosclerosis obliterans.

A therapeutic improvement was achieved in two patients that had been treated with PGI_2 24 and 48 h after a sudden occlusion of central retinal vein but not in the patient that received the treatment on the seventh day of the disease. In 28 patients to whom PGI_2 (5–10 ng kg^{-1} min^{-1}, intravenously) was administered because of arteriosclerosis obliterans of the lower extremities, we did not observe any vasodilatation of retinal blood vessels (our unpublished data). Therefore, it might be that a disaggregatory action of PGI_2 was responsible for the reopening of retinal blood vessels that were occluded with fresh platelet clumps. It is tempting to speculate that the PGI_2-induced release of a plasminogen activator from lungs may also contribute to the effectiveness of PGI_2 in occlusive vascular disease (Hechtman *et al.* 1980).

Central retinal vein occlusion is usually treated with heparin, streptokinase, urokinase, steroidal and non-steroidal anti-inflammatory drugs, dextran, vasodilators, vitamin C or P (Anon 1979; Coscas & Dhermy 1978). According to Rubinstein & Jones (1976) of 143 patients treated pharmacologically, the regression of retinal lesions was complete only in 11. In our ophthalmological clinic, 48 patients with acute occlusion of central retinal vein were treated with heparin, vitamin C and nicotinic acid derivatives. In 32 patients visual acuity showed no change.

Patients with occlusion of the central retinal vein suffer from late complications of the disease such as secondary glaucoma, maculopathy and proliferation of new vessels. These are usually treated with xenon-arc or laser photocoagulation (May *et al.* 1979). The above complications have not so far developed in the patients treated with PGI_2. A rapid improvement and lack of late complications in two patients treated with PGI_2 at the early stage of the disease encourages further studies on the therapeutic use of PGI_2 in acute occlusion of the central retinal vein and, possibly, of other cerebral blood vessels.

PGI_2 has also been successfully used in the treatment of spontaneous angina (Szczeklik *et al.* 1980*b*). There exists an experimental basis for clinical trials with PGI_2 in preventing of rejection of renal transplants (Leithner *et al.* 1980), in treatment of pulmonary embolism (Utsunomiya *et al.* 1980) and in supplementation of heparin during haemodialysis and haemoperfusion (Bunting *et al.* 1979; Weston *et al.* 1979). The effectiveness of PGI_2 in vascular occlusive disease seems to be associated with its anti-aggregatory, disaggregatory and anti-releasing actions on blood platelets. The prevention of activation of the coagulation system derives from the effects of PGI_2 on platelets. The activation of fibrinolytic systems by PGI_2 in the lungs constitutes a new concept of its action (Hechtman *et al.* 1980).

REFERENCES (Gryglewski *et al.*)

Angelo, V. M., Mysliwiec, M. B. & Gaetano, G. 1978 Defective fibrinolytic and prostacyclin-like activity in human atheromatous plaques. *Thromb. Haemostas.* **39**, 535–536.

Anon. 1979 Retinal vein occlusion [editorial]. *Br. J. Ophthal.* **63**, 375.

Bunting, S., Gryglewski, R., Moncada, S. & Vane, J. R. 1976 Arterial walls generate from prostaglandin endoperoxides a substance (prostaglandin X) which relaxes strips of mesenteric and coeliac arteries and inhibits platelet aggregation. *Prostaglandins.* **12**, 897–913.

Bunting, S., Moncada, S., Vane, J. R., Woods, H. F. & Weston, M. J. 1979 Prostacyclin improves hemocompatibility during charcoal hemoperfusion. In *Prostacyclin* (ed. J. R. Vane & S. Bergström), pp. 361–370. New York: Raven Press.

Coffman, J. D. 1979 Intermittent claudication and rest pain: physiological concepts and therapeutic approaches. *Prog. Cardiovasc. Dis.* **22**, 53–71.

Coscas, G. & Dhermy, T. 1978 *Occlusions veineuses rétiniennes.* Paris: Masson.

Dembińska-Kieć, A., Gryglewska, T., Żmuda, A. & Gryglewski, R. J. 1977 The generation of prostacyclin by arteries and by the coronary vascular bed is reduced in experimental atherosclerosis in rabbits. *Prostaglandins* **14**, 1025–1035.

Dembińska-Kieć, A., Rücker, W. & Schönhöfer, P. S. 1979 Atherosclerosis decreased prostacyclin formation in rabbit lungs and kidneys. *Prostaglandins* **17**, 831–837.

Glavind, J., Hartman, S., Clemensen, J., Jessen, K. E. & Dam, H. 1952 Studies on the role of lipid peroxides in human pathology. II. The presence of peroxidized lipids in the atherosclerotic aortas. *Acta path. microbiol. scand.* **30**, 1–6.

Gorman, R. R., Bunting, S. & Miller, O. V. 1977 Modulation of human platelet adenylate cyclase by prostacyclin (PGX). *Prostaglandins* **13**, 377–388.

Gryglewski, R. J. 1979*a* Prostacyclin as a circulatory hormone. *Biochem. Pharmac.* **28**, 3161–3166.

Gryglewski, R. J. 1979 b Is the lung an endocrine organ that secretes prostacyclin? In *Prostacyclin* (ed. J. R. Vane & S. Bergström), pp. 275–278. New York: Raven Press.

Gryglewski, R. J. 1980 Prostaglandins, platelets and atherosclerosis. *C.R.C. Crit. Rev. Biochem.* **7**, 291–338.

Gryglewski, R. J., Bunting, S., Moncada, S., Flower, R. J. & Vane, J. R. 1976 Arterial walls are protected against deposition of platelet thrombi by a substance (prostaglandin X) which they make from prostaglandin endoperoxides. *Prostaglandins* **12**, 685–713.

Gryglewski, R. J., Dembińska-Kieć, A., Chytkowski, A. & Gryglewska, T. 1978 d Prostacyclin and thromboxane A_2 biosynthesis capacities of heart, arteries and platelets at various stages of experimental atherosclerosis in rabbits. *Atherosclerosis* **31**, 385–394.

Gryglewski, R. J., Korbut, R. & Ocetkiewicz, A. 1978 a Reversal of platelet aggregation by prostacyclin. *Pharmac. Res. Commun.* **10**, 185–189.

Gryglewski, R. J., Korbut, R. & Ocetkiewicz, A. 1978 b Generation of prostacyclin by lungs in vivo and its release into arterial circulation. *Nature, Lond.* **273**, 765–767.

Gryglewski, R. J., Korbut, R., Ocetkiewicz, A., Spławiński, J., Wojtaszek, B. & Święs, J. 1978 c Lungs as the generator of prostacyclin-hypothesis on physiological significance. *Naunyn-Schmiedebergs Arch. Pharmac.* **304**, 45–50.

Gryglewski, R. J., Korbut, R. & Spławiński, J. 1979 Endogenous mechanisms which regulate prostacyclin release. *Haemostasis* **8**, 294–299.

Gryglewski, R. J., Radomski, M., Święs, J. & Ocetkiewicz, A. 1980 a Release of prostacyclin into circulation by chemical mediators. In *Symp. A. Einstein*, College of Medicine, 28–31 October 1980. New York: Raven Press. (In the press.)

Gryglewski, R. J., Spławiński, J. & Korbut, R. 1980 b Endogenous mechanisms that regulate prostacyclin release. In *Advances in prostaglandin and thromboxane research* (ed. B. Samuelsson, P. W. Ramwell & R. Paoletti), pp. 777–787. New York: Raven Press.

Gryglewski, R. J., Szczeklik, A. & Niżankowski, R. 1978 e Antiplatelet action of intravenous infusion of prostacyclin in man. *Thromb. Res.* **13** 153–163.

Hartroft, W. S. & Prta, E. A. 1965 Ceroid. *Am. J. med. Sci.* **250**, 324, 344.

Hechtman, H. B., Utsunomiya, T., Vegas, A. M., Grindlinger, G. A., McLoughlin, G. A., Krausz, M. M. & Shepro, D. 1980 Prostaglandin mediation of pulmonary fibrinolytic activity. In *Symp. A. Einstein*, College of Medicine, 28–31 October 1980. New York: Raven Press. (In the press.)

Henriksen, T. S., Evensen, S. A. & Carlander, B. 1979 Injury to cultured endothelial cells induced by low density lipoproteins: protection by high density lipoproteins. *Scand. J. clin. Lab. Invest.* **39**, 369–375.

Kadowitz, P. J., Spannhake, E. W., Levin, J. L. & Hyman, A. 1980 Differential actions of the prostaglandins on the pulmonary vascular bed. In *Advances in prostaglandin and thromboxane research* (ed. B. Samuelsson, P. W. Ramwell & R. Paoletti), pp. 731–743. New York: Raven Press.

Kuehl, F. A., Jr., Humes, J. L., Ham, E. A., Egan, R. W. & Dougherty, H. W. 1980 Inflammation: the role of peroxidase-derived products. In *Advances in prostaglandin and thromboxane research* (ed. B. Samuelsson, P. W. Ramwell & R. Paoletti), pp. 77–86. New York: Raven Press.

Leithner, C., Sinzinger, H., Silberbauer, K. & Klein, K. 1980 The role of prostacyclin in human renal transplant rejection. In *Abstracts of Symposium on Arachidonic Acid Cascade*, 25–27 September 1980, Poznań. Poland.

Marcus, A. J., Weksler, B. B. & Jaffe, E. A. 1978 Enzymatic conversion of prostaglandin endoperoxide H_2 and arachidonic acid to prostacyclin by cultured human endothelial cells. *J. biol. Chem.* **253**, 7138–7141.

Masotti, G., Galanti, G., Poggesi, L., Curcio, A. & Neri Serneri, G. G. 1979 Early changes of the endothelial antithrombotic properties in cholesterol fed rabbits. III. Decreased PGI_2 production by aortic wall [abstract]. *Thromb. Haemostas.* **42**, 423.

May, D. R., Klein, M. L., Peyman, G. A. & Raichand, M. 1979 Xenon-arc panretinal photocoagulation for central retinal vein occlusion: randomised perspective study. *Br. J. Ophthalm.* **63**, 725.

Moncada, S., Gryglewski, R. J., Bunting, S. & Vane, J. R. 1976 a An enzyme isolated from arteries transforms prostaglandin endoperoxides to an unstable substance that inhibits platelet aggregation. *Nature, Lond.* **263**, 663–665.

Moncada, S., Gryglewski, R. J., Bunting, S. & Vane, J. R. 1976 b A lipid peroxide inhibits the enzyme in blood vessel microsomes that generates from prostaglandin endoperoxides the substance (prostaglandin X) which prevents platelet aggregation. *Prostaglandins* **12**, 715–737.

Moncada, S., Korbut, R., Bunting, S. & Vane, J. R. 1978 Prostacyclin as a circulating hormone. *Nature, Lond.* **237**, 767–769.

Mullane, K. M. & Moncada, S. 1980 Prostacyclin release and the modulation of some vasoactive hormones. *Prostaglandins* **20**, 25–49.

Nordøy, A., Svensson, B., Wiebe, D. & Hoak, J. C. 1978 Lipoproteins and the inhibitory effect of human endothelial cells on platelet function. *Circul. Res.* **43**, 527–533.

Pace-Asciak, C. R. & Rangaraj, G. 1977 Distribution of prostaglandin biosynthetic pathways in several rat tissues. Formation of 6-keto prostaglandin F_{1a}. *Biochim. biophys. Acta* **486**, 579–582.

Remuzzi, G., Cavenaghi, A. E., Mecca, G., Donati, M. B. & deGaetano, G. 1978 Human renal cortex generates prostacyclin-like activity. *Thromb. Res.* **12**, 363–366.

Rubinstein, K. & Jones, E. B. 1976 Retinal vein occlusion: long-term prospects 10 years' follow up of 143 patients. *Br. J. Ophthalm.* **60**, 148.

Salmon, J. A., Smith, D. R., Flower, R. J., Moncada, S. & Vane, J. R. 1978 Further studies on the enzymatic conversion of prostaglandin endoperoxide into prostacyclin by porcine aorta microsomes. *Biochim. biophys. Acta,* **523**, 250–262.

Silberbauer, K., Sinzinger, H. & Winter, M. 1979 Prostacyclin activity in rat kidney stimulated by angiotensin II. *Br. J. Path.* **60**, 38–44.

Szczeklik, A. & Gryglewski, R. J. 1978 Thromboxane A$_2$ synthesis in platelets of patients with coronary heart disease. In *Int. Conf. on Atherosclerosis* (ed. L. A. Carlson, C. R. Sirtori & G. Weber), pp. 597–606. New York: Raven Press.

Szczeklik, A. & Gryglewski, R. J. 1980 Low-density lipoproteins (LDL) are carriers for lipid peroxides and invalidate prostacyclin (PGI$_2$) biosynthesis in arteries. *Artery.* (Submitted.)

Szczeklik, A., Gryglewski, R. J. & Grodzińska, L., Serwońska, M. & Marcinkiewicz, E. 1978a Thromboxane generation and platelet aggregation in survivals of myocardial infarction. *Thrombos. Haemostas.* **40**, 66–74.

Szczeklik, A., Gryglewski, R. J., Kostka-Trąbka, E., Niżankowski, R., Skawiński, S., Billewicz, O., Głuszko, P., Szczeklik, J., Piętoń, R., Grodzińska, L., Dembińska-Kieć, A., Bieroń, K. & Telesz, E. 1980a Prostacyclin in treatment of peripheral vascular disease of lower extremities. *Przegl. lek.* (in the press.)

Szczeklik, A., Gryglewski, R. J., Niżankowski, R., Musiał, J., Piętoń, R. & Mruk, J. 1978b. Circulatory and anti-platelet effects of intravenous prostacyclin in healthy men. *Pharmac. Res. Commun.* **10**, 545–556.

Szczeklik, A., Niżankowski, R., Skawiński, S., Szczeklik, J., Głuszko, P. & Gryglewski, R. J. 1979 Successful therapy of advanced arteriosclerosis obliterans with prostacyclin. *Lancet* i, 1111–1114.

Szczeklik, A., Szczeklik, J., Niżankowski, R. & Gluszko, P. 1980b Prostacyclin for acute coronary insufficiency. *Artery.* (In the press.)

Tateson, J. E., Moncada, S. & Vane, J. R. 1977 Effects of prostaglandin X(PGX) on cyclic AMP concentration in human platelets. *Prostaglandins* **13**, 389–397.

Utsunomiya, T., Krausz, M. M., Valery, S. R., Shepro, D. & Hechtman, H. B. 1980 Treatment of pulmonary embolism with prostacyclin. *Surgery* **88**, 25–30.

Vesin, M. F., Khac, L. D. & Harbon, S. 1979 Prostacyclin as an endogenous modulator of adenosine cyclic 3,5-monophosphate levels in rat myometrium and endometrium. *Molec. Pharmac.* **16**, 823–840.

Weston, M. J., Woods, H. F., Ash, G., Bunting, S., Moncada, S. & Vane, J. R. 1979 Prostacyclin as an alternative to heparin for hemodialysis in dogs. In *Prostacyclin* (ed. J. R. Vane & S. Bergström), pp. 349–360. New York: Raven Press.

Whorton, A. R., Smigiel, M., Oates, J. A. & Frölich, J. C. 1977 Evidence for prostacyclin production in renal cortex. *Prostaglandins* **13**, 1021.

Williams, K. I., Dembińska-Kieć, A., Żmuda, A. & Gryglewski, R. J. 1978 Prostacyclin formation by myometrial and decidual fractions of pregnant rat uterus. *Prostaglandins* **15**, 343–350.

Żmuda, A., Dembińska-Kieć, A., Chytkowski, A. & Gryglewski, R. J. 1977 Experimental atherosclerosis in rabbits: platelet aggregability, thromboxane A$_2$ generation and anti-aggregatory potency of prostacyclin. *Prostaglandins* **14**, 1035–1042.

Żygulska-Mach, H., Kostka-Trąbka, E. & Gryglewski, R. J. 1980 Prostacyclin in central retinal vein occlusion. *Lancet* i, 1075.

Phil. Trans. R. Soc. Lond. B **294**, 389–398 (1981)
Printed in Great Britain

Platelets and artificial surfaces: the effects of drugs

By E. W. Salzman,[†] Destiny Brier-Russell[†],
J. Lindon[†] and E. W. Merrill[‡]

† *Department of Surgery, Beth Israel Hospital and Harvard Medical School, and the Charles A. Dana Research Institute, Beth Israel Hospital, Boston, Massachusetts 02215, U.S.A.*
‡ *Department of Chemical Engineering, Massachusetts Institute of Technology, Cambridge, Massachusetts, U.S.A.*

[Plate 1]

Contact of blood with a foreign surface activates platelets and leads to their consumption. This property is shared by most non-biological materials, including air, but can be reduced by an optimal balance of hydrophobicity and hydrophilicity, minimal capacity for hydrogen bonding, avoidance of crystallinity, maintenance of polymer backbone mobility, and other manipulations of the chemistry of the polymer. None the less, no totally non-thrombogenic artificial surface has been developed. Attention has therefore turned to suppression of platelet–surface interaction by drugs that alter platelet function. Agents that block cyclo-oxygenase inhibit surface-induced secretion and aggregation but have no effect on platelet adhesion. Drugs that increase platelet cyclic AMP levels have a dose-related effect, which at high concentrations can eliminate adhesion to surfaces. The most successful agent, prostacyclin, has achieved total protection of platelets during cardiopulmonary bypass, with preservation of normal platelet number and function. Associated vasodilatation is a notable side effect, and hypotension may prove to be a significant problem in clinical practice. The development of more selective analogues with minimal vasodepressor activity is to be encouraged.

Blood–surface interactions

Exposure of the blood to artificial surfaces leads frequently to thromboembolic complications in patients with artificial heart valves, arterial grafts, and other prosthetic devices, and in patients undergoing extracorporeal circulation, including cardiopulmonary bypass and haemodialysis. Blood platelets are particularly susceptible to the effects of contact of blood with an artificial surface, which may result in altered platelet function, shortened platelet survival, thrombocytopenia, or gross thromboembolism. In spite of substantial efforts to develop thrombo-resistant surfaces, present-day biomaterials are not totally bland in contact with the blood. The widespread successful clinical use of artificial organs is therefore dependent on skilful engineering and appreciation of fluid mechanics and is in large part attributable to the patient's tolerance to microembolism and his capacity to compensate for increased consumption of haemostatic elements.

At its extreme, the situation is illustrated by the haematological effects of cardiopulmonary bypass (Bachmann *et al.* 1975; McKenna *et al.* 1975). Patients undergoing open-heart operations with the support of a pump oxygenator invariably develop a bleeding tendency characterized by thrombocytopenia, defective platelet function (manifested by a reduction in the aggregation response to ADP and other stimuli), evidence of platelet activation (demonstrated by increased

[173]

circulating levels of plasma thromboxane B_2 (Davies et al. 1980), platelet factor 4 (Hennessey et al. 1977) and other platelet products (Addonizio 1980), and incoagulability of the blood as a result of heparin anticoagulation.

The first event observed upon contact of the blood with an artificial surface is adsorption of plasma proteins on the surface (Baier & Dutton 1969). The small size and high concentration of plasma protein molecules compared with blood cells dictate that protein adsorption must occur before formed elements can diffuse to the surface (Salzman 1971). Thus, the platelet never encounters a bare surface but only a film of blood constituents deposited on it. It seems likely that the composition of the adsorbed protein coat and changes in configuration of protein molecules secondary to the adsorption process are critical in transmitting to blood elements a message regarding the nature of the underlying surface and thus in determining the subsequent events. The details of these interactions are not well understood.

Initial conditioning of the surface by the adsorbed film of plasma proteins is quickly followed by adhesion of platelets. The adsorbed platelets spread out on the surface, a gross distortion of platelet morphology that is analogous in many respects to the shape change that precedes the primary phase of platelet aggregation induced in vitro by ADP (Salzman et al. 1977). The formation of an aggregate of platelets on the surface subsequently occurs by accretion. The reaction may be augmented by secretion of platelet constituents such as ADP and serotonin by platelets adhering to the surface or to other platelets, and further aggregation of non-adherent platelets in the bulk fluid phase may ensue. The process has many features in common with formation of a haemostatic plug or intravascular thrombus but has a number of important distinctive features.

1. The intensity of the platelet response varies depending on the surface. Although there is evidence that platelets adhere to virtually all artificial surfaces (Friedman et al. 1970), platelet adhesion can be reduced or even prevented by manipulation of the adsorbed plasma protein film on the surface. Furthermore, the degree to which platelet–surface interaction leads to platelet aggregation and secretion varies with the nature of the surface, being influenced by features such as contour (i.e. roughness on a scale the size of a blood cell), crystallinity, hydrophobicity, hydrophilicity, capacity for hydrogen bonding, and possibly the flexibility of the molecular backbone, in polymers.

2. An artificial surface lacks the capacity of the natural endothelial cell for active inhibition of platelet interactions afforded by local production of prostacyclin and ADP-hydrolysing enzymes (Moncada et al. 1976).

INFLUENCE OF THE SURFACE

We have studied the contribution of the nature of a surface to the events that follow its contact with blood in a model system in vitro (Lindon et al. 1978) in which whole blood anti-coagulated with citrate is pumped from below through a column of beads composed of or coated with the material to be studied. The system has a very large surface/volume ratio (e.g. 1500 cm² for 3 ml of blood) and is thus a severe test of the compatibility of a material with the blood. Platelets are retained within the column by adhesion to the beads, followed by development of aggregates as further platelets adhere to the initial platelet layer. Comparison of the platelet count in effluent blood with the platelet count in blood before surface contact reflects both platelet adhesion and aggregation. The secretion of platelet constituents can also be measured.

As an illustration of the importance of surface composition, consider the segmented polyurethanes, inhomogeneous block copolymers consisting of a continuous 'soft segment' phase composed of linear polyethers held together by partial crystallization of 'hard segment' areas containing the intensely hydrogen-bonding urea or urethane moieties. Such polymers are widely used for angiographic catheters and other clinical applications because of their favourable

TABLE 1. HYDROPHILICITY AND PLATELET REACTIVITY

polyurethane	n	a or c	percentage H_2O	p.r.i.†
PEO	46	a	64	0.95
PEO	28	a	33	0.88
PTMO	28	a	28	0.71
PTMO	56	c	5	0.45
HSA	5	c	±0	0.20

Abbreviations: a, amorphous; c, crystalline; PEO, polyethylene oxide soft segment; PTMO, polytetramethylene oxide soft segment; HSA, hard segment analogue; n, number of structural units.

† Platelet recovery index: ratio of platelets in effluent to platelets entering the bead columns. For a bland surface, p.r.i. = 1; for a surface that retains all platelets presented to it, p.r.i. = 0.

mechanical properties and relative blandness in contact with blood. In a series of polyurethanes varying in composition of the hard and soft segments, we observed (Sa da Costa *et al.* 1980) that reactivity with platelets increased as the fractional concentration of the hard segment phase at the blood contacting surface. The most successful polyurethanes in practical clinical use can be shown by electron spectroscopy for chemical analysis to lack nitrogen (an indicator of the hard segment) within 5 nm of the blood-contacting interface. Furthermore, a series of model polyurethanes that vary in composition of the soft segment have decreasing platelet reactivity as the capacity of the polymer to imbibe water increases (table 1).

Experiments such as these lead to the following generalization: for thromboresistance, the surface of a polyurethane destined to come in contact with the blood should be formed against a hydrophobic interface, such as air, which encourages phase separation and promotes the formation of a surface composed chiefly of the relatively hydrophobic soft segments, the highly reactive hard segment phases being buried below. The composition of the soft segment phase should be selected to be as hydrophilic as possible, short of actually having the capacity for hydrogen bonding or polar interactions.

The undesirable effects of surface hydrophobicity are not limited to polyurethanes. We studied (Brier-Russell *et al.* 1981) a series of alkyl acrylates and methacrylates whose alkyl side chains varied in length from one carbon (polymethylacrylate, polymethylmethacrylate) to 12 (polylaurylacrylate, polylauryl methacrylate). Platelet reactivity varied directly with the length of the alkyl side chains and thus with the capacity of the polymer for hydrophobic interactions (figure 1). Polymethylacrylate was one of the least reactive materials we have studied. While not hydrophilic, it is the least hydrophobic of the acrylate and methacrylate series. Its blandness is also demonstrable *in vivo*. To study platelet–surface interactions in living animals, we have measured (Lindon *et al.* 1980) the lifespan of ^{51}Cr-labelled or ^{111}In-labelled platelets in sheep bearing arteriovenous shunts in the form of tubing. The survival time of platelets in animals with a polymethylacrylate arterio-venous shunt 150 cm long is no shorter than in control animals.

Pharmacological control of platelet–surface interactions

Experiments such as the foregoing may lead to an increased understanding of a theoretical basis for the interaction of blood with artificial surfaces. However, until truly non-thrombogenic surfaces are available, the use of prosthetic devices in contact with the blood will of necessity be supplemented instead by anticoagulant drugs and agents that alter platelet function to prevent thromboembolic complications and consumption or alteration of blood elements.

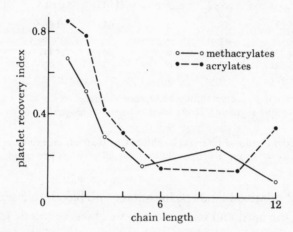

FIGURE 1. Platelet recovery after passage of citrated whole blood through a column of acrylate- or methacrylate-coated beads, in which the length of the alkyl side chain is varied from one (polymethylacrylate and polymethylmethacrylate) to 12 (polylaurylacrylate and polylaurylmethacrylate). From Brier-Russell *et al.* (1981).

Conventional anticoagulation has a limited ability to protect against the haematological consequences of blood–surface interaction, in which platelets play a predominant role. The administration of heparin during coronary angiography reduces thromboembolic complications, but the effects of cardiopulmonary bypass and haemodialysis on the blood occur despite the universal use of heparin with these procedures. In patients with prosthetic heart valves, anticoagulation with vitamin K antagonists reduces the frequency of thromboembolic events but does not totally eliminate them. Anticoagulants do not inhibit platelet reactions except those induced by thrombin; in fact, there is evidence (Salzman *et al.* 1980) that heparin actually enhances platelet reactivity, inducing the aggregation of platelets itself and augmenting the effects of other aggregating agents such as ADP.

In the resultant search for more effective pharmacological aids in the suppression of blood–surface interactions, drugs that alter platelet function have received increasing attention. A host of agents suppress platelet activity by various mechanisms, but for practical purposes at present the drugs available are those that either block the activity of platelet arachidonic acid cyclo-oxygenase or increase the platelet content of cyclic AMP. Decalcifying agents such as EDTA and 'membrane-stabilizing agents' such as local anaesthetics, which alter the calcium homoeo-stasis of the platelet, are highly effective *in vitro* but have limited application *in vivo* because of their lack of selectivity and their effects on other organs. Regional use of such drugs during haemodialysis in experimental animals has been reported (Scharschmidt *et al.* 1977), but does not appear to have been studied in man.

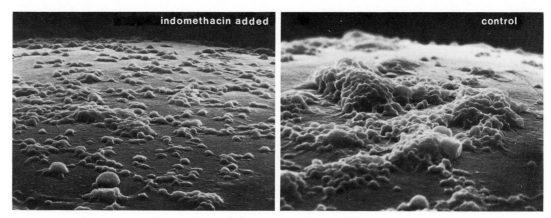

FIGURE 2. Suppression of platelet aggregation by 10^{-4} M indomethacin. Platelet adhesion to the bead surface is not inhibited. From Salzman *et al.* (1977).

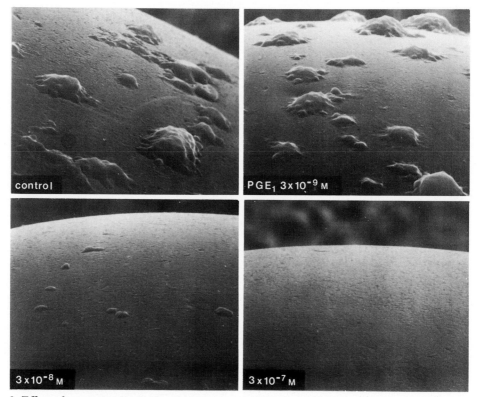

FIGURE 3. Effect of prostaglandin E_1 (3×10^{-9} M to 3×10^{-7} M) on platelet interaction with polystyrene beads.

Inhibitors of platelet cyclo-oxygenase

Non-steroidal anti-inflammatory agents such as aspirin and indomethacin and the uricosuric drug sulphinpyrazone inhibit the generation of thromboxane A_2 by platelets and thus prevent platelet aggregation by this substance, which appears to mediate the effect of many platelet stimulants. Alternative pathways to platelet activation are available to thrombin and collagen, so drugs such as aspirin usually do not produce an intolerable interruption of haemostasis. The formation of platelet aggregates on artificial surfaces is markedly reduced, and secretion of platelet products is largely eliminated. The combination of oral anticoagulants with sulphin-pyrazone or aspirin has proved to be more effective to prevent thromboembolism in patients with prosthetic heart valves then has Warfarin alone (Dale *et al.* 1977; Steele & Genton 1976). Lindsay *et al.* (1972) found reduced platelet consumption during haemodialysis in patients who received aspirin. Kaegi *et al.* (1975) reported that the occlusion of arterio-venous shunts employed for haemodialysis was prevented by the administration of sulphinpyrazone.

Unfortunately, these encouraging results must be tempered by the serious shortcomings of non-steroidal anti-inflammatory agents in extracorporeal circulation. Blood loss is significantly increased in patients who undergo cardiopulmonary bypass after the administration of aspirin (Torosian *et al.* 1978), and increased blood loss has also been observed during haemodialysis after aspirin ingestion. Aspirin and drugs that act similarly lack the property of prompt reversibility of action that is essential to the successful use of platelet-active agents during cardiopulmonary bypass. Otherwise the protection against platelet consumption afforded by paralysis of platelet function during extracorporeal circulation would be vitiated by the persistant bleeding tendency induced by the drug, whose effect must be reversed at the conclusion of bypass for haemostatic competence. Furthermore, inhibitors of platelet cyclo-oxygenase block platelet aggregation but do not prevent the adhesion of platelets to artificial surfaces (figure 2, plate 1). The vast surface areas of membrane oxygenators and dialysers may provide a capacious platelet sink even in the absence of platelet aggregation. Also, even without aggregation, the adhesion of individual platelets may seriously interfere with the function of a device designed for transfer of gases or solutes by compromising the area available for diffusion.

Drugs that raise platelet cyclic AMP levels

The inhibition of platelet activity by elevation of cyclic AMP may be brought about by the activation of adenylate cyclase or the inhibition of phosphodiesterase or more directly by the incubation of platelets with a cyclic AMP derivative, such as dibutyryl cyclic AMP, able to cross the cell membrane. *In vitro*, the platelet response to cyclic AMP elevation is dose-dependent. With increasing concentrations of inhibitor, there is at first suppression of platelet secretion and reduction in the size of aggregates, then elimination of aggregation with persistance of adhesion, and finally prevention of adhesion of solitary platelets to the surface (figure 3, plate 1). The mechanism of these reactions is not completely understood. It is known that cyclic AMP can activate a calcium pump mechanism in platelets (Käser-Glanzmann *et al.* 1977) and presumably through this action can lower cytoplasmic calcium levels. Such an action would inhibit the activity of the calcium-dependent enzymes phospholipase A_2 and phospholipase C and arachidonic acid cyclo-oxygenase, thus blocking the production of thromboxane A_2. That there are other important effects of cyclic AMP is suggested (Steer & Salzman 1980) by the fact that increased cyclic AMP inhibits platelet reactions that do not appear to require metabolism of arachidonic acid, such as the action of the thromboxane A_2 itself or its synthetic analogues, the 'primary phase' of platelet aggregation induced by ADP, and the adhesion of platelets to artificial surfaces. There is evidence (Hathaway *et al.* 1980) that cyclic AMP is required for the phosphorylation of myosin light chain kinase, which could account for a direct effect of elevated cyclic AMP levels on the contractile activity of the platelet.

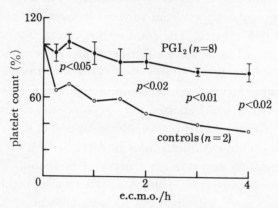

FIGURE 4. Effect of prostacyclin (PGI_2) on consumption of platelets during veno-venous bypass for extracorporeal membrane oxygenation (e.c.m.o.) in lambs. Platelet counts expressed as a percentage of pre-e.c.m.o. levels. From Coppe *et al.* (1979).

The phosphodiesterase inhibitor dipyridamole has been extensively studied as an anti-thrombotic drug, most effectively when administered in conjunction with aspirin, and has been found to offer some protection against prosthetic valve-associated thromboembolism (Sullivan *et al.* 1968) and platelet consumption during cardiopulmonary bypass or haemodialysis (Becker *et al.* 1972; Nuutinen *et al.* 1977). It has been suggested (Whittle 1978) that the action of dipyridamole is based on its ability to enhance the elevation of platelet cyclic AMP induced by natural or exogenous stimulants to adenylate cyclase, such as the prostaglandins.

There are several reported studies of the use of prostaglandin E_1 in *ex vivo* models of cardio-pulmonary bypass and in animals, and a more limited experience in patients has been described. In monkeys, PGE_1 (0.2–5 µg kg^{-1} min^{-1}) significantly reduced consumption of platelets during cardiopulmonary bypass, ameliorated the defect in platelet aggregation that otherwise occurred, and maintained a normal bleeding time (Addonizio *et al.* 1978). However, administration of PGE_1 to patients during bypass was unsatisfactory because of profound vasodilatation and hypotension that made it impossible to give enough of the drug to prevent platelet consumption (van den Dungen *et al.* 1980; Ellison *et al.* 1980). Administration of PGE_1 (0.1 µg kg^{-1} min^{-1}) did not significantly affect platelet number or function, compared with a control group receiving no prostaglandin. There was no difference in post-operative blood loss in the two groups of patients.

Exploration of the use of prostacyclin (PGI_2) in extracorporeal circulation has been more encouraging. Several authors (Coppe *et al.* 1979, 1981; Addonizio *et al.* 1979; Longmore *et al.* 1979; Plachetka *et al.* 1980) have reported reduction of platelet consumption *in vitro* and during veno-venous bypass or total cardiopulmonary bypass in lambs and dogs (figure 4), and similar observations have been reported with haemodialysis (Turney *et al.* 1980) and charcoal haemo-perfusion (Gimson *et al.* 1980). A defect in platelet aggregation is regularly induced by cardiopulmonary bypass and is attributed (Beurling-Harbury *et al.* 1978) to continued circulation of platelets that had previously been partly activated and thus partly exhausted by contact with the extracorporeal circuit. This functional defect was reduced or in some cases totally eliminated by infusion of prostacyclin (figure 5). The dose required in lambs was around 1 μg kg⁻¹ min⁻¹, and that in dogs even higher, and was accompanied by significant hypotension. Prostacyclin

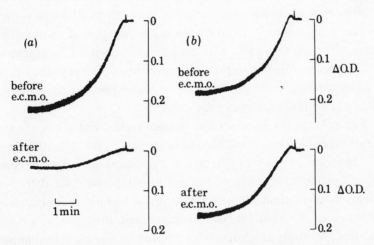

FIGURE 5. Reduction in platelet aggregation in response to ADP-induced extracorporeal membrane oxygenation. ADP concentration, 5 μM. (*a*) Control animals; (*b*) animals receiving PGI₂. Platelet responsiveness was preserved in the animals receiving PGI₂.

is labile, with a half-life in blood of only a few minutes. During veno-venous bypass (Coppe *et al.* 1979), its regional administration was possible by infusion into the venous outflow line, confining the effect of the drug to the extracorporeal circuit. Thus, during bypass the ability of platelets to aggregate could be totally inhibited in the extracorporeal circuit, while simultaneous blood samples drawn from the pulmonary artery displayed a nearly normal platelet aggregation response. Unfortunately, the more rapid flow rates required for total cardiopulmonary bypass made it impossible to limit the effect of prostacyclin to the extracorporeal circuit, which magnified the problem of prostaglandin-induced hypotension.

Several centres have reported clinical trials of prostacyclin infusion in cardiopulmonary bypass in man. The reports (Walker *et al.* 1980; Radegran *et al.* 1980; Bunting *et al.* 1981; Pokar *et al.* 1981) describe a total of nearly 100 patients receiving prostacyclin infusions during extracorporeal circulation for open-heart operations. Since man is more sensitive to PGI₂ than are most experimental animals, lower doses of the agent have been possible, 20–50 ng kg⁻¹ min⁻¹ being customary. Partial prevention of platelet consumption has been achieved in all of these studies, with significantly higher platelet concentrations circulating immediately after bypass. There is evidence of reduced platelet activation, including lower levels of plasma β-thromboglobulin and platelet factor 4 than in controls, less accumulation of circulating debris on arterial filters, and prevention of the usual increase in screen filtration pressure attributed to circulating platelet aggregates. A reduced frequency of post-bypass psychiatric changes has been claimed, presumably by prevention of microembolization to the brain.

Total prevention of platelet loss has not been achieved at these rates of prostacyclin infusion, nor has there been a consistant improvement in post-bypass platelet function. Improved results might be obtained with higher doses of prostacyclin, but this is impractical because of the serious hypotensive effects of vasodilation induced by the drug, which has limited the tolerable dose. Decreased urine output in patients receiving prostacyclin was reported and is not unexpected, considering the reduction in perfusion pressure induced by the drug. Reduction in the dose of heparin required has been reported by several authors, as judged by the activated clotting time or other coagulation tests. Heparin sparing has been explained by the absence of platelet secretion of the heparin antagonist, platelet factor 4, in the presence of prostacyclin (Bunting et al. 1979). No deaths have been blamed on the administration of prostacyclin during cardiopulmonary bypass, although one patient in the series reported by Radegran et al. (1980) died of an intra-operative myocardial infarction while receiving prostacyclin. Several authors make mention of the significant effects of prostacyclin on blood pressure and the need for aggressive fluid administration or administration of vasopressors.

Hypotensive side effects may be a serious barrier to the wider use of prostacyclin during cardiopulmonary bypass. Although the thrombocytopenia and alteration in platelet function that complicate cardiopulmonary bypass are a significant source of haemorrhagic complications, practising cardiac surgeons have learned to compensate for defective haemostasis in open-heart patients by meticulous attention to surgical technique and an aggressive attitude toward re-exploration of the chest, should haemorrhagic drainage be excessive in the early post-operative period. No study of prostacyclin infusion during cardiopulmonary bypass in man has yet shown preservation of normal platelet function or unequivocal evidence of reduction in intra-operative or post-operative blood loss. It seems likely that to achieve these goals it will be necessary to accomplish a total paralysis of platelet function during contact of the blood with the extracorporeal circuit. The heparin-sparing effect of prostacyclin is of interest but is not of obvious clinical benefit to the patient.

The development of open-heart surgery is one of medicine's great achievements of the past three decades. Complicated operations on the heart and great vessels are routinely performed with minimal mortality, to which haemorrhage makes only a small contribution. The introduction of serious hypotensive cardiac, renal or cerebral side effects of a new drug, even if infrequent, would be intolerable in current practice. Development of more selective agents with the ability to stimulate platelet adenylate cyclase but without the vasodilating effects of prostacyclin would seem to be essential before this approach to cardiopulmonary bypass can be adopted more widely.

This work was supported by N.I.H. grants no. HL 25066 and HL 20079.

REFERENCES (Salzman et al.)

Addonizio, V. P., Macarak, E. J., Nicolaou, K. C., Edmunds, Jr, L. H. & Colman, R. W. 1979 Effects of prostacyclin and albumin on platelet loss during in vitro simulation of extracorporeal circulation. Blood 53, 1033–1042.

Addonizio, V. P., Smith, J. B., Strauss, J. F., Colman, R. W. & Edmunds, Jr, L. H. 1980 Thromboxane synthesis and platelet secretion during cardiopulmonary bypass with bubble oxygenator. J. thorac. cardiovasc. Surg. 79, 91–96.

Addonizio, Jr, V. P., Strauss, J. F., Macarak, E. J., Colman, R. W. & Edmunds, Jr, L. H. 1978 Preservation of platelet number and function with prostaglandin E$_1$ during total cardiopulmonary bypass in rhesus monkeys. Surgery 83, 619–625.

Bachmann, F., McKenna, R., Cole, E. R. & Najafi, H. 1978 The hemostatic mechanisms after open-heart surgery. I. Studies on plasma coagulation factors and fibrinolysis in 512 patients after extracorporeal circulation. J. thorac. cardiovasc. Surg. 70, 76–85.

Baier, R. E. & Dutton, R. C. 1969 Initial events in interactions of blood with a foreign surface. *J. biomed. Mater. Res.* **3**, 191–206.

Becker, R. M., Smith, M. R. & Dobell, A. T. C. 1972 Effect of dipyridamole on platelet function in cardiopulmonary bypass in pigs. *Surg. Forum* **23**, 169.

Brier-Russell, D., Salzman, E. W., Lindon, J., Handin, R., Merrill, E. W., Dincer, A. K. & Wu, J. 1981 *In vitro* assessment of interaction of blood with model surfaces: acrylates and methacrylates. *J. Colloid Interface Sci.* (In the press.)

Beurling-Harbury, C. & Galvan, C. A. 1978 Acquired decrease in platelet secretory ADP associated with increased postoperative bleeding in post-cardiopulmonary bypass patients and in patients with severe valvular heart disease. *Blood* **52**, 13–23.

Bunting, S. & Moncada, S. 1979 Prostacyclin, by preventing platelet activation, prolongs activated clotting time in blood and platelet rich plasma and potentiates the anticoagulant effect of heparin. *Proc. Br. pharmac. Soc.* 268P.

Bunting, S., O'Grady, J., Moncada, S. & Vane, J. R. 1981 Prostacyclin improves biocompatibility of cardiopulmonary bypass apparatus in man. (In preparation.)

Coppe, D., Sobel, M., Seamans, L., Levine, F., Salzman, E. W. 1981 Prostacyclin preserves platelet function and number during cardiopulmonary bypass. *J. thorac. cardiovasc. Surg.* **81**, 274–278.

Coppe, D., Wonder, T., Snider, M. & Salzman, E. W. 1979 Preservation of platelet number and function during extracorporeal membrane oxygenation by regional infusion of prostacyclin. In *Prostacyclin* (ed. J. R. Vane & S. Bergstrom), pp. 371–382. New York: Raven Press.

Dale, J., Myhre, E., Storstein, O., Stormorken, H. & Efskind, L. 1977 Prevention of arterial thromboembolism with acetylsalicylic acid. *Am. Heart J.* **94**, 101–111.

Ellison, N., Addonizio, V. P., Niewiarowski, S., MacVaugh III, H., Harken, A. H., Colman, R. W. & Edmunds, Jr, L. H. 1980 Platelet protection during cardiopulmonary bypass with albumin primes and prostaglandin E_1 infusion. *Anesthesiology* **53**, S168.

Friedman, L. I., Liem, H., Grabowski, E. F., Leonard, E. F. & McCord, C. W. 1970 Inconsequentiality of surface properties for initial platelet adhesion. *Trans. Am. Soc. artif. intern. Org.* **16**, 63–73.

Gimson, A. E. S., Langley, P. G., Huges, R. D., Canalese, J., Williams, R., Woods, H. F. & Weston, M. J. 1980 Prostacyclin to prevent platelet activation during charcoal haemoperfusion in fulminant hepatic failure. *Lancet* i, 173–175.

Hathaway, D. R., Eaton, C. R. & Adelstein, R. S. 1980 Regulation of human platelet myosin kinase by calcium-calmodulin and cyclic AMP. In *The regulation of coagulation* (ed. K. G. Mann & F. B. Taylor, Jr), pp. 271–276. New York: Elsevier/North-Holland.

Hennessy, Jr, V. I., Hicks, R. E., Niewiaroski, S., Edmunds, Jr, L. H. & Colman, R. W. 1977 Function of human platelets during extracorporeal circulation. *Am. J. Physiol.* **232**, H622–628.

Kaegi, A., Pineo, G. F., Shimizu, A. Trivedi, H., Hirsh, H. & Gent, M. 1975 The role of sulfinpyrazone in the prevention of arterio-venous shunt thrombosis. *Circulation* **52**, 497–499.

Kaser-Glanzmann, R., Jakabova, M., George, J. N. & Luscher, E. F. 1977 Stimulation of calcium uptake in platelet membrane vesicles by adenosine 3′,5′-cyclic monophosphate and protein kinase. *Biochim. Biophys. Acta.* **466**, 429–440.

Lindon, J. N., Collins, R. E. C., Coe, N. P., Jagoda, A., Brier-Russell, D., Merrill, E. W. & Salzman, E. W. 1980 *In vivo* assessment of thromboresistant materials by determination of platelet survival. *Circuln Res.* **46**, 84–90.

Lindon, J. N., Rodvien, R., Brier, D., Greenberg, R., Merrill, E. W. & Salzman, E. W. 1978 *In vitro* assessment of interaction of blood with model surfaces. *J. lab. clin. Med.* **92**, 904–915.

Lindsay, R. M., Prentice, C. R. M., Ferguson, D., Burton, J. A. & McNicol, G. P. 1972 Reduction of thrombus formation on dialyser membrane by aspirin and RA 233. *Lancet* ii, 1287–1290.

Longmore, D. B., Bennett, G., Gueirrara, D., Smith, M., Buntin, S., Moncada, S., Reed, P., Read, N. G. & Vane, J. R. 1979 Prostacyclin: a solution to some problems of extracorporeal circulation. *Lancet* i, 1002–1005.

McKenna, R., Bachmann, F., Whittaker, B., Gilson, J., Weinberg, M. 1975 The hemostatic mechanism after open-heart surgery. III. Frequency of abnormal platelet functions during and after extracorporeal circulation. *J. thorac. cardiovasc. Surg.* **70**, 298–309.

Michelson, E. L., Morganroth, J., Torosian, M. & MacVaugh III, H. 1978 Relation of preoperative use of aspirin to increased mediastinal blood loss after coronary artery bypass graft surgery. *J. thorac. cardiovasc. Surg.* **76**, 694–697.

Moncada, S., Gryglewski, R., Bunting, S. & Vane, J. R. 1976 An enzyme isolated from arteries transforms prostaglandin endoperoxides to an unstable substance that inhibits platelet aggregation. *Nature, Lond.* **263**, 663–665.

Nuutinen, L. S., Pihlajaiemi, R., Saarela, E., Karkola, P. & Hollmen, A. 1977 The effect of dipyridamole on the thrombocyte count and bleeding tendency in open-heart surgery. *J. thorac. cardiovasc. Surg.* **74**, 295–298.

Plachetka, J. R., Salomon, N. W., Larson, D. F. & Copeland, J. G. 1980 Platelet loss during experimental cardiopulmonary bypass and its prevention with prostacyclin. *Ann. thorac. Surg.* **30**, 58–63.

Pokar, H., Bleese, M., Fischer-Dusterhoff, H. & Tilsner, V. 1981 Summary of interim report of a trial of prostacyclin in the prevention of postoperative neurological disturbances after open heart surgery and effects on platelet numbers and platelet activation. (In preparation.)

Radegran, K. & Papaconstantinou, C. 1980 Prostacyclin infusion during cardiopulmonary bypass in man. *Thromb. Res.* **19**, 267–270.

Sa da Costa, V., Brier-Russell, D., Trudel, G. E., Waugh, D. F., Salzman, E. W. & Merrill, E. W. 1980 Polyether-polyurethane surfaces: thrombin adsorption, platelet adsorption, and ESCA scanning. *J. Colloid Interface Sci.* **76**, 594.

Salzman, E. W. 1971 Role of platelets in blood–surface interactions. *Fedn Proc. Fedn Am. Socs exp. biol.* **30**, 1503.

Salzman, E. W., Lindon, J. N., Brier, D. & Merrill, E. W. 1977 Surface induced platelet adhesion, aggregation, and release. *Proc. N.Y. Acad. Sci.* **283**, 114–127.

Salzman, E. W., Rosenberg, R. D., Smith, M. H., Lindon, J. N. & Favreau, L. 1980 Effect of heparin and heparin fractions on platelet aggregation. *J. clin. Invest.* **65**, 64.

Scharschmidt, B. F., Martin, J. F., Shapiro, L. J., Plotz, P. H. & Berk, P. D. 1977 The use of calcium chelating agents and prostaglandin E_1 to eliminate platelet and white blood cell losses resulting from hemoperfusion through uncoated charcoal, albumin–agarose gel, and neutral and cation exchange resins. *J. Lab. clin. Med.* **89**, 110–119.

Steele, P. & Genton, E. 1976 Thromboembolism and platelet survival time before and after valve surgery. *Adv. Cardiol.* **17**, 189–198.

Steer, M. L. & Salzman, E. W. 1980 Cyclic nucleotides in hemostasis and thrombosis. In *Advances in cyclic nucleotide research*, vol. 12 (ed. P. Greengard & G. A. Robison), pp. 71–92. New York: Raven Press.

Sullivan, J. M., Harken, D. E. & Gorlin, R. 1968 Pharmacologic control of thromboembolic complications of cardia valve replacement. A preliminary report. *New Engl. J. Med.* **279**, 576–580.

Torosian, M., Michelson, E. L., Morganroth, J. & MacVaugh III, H. 1978 Aspirin- and coumadin-related bleeding after coronary-artery bypass graft surgery. *Ann. intern. Med.* **89**, 325–328.

Turney, J. H., Williams, L. C., Fewell, M. R., Parsons, V. & Weston, M. J. 1980 Platelet protection and heparin sparing with prostacyclin during regular dialysis therapy. *Lancet* ii, 219–222.

van den Dungen, J. J. A. M., Velders, A. J., Karliczek, G. F., Homan van der Heide, J. N. & Wildevuur, C. R. H. 1980 Platelet preservation during cardiopulmonary bypass (CPB) with prostaglandin (PGE_1) and prostacyclin (PGI_2). *Trans. Am. Soc. artif. intern. Org.* **26**, 481–485.

Walker, I. D., Davidson, J. F., Faichney, A., Davidson, K. G. & Wheatley, D. J. 1980 Prostacyclin in cardiopulmonary bypass surgery [abstract]. In *6th Int. Cong. Med. League Against Thrombosis*, p. 141.

Whittle, B. J. R., Moncada, S. & Vane, J. R. 1978 Comparison of the effects of prostacyclin (PGI_2), prostaglandins E_1 and D_2 on platelet aggregation in different species. *Prostaglandins* **16**, 373–388.

Phil. Trans. R. Soc. Lond. B **294**, 399–412 (1981)

Printed in Great Britain

Experience with prostacyclin in cardiopulmonary bypass in dog and man

By D. B. Longmore

The National Heart Hospital, Westmoreland Street, London W1M 8BA, *U.K.*

[Plate 1]

The activation and disruption of platelets resulting from contact with bypass equipment is responsible for bleeding problems after open-heart surgery and for vascular injury leading to cerebral damage. This paper presents experimental and clinical evidence for the benefits of the preservation of platelets by prostacyclin (PGI_2) during cardiopulmonary bypass operations.

Work with dogs showed that PGI_2 was more effective than heparin in maintaining the numbers and aggregability of the platelet population, but by far the most effective was a combination of the two agents.

A subsequent double-blind clinical trial on 24 patients undergoing coronary vein grafts, in which the combination was compared with heparin alone, confirmed these findings in man. In the presence of PGI_2, platelet numbers and aggregability were preserved, with a consequent reduction in blood loss. Significantly fewer reinforcing doses of heparin were required by the PGI_2 group. The integrity of platelets in the presence of PGI_2 was reflected by the lack of micro-aggregates and fibrin deposits on arterial line filters. In both the human and dog studies, PGI_2 was shown, by the cultured foetal mouse heart test, to prevent the release of circulating cardiotoxic factors during bypass.

The known vasodilator effect of PGI_2 was observed but caused no clinical problems. An unexpected feature was the maintenance of perfusion pressure without the need for additional fluid. This may indicate that PGI_2 reduces capillary permeability.

Introduction

The discovery of prostacyclin (PGI_2) in 1976 (see Moncada & Vane 1978), the most powerful inhibitor of platelet function described so far, was of immediate interest to those of us who are concerned about the unsatisfactory results of contemporary cardiopulmonary bypass procedures. Many of the problems after open-heart surgery are attributable to deficiencies of the haemostatic system. Post-operative bleeding, embolism and thrombosis are occasionally a threat to life and very commonly a cause of post-operative morbidity. Heparin anticoagulation and protamine reversal is still the only technique available for routine use in open-heart surgery. For many years this combination has been recognized as less than satisfactory (Bass & Longmore 1969; Åberg 1974).

The adverse effects of protamine, a family of basic polypeptides, are well known (Larkin *et al.* 1978; Ellison *et al.* 1978; Velders 1980). The use of heparin, a family of complex polysaccharides, while preventing gross coagulation of blood, does not inhibit the first stages of the clotting cascade. Platelets are activated and destroyed as a result of the contact between blood and the artificial surfaces of the heart–lung machine. Heparin may itself exacerbate such destruction (Wolf 1967).

After open-heart surgery, the patient's recovery is always very much slower than after closed-heart or general surgery. Post-operative complications include varying degrees of psycho-pathological disturbances. Some patients are unable to work or live in harmony with their families after contemporary open-heart surgery. Surgical life-saving triumphs are all too commonly marred by disabling complications. These complications are more serious than might be expected from the loss of some platelets. Platelet adhesion to the extracorporeal apparatus and aggregation, not prevented by heparin, leads to the release of platelet granular constituents. ADP, 5-hydroxytryptamine and the small proteins β-thromboglobulin (βTG) and platelet factor 4 (PF4) are released into the circulation.

Some of the released substances are procoagulant (Broekman *et al.* 1975), and when caused by abnormal platelet activation may seriously disturb the chemical balance regulating normal endothelial repair in haemostasis. There is evidence supporting the theory that the heparin-neutralizing activity present in blood is due to PF4 released from platelets (Niewiarowski *et al.* 1976). βTG is a significant component of this protein secretion and may inhibit local production of PGI_2 (Hope *et al.* 1979).

During cardiopulmonary bypass, haemodiluting fluids used in the prime and administered to the patient pass rapidly into the extravascular space, suggesting to us that there is increased capillary permeability. We do not know whether this is related to release of 5-hydroxytryptamine and other substances from adherent and disrupting platelets.

Dog experiments

We set out in 1978 to establish in the dog whether the use of PGI_2 would eliminate anti-coagulant-related complications of bypass. Initially we undertook three series of experiments (Longmore *et al.* 1979), using PGI_2 alone, a control group with heparin alone and a series with routine heparinization together with PGI_2.

In all three sets of experiments similar anaesthetic and surgical techniques were used. A simple bypass circuit was used with gravity drainage from an 8 mm atrial basket to a Bentley paediatric Q110 bubble oxygenator. This was connected to a single-roller pulsatile arterial pump with a finely adjustable driven roller to avoid trauma to the blood. A special feature of the bypass circuit was the inclusion of two filters in series in the arterial line. Pressure take-off points proximal to the first filter, between the filters, and distal to the second filter were used to detect clogging of the filters. Scanning electron microscopy of both sides of both filters was used to determine whether material found on the filter surfaces was deposited on or generated by the filters.

Bypass with PGI_2 alone

With the use of the circuit described above, PGI_2 alone was used for 1 h bypass in 14 beagles. Remarkably, we achieved long-term survival in all but the first in which there was a technical failure unrelated to the use of PGI_2. During the surgery in this group, the wounds were dry, appearing as they are in conventional operations performed without extracorporeal circulation and heparinization. There was no measurable blood loss during or after the surgery. Nevertheless, the plasma fibrinogen was reduced and there was frank clot in those regions of the extracorporeal circulation in which there was stasis. There were clots on both filters.

At this stage of the development of oxygenators, reservoirs and filters, the designs for heat exchange and debubbling depend on blood standing in contact with heat exchange surfaces and in holding areas. Until a new generation of apparatus, already designed on different principles, becomes acceptable it will probably not be possible to use PGI_2 on its own.

Heparin alone

We undertook two further sets of experiments on greyhounds. In the first six control experiments the dogs were given heparin 300 i.u./kg intravenously (i.v.) 5 min before starting a 2 h bypass.

Heparin plus PGI₂

A further eight experiments were undertaken by using the same heparin routine and prostacyclin at 10 ng kg^{-1} min^{-1} i.v. for 15 min before bypass and then 1 µg kg^{-1} min^{-1} into the venous return line near to the heart so that the PGI₂ was in maximum concentration in the oxygenator for the 2 h of bypass. All dogs were given protamine sulphate in a 1:1 ratio to the total heparin dose at the end of bypass.

Blood samples were taken after induction of anaesthesia, when the PGI₂ infusion was started, at the beginning of bypass, every 15 min during and after bypass, and after protamine administration until recovery. These samples were used for haemotocrit determination, platelet counts (phase contrast microscopy), and testing on foetal hearts. Platelet-rich plasma was obtained by centrifugation of citrated blood at 1000 g. Aggregation was induced by adenosine diphosphate (20–100 µmol/l) and measured as the increase in light transmission over 2 min in a Born-type aggregometer (Payton dual-channel). Total clotting fibrinogen, thrombin-clotting time, as well as the above measurements, were estimated at the same times and 24 h after operation.

Filters were rapidly removed after bypass and fixed for scanning electron microscopy. During the bypass and during wound closure any bleeding was noted. The pressure differential across the two filters in the arterial line was recorded every 5 min during bypass.

To study possible changes in the plasma proteins and any toxic substances that might be released from damaged platelets, foetal mouse hearts in organ culture were used (Wildenthal 1970, 1971 a, b; Hughes & Longmore 1972; Longmore & Smith 1980). Foetal hearts were taken from Theier's (T.O.) pure-strain mice that had been mated 15 days previously; 15 control and 15 test hearts were each cultured in 2 ml of 'Wellcome' 199 culture medium and 1 ml of plasma with cortisol (1 µg/ml) and insulin (50 µg/ml). The plasma was obtained from samples of blood drawn from the oxygenator just before the end of bypass. The hearts were cultured in 95 % O₂ and 5 % CO₂ at 37 °C. They were examined under a dissecting microscope every 24 h and returned to the incubator when the beating rate had been recorded.

Results of preliminary dog experiments

The results of the dog experiments were unequivocal. In the series with heparin only the wounds remained wet throughout the operation. There was some post-operative oozing from the chest wound. All the dogs recovered slowly. One died 6 h post-operatively of haemorrhage. Two more died within 24 h. The platelet count, corrected for haemodilution (figure 1), fell to below 50 % during the bypass and even further to 35 % after protamine was given. The few platelets remaining in the circulating blood after the protamine injection were incapable of aggregation (figure 2). The plasma fibrinogen was reduced. The pressure differential across the filters in three of the dogs showed a fluctuating pattern: building up, falling, and then building up again.

In the protein-denaturation studies on mouse foetal hearts, there was a significant depression of beating-rate and reduction of survival time (compared with the control plasmas) in hearts receiving plasma from dogs bypassed with heparin alone (figure 3). Scanning electron microscopy

scopy showed a build-up of platelet aggregates on both sides of both filters. The platelets covering the surfaces were breaking down and fibrin strands were forming with red and white cells enmeshed (figure 4*a*, plate 1).

In contrast, in the series combining heparin and PGI_2, there was no fall in platelet count, no change in platelet activity, and no fall in plasma fibrinogen. Furthermore, there was no increase

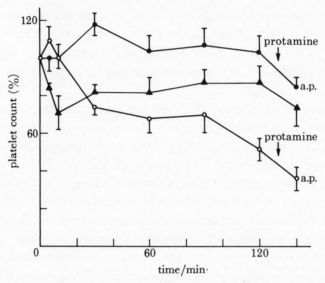

FIGURE 1. Platelet counts during 2 h bypass operations on dogs with heparin alone (○), PGI_2 alone (▲) and a combination of the two (●). A.p., after protamine.

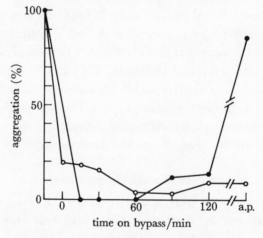

FIGURE 2. Aggregability of dog platelets to ADP during bypass with heparin alone (○) and with heparin plus PGI_2 (●). The ability of platelets to aggregate after a conventional bypass is about 10 % of control. This was improved to over 80 % with heparin and PGI_2. A.p., after protamine.

in pressure across the filters during the 2 h of bypass. Platelet aggregation returned to normal within 30 min of the end of prostacyclin infusion. Electron microscopy showed that the filter mesh had only a few adhering platelets. The platelets that had adhered did not appear to have broken down. There were no fibrin strands formed (figure 4*b*). Plasma taken at the end of bypass from these dogs had no significant effect on the beating rate and survival time of the foetal hearts.

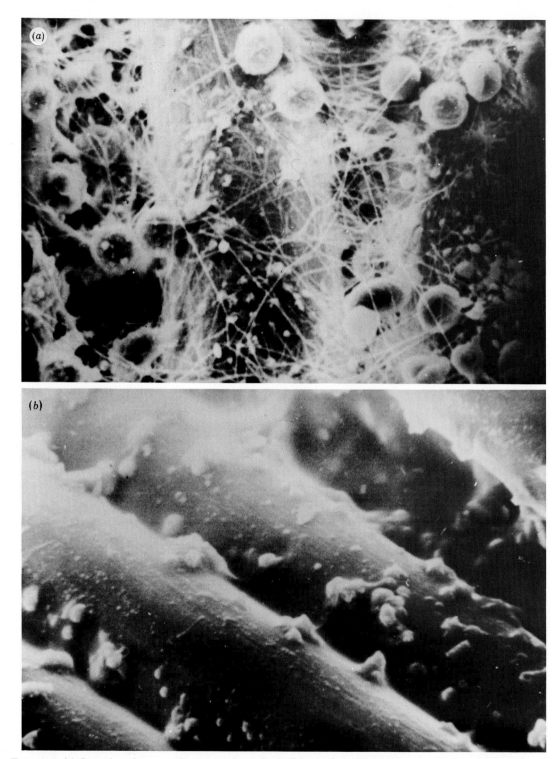

FIGURE 4. (*a*) Scanning electron microscopy showed a build-up of platelet aggregates, fibrin strands and red and white cells on the filter from the bypass with heparin alone. (*b*) Scanning electron microscopy showed few platelet aggregates and no fibrin strands when PGI_2 was used in combination with heparin.

The advantageous effects of prostacyclin in the experiments were not accompanied by any apparent disadvantages. The remarkably low mortality rate in the PGI_2 dog series strongly suggested that the use of PGI_2 in human bypass would be safe. It is well known that the dog is less able than man to withstand the trauma of cardiopulmonary bypass.

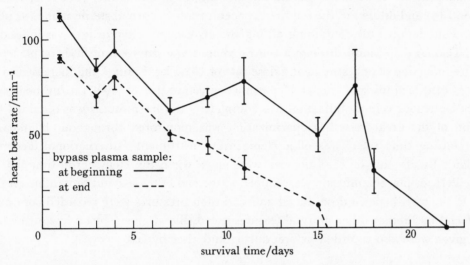

FIGURE 3. Influence of dog plasma on heart rate and survival time of cultured foetal mouse hearts, showing the reduction of these by plasma from the 'heparin only' group. This difference was not seen in the presence of PGI_2.

THE CLINICAL TRIAL

Encouraged by the positive results obtained in the dog laboratory, we undertook a double-blind trial in man, by using PGI_2 in combination with routine heparinization (Longmore *et al.* 1981). This trial was designed to establish whether the beneficial effects of PGI_2 seen in the dog would translate to the human. In addition we also set out to establish whether there would be any measurable clinical benefits from the improved haematological picture obtained when PGI_2 was used. We concentrated on post-operative bleeding and multi-organ damage including brain damage.

Patients and clinical aspects

The study was carried out on 24 male patients between ages of 36 and 64 years (mean 52 years) in which 12 received PGI_2 and 12 received placebo. One patient (subsequently found to be receiving placebo) was excluded from this study because he had to be returned to theatre with cardiac tamponade. Patients undergoing coronary vein grafts were chosen because they are a homogeneous group operated on with a closed heart. The operating techniques used utilise minimal suction and cause minimal tissue damage. Thus, as in the preliminary study on dogs, most activation of platelets would be due to the traumatic passage of blood through the extracorporeal apparatus. The patients were operated on by Mr Donald Ross, Mr Magdi Yacoub and Mr Graeme Bennett at the National Heart Hospital, using similar techniques. A common anaesthetic protocol was used in every case.

In all the patients a routine bypass circuit with a Bos 10 Bentley oxygenator and Sarn's pumps was primed with 2 l of Hartmann's solution and 3000 i.u. heparin added. Flow rates varied between 2.2 and 2.4 l m² min⁻¹. Three suckers were available for the surgeons. These discharged into a Bentley cardiotomy reservoir with a 40 μm in-line filter. No arterial line filtration was used. PGI₂ (synthesized by Upjohn Co. and formulated by the Wellcome Foundation Ltd), reconstituted from the freeze-dried sodium salt (0.5 mg) in glycine buffer (pH 10.5, Wellcome Foundation Ltd) and diluted to the required concentration in normal sterile saline (or placebo (Wellcome Foundation Ltd) containing all ingredients except active drug), was infused by a peristaltic Tekmar drip pump through a central venous line. Infusion of PGI₂ or placebo was started after induction of anaesthesia at a dose rate of 10 ng kg⁻¹ min⁻¹ and increased to 20 ng kg⁻¹ min⁻¹ at the beginning of bypass. Heparin was given routinely (9000 i.u./m² body surface area) after saphenous vein mobilization was completed, and haemostasis was obtained before cannulation of the great vessels. Heparinization was monitored throughout by measuring activated clotting time by means of a Hemochron instrument (International Technidyne Corporation). Reinforcing doses of heparin were given when the Hemochron time fell below 350 s. The PGI₂ or placebo infusion was stopped at the end of bypass and protamine given in a 1:1 ratio to the total heparin dose. Blood and perfusion pressures were recorded continuously and any facial flushing or other unusual features noted. Blood given, blood loss, urine output and fluid given were also recorded before, during and after bypass.

TABLE 1. SAMPLING PROTOCOL

1. During the 24 h pre-operative period (psychometric and neurology tests only)
2. Immediately after induction of anaesthesia to obtain control levels
3. 30 min after beginning of infusion of PGI₂ or placebo
4. 5 min after heparin administration
5. 5 min after start of bypass (when adequate mixing of priming fluid and blood has taken place (foetal heart test only)

6a.
6b.
6c.   } Every 30 min on bypass
6d.

7. At the end of bypass before cardioactive drugs are administered (foetal heart test only)
8. 15 min after protamine administration
.9 2 h after bypass
10. 6 h after bypass (CK and BTG assays only)
11. 24 h after bypass
12. 3 days after bypass (CK and BTG assays and psychometric testing).
13. 6 days after bypass (psychometric and neurological tests)

Haematological and biochemical tests

Blood samples were taken from the radial arterial line or, during bypass, from the arterial reservoir of the pump circuit via a fine catheter.

Sampling times covered the period from induction of anaesthesia to the day after surgery (table 1). Samples were taken at times 2, 3, 4, 6a, 6b, 6c, 8, 9, 10 and 11 for the following haematological tests: haematocrit, haemoglobin, white blood cell count, platelet count, platelet aggregation, prothrombin time, thrombin time, partial thromboplastin time, fibrinogen, anti-thrombin III, and β-thromboglobulin.

β-Thromboglobulin levels were measured by radioimmunoassay with the double antibody (Ludlaim *et al.* 1975).

In addition to these investigations, creatine kinase (including MB isoenzymes) levels were also measured at times 9, 10, 11 and 12.

Post-operative urine samples were collected for creatinine clearance studies. The urine samples were divided into three to avoid loss through accidental spillage or nurses discarding the samples. Platelet aggregability was measured by the Born (1962) technique with a Payton aggregometer. The latter was measured in platelet-rich plasma within 2 min of the blood sample being withdrawn. The degree of aggregability was related to the maximum aggregation attainable with ADP in each specimen.

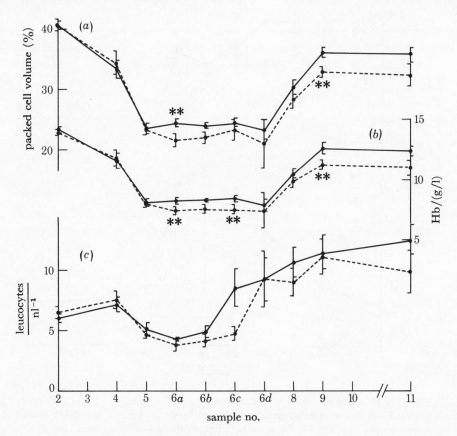

FIGURE 5. Values of haematocrit (a), haemoglobin (b) and white cell count (c) up to 24 h after bypass with (———) and without (– – –) PGI$_2$. These indicate the effect of haemodilution. The steady rise in leucocyte count is to be expected as a result of surgical intervention. **, $p < 0.05$; bars indicate standard error.

The foetal heart test was used as in the dog experiments on samples taken at times 5 and 7.

Psychometric testing was undertaken at times 1, 12 and 13. These tests are designed to detect any post-operative cerebral dysfunction. The testing plan at each testing time (Bethune 1980) included short-term memory recall, the 'Tooting Bec' questionnaire, a digital test, a number connection test and questions relating to the distant past. The complete test takes 20–25 min. At sample times 1 and 13, a routine clinical neurological examination with the use of a fixed protocol, including assessment of cranial nerve function, cerebellar function, muscle power, reflexes and coordination, was undertaken.

RESULTS

Haemoglobin and haematocrit, but not white cell count, showed slight but occasional significant differences between the placebo and active groups ($p < 0.05$; see figure 5). The results in the PGI$_2$ group were higher at times during the bypass and consistently higher after bypass. These three variables also indicate the extent of haemodilution at various stages throughout and after bypass. This indication of dilution can be used to apply a correction factor to other measurements such as platelet counts.

There was no significant difference between the control and test group for prothrombin time, partial thromboplastin time, fibrinogen, antithrombin III, creatine kinase and CK and MB isoenzymes, and β-thromboglobulin.

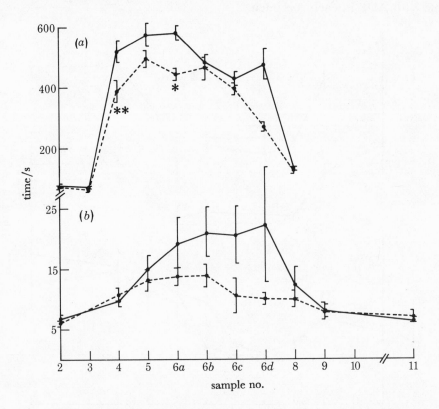

FIGURE 6. The variation of Hemochron value (a) and thrombin time (b) with (——) and without (– – –) PGI_2. Both variables were lower in the placebo group throughout bypass in spite of the higher dosage of heparin required by these patients. *, $p < 0.01$; **, $p < 0.05$; bars indicate standard error.

In the PGI_2 group the Hemochron times varied between 400 and 800 s during bypass. The patients receiving heparin alone showed a very significant lower Hemochron time ($p < 0.01$ in early bypass; figure 6). Some of the placebo group of patients fell below 400 s towards the end of bypass and required an extra reinforcing dose of heparin with a correspondingly increased dose of protamine.

The thrombin times were slightly raised in the PGI_2 group from the time of administration of the heparin dose until 6 h after bypass, when they became the same as in the heparin group.

Platelet counts were consistently higher throughout bypass in the PGI_2 patients than in the placebo group ($p < 0.01$). Figure 7 relates the platelet count and the platelet aggregation.

Platelet aggregation was reduced to 20 % of initial values by PGI_2 throughout the period of its administration. In the prostacyclin group the platelet aggregation had recovered to 70 % of the initial value 2 h after bypass. In the placebo group, platelet aggregability decreased gradually during bypass to approximately 30 % of initial values and only partly recovered 2 h after bypass. By 24 h after bypass there was no significant difference.

TABLE 2. SUMMARY OF CLINICAL MEASUREMENTS
(means ± s.e.m.)

	PGI$_2$	placebo
mean blood pressure after cannulation/mmHg		
systolic	81 ± 6	123 ± 9
diastolic	55 ± 4	88 ± 5
mean heart rate/min^{-1}		
after cannulation	85 ± 5	93 ± 5
after protamine given	96 ± 6	90 ± 4
mean blood usage/ml		
during operation	596 ± 226	909 ± 260
after operation (18 h)	1073 ± 200	1495 ± 311
total across operation	1669 ± 303	2404 ± 485
blood loss/ml		
0–6 h	250 ± 29	499 ± 103
6–18 h	103 ± 8	273 ± 67
> 18 h	132 ± 18	138 ± 23
total	485 ± 48	910 ± 172
mean administration of other fluids/ml		
during operation	3095 ± 357	3384 ± 471
after operation (18 h)	841 ± 46	846 ± 44
total	3936 ± 346	4211 ± 454
mean urine output/ml		
during operation	1120 ± 108	1435 ± 229
after operation	1992 ± 337	1637 ± 115
total	3112 ± 426	3072 ± 221

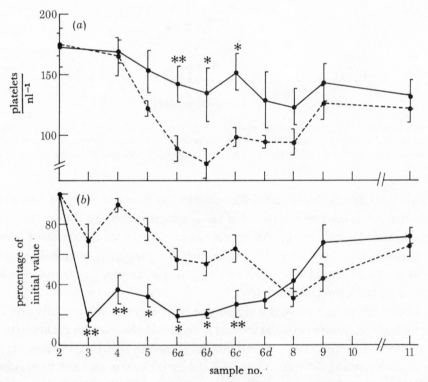

FIGURE 7. Variation of platelet count (a) and platelet aggregability (b) to ADP with (——) and without (– – –) PGI$_2$. Note the protection of the platelet population in the presence of PGI$_2$, and also that their aggregability is markedly diminished **during** bypass, recovering to *ca.* 70 % 6 h later, whereas in the placebo group it is only 45 % at this critical post-operative time. *, $p < 0.01$; **, $p < 0.05$; bars indicate standard error.

Clinical measurements

The clinical measurements are summarized in table 2. As expected, prostacyclin induced some hypotension, but this caused no difficulties in the clinical management of the patients. Only two patients required small doses of vasopressors. Our protocol allowed for any fall in blood pressure to be treated by the administration of additional fluid. In fact less fluid was required by the PGI_2 group. In spite of the lower blood pressures before bypass in the PGI_2 groups, the urine outputs were not significantly different in the two groups.

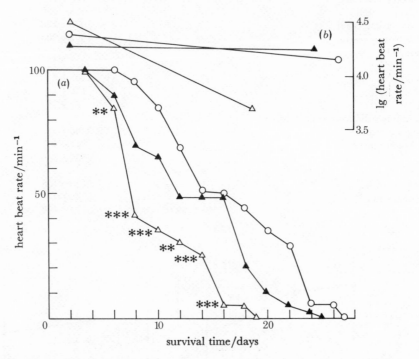

FIGURE 8. Reduction of heart rate and survival time (*a*) of cultured foetal mouse hearts; (*b*) linear regression analysis. The hearts exposed to plasma from the placebo group (△) show a significant depression of beating rate and survival time compared with that from a normal control (○) and the PGI_2 group (▲). **, $p < 0.05$; ***, $p < 0.001$.

We were unable to detect significant differences in the cerebral function and neurological status between the two groups of patients. No patient in either group showed any permanent detectable psychopathological change. All became more skilful with the repeated tests, showing an apparent improvement by 6 days after operation. Importantly, over half of the placebo group complained of inability to focus their eyes and to read newspaper print for 48 h. None of the PGI_2 group suffered from this disability.

The foetal heart culture test showed a significant depression of the foetal hearts exposed to plasma taken from blood samples no. 7 at the end of bypass in the placebo group, with reduction of the beating rate and survival time ($p < 0.001$) as shown in figure 8. Median survival times (l.t.$_{50}$) showed no significant difference between the foetal hearts exposed to plasma proteins from the PGI_2 group and plasma obtained from a normal volunteer, whereas there were marked differences with the placebo sample. The creatinine clearance test showed no significant difference between the two groups.

DISCUSSION

The three known effects of prostacyclin were confirmed with this study: stabilization of the platelet in the extracorporeal circulation, the heparin sparing effect and the vasodilator effect. In addition to these effects of PGI_2, our studies suggest that PGI_2 reduces the capillary damage leading to increased capillary permeability that takes place during cardiopulmonary bypass. The mechanism of this may be related to the reduction of platelet granule release. This mechanism is suggested by the foetal heart studies.

Foetal heart test

The foetal hearts showed significantly better survival times and beating performance when exposed to plasma from patients who had received PGI_2 compared with those who had received placebo. This is probably due to a reduction in the amount of platelet granular substances liberated when prostacyclin is administered. In our previous studies without the use of PGI_2 (Longmore *et al.* 1980) we have always shown depression of beating rate and survival time in foetal hearts when they are exposed to plasma taken at the end of bypass. The corresponding plasma from the PGI_2 patients was comparable with the control blood drawn from the healthy volunteer. It has been argued that the cause of the depression of the foetal hearts that follows a normal bypass may be associated with mechanical damage to proteins or may be due to protein damage following granule release from platelets. The beneficial effects of PGI_2 suggests the latter mechanism, as does the possible change in capillary permeability.

The β-thromboglobulin results do not help to resolve this problem. Plasma β-thromboglobulin concentration was increased in samples from both groups during and after surgery. This suggests a high level of platelet activation, but massive *in vitro* liberation of βTG may take place in the long cannulae through which blood samples were withdrawn.

Platelet aggregation and reduction of blood loss

The PGI_2 effect on platelet aggregation in the human clinical trial was less profound than in the experiments on dogs. Nevertheless, there was virtually complete preservation of the platelet population throughout cardiopulmonary bypass. Importantly, the platelet function returned almost to normal after bypass with a concomitant halving of blood loss. No patient in the PGI_2 series bled sufficiently to cause anxiety post-operatively. The total blood loss was so small that administration of blood after bypass would appear to be superfluous when PGI_2 is used.

Heparin sparing effect

The heparin sparing effect previously described in experimental renal dialysis by Woods *et al.* (1978) was confirmed. The effect of this was to reduce the amount of additional heparin required towards the end of bypass to maintain an acceptable Hemochron level. The amount of protamine required in the PGI_2 group was correspondingly less.

The vasodilator effect of PGI_2

The vasodilator effect of the pre-perfusion dose of 10 ng kg^{-1} min^{-1} was variable. It was troublesome enough to indicate the need for small doses of vasopressor agents in only two patients. In all other cases in this series, the anaesthetist was unable to determine whether prostacyclin was present although he was looking for hypotension and facial flushing. We expected that the hypotensive effects of PGI_2 might require the administration of more fluids during bypass to maintain the blood pressure; even when the dose of PGI_2 was doubled to 20 ng kg^{-1} min^{-1} at the beginning of bypass this was not so. There was no significant difference between the flow rates in the two groups, although it is our practice to increase the flow rather than administer vasopressors when the perfusion pressures are low.

We also considered the theoretical possibility that any hypotension before the bypass started could cause a reduction in renal perfusion and urine flow. If this was followed by an increase in urine flow towards the end of bypass, it might be difficult to administer sufficient potassium in the depleted patient. We did not experience this problem. In two patients in the PGI_2 group, the urine flow was reduced before bypass, but within the first few minutes of bypass, urine started to flow. No difficulties in the management of the serum potassium was experienced in these patients.

In this series, Bos 10 bubble oxygenators were used because we were not certain what the effects of PGI_2 would be on the deposition of the layer of blood products on the surface of 'Celgard' microporous membranes upon which oxygenation depends in some membrane oxygenators. In a subsequent pilot study of membrane oxygenators, using dogs, we find by scanning electron micrography that in spite of the presence of prostacyclin, this essential layer is deposited although it is thinner. There would appear to be no contra-indication to the use of PGI_2 with membrane oxygenators. We are investigating this further.

We were disappointed that the reduction in the amount of brain damage that sometimes occurs in cardiopulmonary bypass owing to platelet aggregates and intravascular clotting was not obvious in this trial. We used the memory recall tests devised by Bethune (1980). In all our patients, 3 days after operation there was a demonstrable impairment of cerebral function, but by 6 days after operation no patient showed any cerebral dysfunction according to the test. Bethune now feels that the test is not sufficiently sensitive for this purpose. The International Group (Katz et al. 1978) studying cerebral damage after open-heart surgery is proposing to use a combination of memory recall, conceptual logic analogue testing and word rotation tests; this is more sensitive. We obtained some difficulty in obtaining the patients' attention in the busy pre-operative period and feel that a long and complex test is undesirable and might distress the patient at that time. Over half of the placebo patients complained of visual disturbances that were not experienced by the PGI_2 group. Further investigation is required to find whether PGI_2 will eliminate all multi-organ and cerebral complications.

CONCLUSION

In spite of the theoretical possible disadvantages of the vasodilator effects of PGI_2 referred to by Salzman (this symposium), both animal studies and a carefully conducted double-blind human clinical trial show them to be irrelevant and far outweighed by the real measured advantages of its use.

Exploitation of the beneficial effects of PGI_2 in extracorporeal circulation probably presents the most important potential advance in open-heart surgery in the 23 years since it first became routine.

There are, however, two coincidental advances, which probably make the discovery of PGI_2 even more important. These are in the unrelated field of computer-enhanced non-invasive instruments for the early diagnosis of cardiovascular disease (Longmore et al. 1976) and the discovery of growth-limiting substances of the arterial wall smooth muscle cells (Florentin *et al.* 1973; Nam *et al.* 1974; Thomas *et al.* 1976). We may soon enter a new era in the management of cardiovascular disease, with early diagnosis of atherosclerosis, inhibition of untoward platelet activity blocking vessels and stimulating smooth muscle proliferation (Stemerman 1979), and control of hyperplastic smooth muscle. PGI$_2$ is an important first member of a family of substances that may well enable medicine to influence the progress of the disease process which causes over half of all deaths and morbidity in the Western World.

I wish to acknowledge the contribution of my surgical and anaesthetic colleagues, and in particular Mr Graeme Bennett, who was present at nearly every case presented in this series, either as one of the surgical team or with Mr Donald Ross and Mr Magdi Yacoub, as a co-ordinator and organizer for the sampling protocols. Without his help this work would not have been possible.

I thank Dr Pat Hoyle, Miss Amanda Gregory and Miss Merilyn Smith who were responsible for the haematological, psychometric and foetal heart testing. I also thank Dr Jean Dawes for help with the undertaking of β-thromboglobulin studies.

We were helped in the laboratories of the National Heart Hospital by Mr Michael Stephens, Miss Linda Townsend, Mr Robert Clitherow and Mr Brian Willis.

I would like to thank the Board of Governors of the National Heart and Chest Hospitals for generous financial support and the staff of the Wellcome Research Laboratories for help and advice.

REFERENCES (Longmore)

Äberg, T. 1974 Effect of open heart surgery in intellectual function. *Scand. J. thorac. cardiovasc. Surg., Suppl.* **15**, 1–63.

Bass, R. M. & Longmore, D. B. 1969 Cerebral damage during openheart surgery. *Nature, Lond.* **222**, 30–33.

Bethune, D. W. 1980 Psychometric testing in the evaluation of post-operative cardiac patient. In *Towards safer cardiac surgery* (ed. D. B. Longmore), pp. 613–617. Medical Technical Press.

Born, G. V. R. 1962 Aggregation of blood platelets by adenosine diphosphate and its reversal. *Nature, Lond.* **194**, 927–929.

Ellison, N., Edmunds, L. H., Jr & Colman, R. W. 1978 Platelet aggregation following heparin and protamine administration. *Anesthesiology* **48**, 65–68

Florentin, R. A., Nam, S. C., Janakidevi, K., Lee, K. T., Reiner, J. M. & Thomas, W. A. 1973 Population dynamics of arterial smoothmuscle cells. II. *In vivo* inhibition of entry into mitosis of swine arterial smooth-muscle cells by aortic tissue extracts. *Arch. Path.* **95**, 317–320.

Hope, W., Martin, T. J., Chesterman, C. N. & Morgan, F. J. 1979 Human β-thromboglobulin inhibits PGI$_2$ production and binds to a specific site in bovine aortic endothelial cells. *Nature, Lond.* **282**, 210–212.

Hughes, D. M. & Longmore, D. B. 1972 Relationship between the stage of development of foetal hearts and their survival in organ culture. *Nature Lond.* **235**, 334–336.

Katz, J., Longmore, D. B. & Speidel, H. 1980 *Secretariat, International Study Group on Cerebral and Psychopathological Dysfunction following Cardiac Surgery* Milwaukee County Mental Health Complex, 9191 Watertown Plank Road, Milwaukee, Wisconsin 53226, U.S.A.

Larkin, J. D., Blocker, T. J., Strong, D. M. & Yocum, M. W. 1978 Anaphylaxis to protamine sulphate mediated by complement-dependent IgG antibody. *J. Allergy clin. Immunol.* **61**, 102–107.

Longmore, D. B. & Smith, M. A. 1980 Toxins in open heart surgery. In *Towards safer cardiac surgery* (ed. D. B. Longmore), pp. 447–473. Medical Technical Press.

Longmore, D. B., Bennett, G., Gueirrara, D., Smith, M., Bunting, S., Moncada, S., Reed, P., Read, N. G. & Vane, J. R. 1979 Prostacyclin: a solution to some problems of extracorporeal circulation. *Lancet* i, 1002–1005.

Longmore, D. B., Bennett, G., Hoyle, P. M., Smith, M. A., Gregory, A., Osivand, T. & Jones, W. A. 1981 Prostacyclin administration during cardiopulmonary bypass in man. *Lancet* i, 800–804.

Longmore, D. B., Turk, J. L. & Lockey, E. 1978 *Scientific Manifesto of H.E.A.R.T.*, 47 Wimpole Street, London, W.1, U.K.

Ludlam, C. A., Moore, S., Bolton, A. E., Pepper, D. S. & Cash, J. D. 1975 The release of a human platelet specific protein measured by a radioimmunoassay. *Thromb. Res.* **6**, 543–548.

Moncada, S. & Vane, J. R. 1978 Unstable metabolites of arachidonic acid and their role in haemostasis and thrombosis. *Br. med. Bull.* **34**, 129–135.

Nam, S. C., Florentin, R. A., Janakidevi, K., Lee, K. T., Reiner, J. M. & Thomas, W. A. 1974 Population dynamics of arterial smooth-muscle cells. III. Inhibition by aortic tissue extracts of proliferative response to intimal injury in hypercholesterolemic swine. *Expl molec. Pathol.* **21**, 259–267.

Stemerman, M. B. 1979 Hemostasis, thrombosis and atherogenesis. *Atherosclerosis Rev.* **6**, 105–146.

Thomas, W. A., Janakidevi, K., Florentin, R. A., Lee, K. T. & Reiner, J. M. 1976 Search for arterial smooth-muscle cell chalone(s). Chapter 20 In *Chalones* (ed. J. H. Houck), ch. 20. New York: North-Holland.

Velders, A. J., van den Dungen, J. J. A. M., Westerhof, N. J. W. & Wildevuur, C. R. H. 1980 Platelet damage by protamine administration: protection by reducing protamine or by prostacyclin (PGI_2) treatment. *Eur. surg. Res.* **12** (suppl. 1), 50–51.

Wildenthal, K. 1971a Factors promoting the survival and beating of intact foetal mouse hearts in organ culture. *J. molec. Cell Cardiol.* **1**, 101–104.

Wildenthal, K. 1971b Long-term maintenance of spontaneously beating mouse hearts in organ culture. *J. appl. Physiol.* **30**, 153–157.

Wolf, P. 1967 The nature and significance of platelet products in human plasma. *Br. J. Haemat.* **13**, 269–288.

Woods, H. F., Ash, G., Weston, M. J., Bunting, S., Moncada, S. & Vane, J. R. 1978 Prostacyclin can replace heparin in haemodialysis in dogs. *Lancet* ii, 1075–1077.